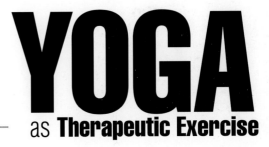

YOGA
as Therapeutic Exercise

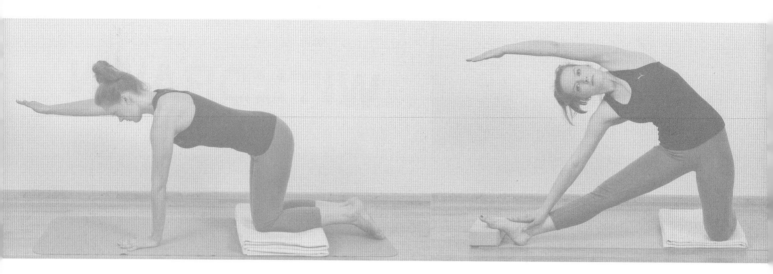

For Elsevier

Commissioning Editor: Claire Wilson

Development Editor: Sheila Black

Project Manager: Jagannathan Varadarajan

Senior Designer: Stewart Larking

Illustration Manager: Gillian Richards

Illustrator: Graeme Chambers

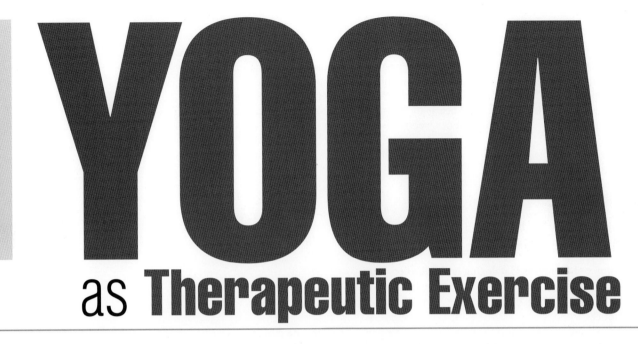

YOGA
as Therapeutic Exercise

A Practical Guide for Manual Therapists

Luise Wörle BSc(Hons) Osteopathy MA
Yoga Teacher and Teacher Trainer, long-standing student of Yogācārya B.K.S. Iyengar, Munich, Germany

Erik Pfeiff DiplPsych
Clinical Psychologist and Psychotherapist, Manual Therapist; Advanced Aikido Teacher, Munich, Germany

Photography by
Wilfried Petzi
Munich, Germany

Forewords by
Yogācārya B.K.S. Iyengar
Ramāmaṇi Iyengar Memorial Yoga Institute, Pune, India

Professor Laurie Hartman DO PhD
Associate Professor of Osteopathic Technique, British School of Osteopathy, London, UK

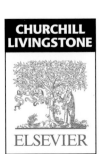

Edinburgh London New York Oxford Philadelphia St Louis Sydney Toronto 2010

CHURCHILL
LIVINGSTONE
ELSEVIER

ISBN 978-0-7020-3383-4

British Library Cataloguing in Publication Data
A catalogue record for this book is available from the British Library

Library of Congress Cataloging in Publication Data
A catalog record for this book is available from the Library of Congress

Notices
Knowledge and best practice in this field are constantly changing. As new research and experience broaden our understanding, changes in research methods, professional practices, or medical treatment may become necessary.

Practitioners and researchers must always rely on their own experience and knowledge in evaluating and using any information, methods, compounds, or experiments described herein. In using such information or methods they should be mindful of their own safety and the safety of others, including parties for whom they have a professional responsibility.

With respect to any drug or pharmaceutical products identified, readers are advised to check the most current information provided (i) on procedures featured or (ii) by the manufacturer of each product to be administered, to verify the recommended dose or formula, the method and duration of administration, and contraindications. It is the responsibility of practitioners, relying on their own experience and knowledge of their patients, to make diagnoses, to determine dosages and the best treatment for each individual patient, and to take all appropriate safety precautions.

To the fullest extent of the law, neither the Publisher nor the authors, contributors, or editors assume any liability for any injury and/or damage to persons or property as a matter of products liability, negligence or otherwise, or from any use or operation of any methods, products, instructions, or ideas contained in the material herein.

 ELSEVIER your source for books, journals and multimedia in the health sciences
www.elsevierhealth.com

Working together to grow libraries in developing countries

www.elsevier.com | www.bookaid.org | www.sabre.org

ELSEVIER   BOOK AID International   Sabre Foundation

The Publisher's policy is to use **paper manufactured from sustainable forests**

Printed in China

Contents

The majority of people live on their emotions. This leads to disturbance of their body hormones, as well as to economic and mental stress, all of which create imbalance in physico-physiological, physio-psychological and psycho-neurological systems.

In yogic science, the āsanas and prāṇāyāmas are particularly helpful in generating and distributing life-saving energy wherever and whenever it is needed, so that each cell in the body revibrates with sound health, satisfaction, contentment, and a composed state of attention and awareness in the brain and mind.

Luise Wörle and Erik Pfeiff's work, *Yoga as Therapeutic Exercise – A Guide for Manual Therapists*, may serve as a handbook to help suffering humanity to achieve better health and a better way of living.

Luise has undergone training at my Institute in Pune, India, on remedial classes and has undertaken this work in presenting the curative aspects of yoga for developing a sound, healthy immune system.

Yoga is a powerful preventive system. It has the power to eradicate psychosomatic or somatopsychic diseases completely. In cases where a complete cure is not possible, this method develops that enduring power and keeps the disease in check.

Luise Wörle and Erik Pfeiff have covered the subject well and I am sure that this manual will add further knowledge to increase understanding of the subject as a healing art and science.

B.K.S. Iyengar

Luise Wörle is a yoga teacher of considerable experience, who became interested in Osteopathy after translating for me at many conferences. She qualified as an osteopath in 2005.

Erik Pfeiff is a manual therapist and psychotherapist; dedicated to his own yoga practice, he has also contributed many of the basic ideas in this book.

Throughout three decades of cooperation, Luise and Erik have taught many patients to practice yoga and have observed the benefits of this for greater treatment success. They have also taught patients how to develop mindfulness and the sensitivity to adjust their individual practice to their capacity and conditions.

This book links the manual therapist's diagnostic tools to a wide variety of basic exercises and guides the reader, in small steps, into a more complex task and a deeper understanding of the practice.

The authors' understanding of the theory of osteopathy and their knowledge of yoga has proved extremely useful to their teaching. The tests and diagnoses help design and programme the work the patient needs to do to achieve a good result. Patients quickly become and remain motivated, as the results soon become apparent. The use of breathing, which

is a special part of yoga, has been a major part of this work, as have modifications of the basic exercises. Why should patients exercise at all? This book illustrates what can be done with exercises designed for individual patients. Supervision of exercise to ensure accuracy is emphasised. Most patients will feel the benefit of the exercises and a sense of achievement, knowing that it is their work and cooperation that gets results.

Luise has done an enormous amount of work and drawn on her knowledge, experience and beliefs to write this book for patients and practitioners. It stands alone as a classic manual for patients and practitioners alike.

I congratulate both authors on this enormous task and hope that they will both carry on developing and improving approaches to patients' pain and recovery in their work and practice.

This first-class book will enable a wide range of therapists to help make the benefits of improved posture and movement patterns available to their patients.

Professor Laurie Hartman DO PhD

Although my childhood was marked by poverty and poor health, I have many happy memories of that time. I owe this to my parents and their wonderful ability to live with a positive mental attitude and to pass it on to other people. For this precious legacy I am grateful to them with all my heart.

As a teenager I developed a great enthusiasm for movement and dance in spite of always getting the lowest grades in physical education. In 1970 I happened to attend a yoga class and, the very next day, had the distinct feeling that something inside me had changed fundamentally; I therefore continued attending the class. Later I was told that my yoga teacher practiced according to B.K.S. Iyengar's book *Light on Yoga*, and I was filled with the desire to get to know Mr Iyengar personally. This wish to be taught by someone I felt was the best yoga teacher for me came true.

Following my regular practice, it was not long before the opportunity arose for me to give lessons myself. This experience changed my understanding of yoga. Gradually it became my aim not only to convey positions and movements to my students but also to foster their own understanding and sensitivity. Out of this grew a particular method of practicing yoga and a framework of hints and tips, in which feelings could be related to practice. This led to the development of a yoga system involving mindfulness.

Informed by respect for the human body's ingenuity and by the possibilities of exploring it deeply in different yoga positions, I wanted to learn more about its scientific and medical foundations. This finally led me to a BSc in Osteopathy. All these experiences have found their way into this book.

Luise Wörle
Munich 2010

In 1980, when I returned to Germany after completing additional training in Ida Rolf's Structural Integration methods, I was contacted by Luise Wörle. She asked if I would be interested in attending one of her yoga seminars in order to explore possible connections between the practice of yoga and manual therapy. This was the beginning of a collaboration that has now stretched over three decades, consisting of many fruitful conversations and jointly conducted seminars. The aims and principles that became more and more evident during this work have stimulated an evolutionary process in my understanding of yoga practice. In the end, a therapeutic approach emerged that has helped me in my daily professional practice when trying to guide patients towards becoming proactive and assuming more responsibility for themselves.

In this book we propose to encourage the student's or patient's own activity through simple yoga exercises in order to activate self-healing forces. It is a manual for beginning to practice yoga regardless of physical problems or constraints that, for the present, make certain movements impossible. The crucial point is to persevere in practicing step by step, thereby assuming responsibility for one's own health while being happy with one's progress, however small. In this way, the book can be useful to individual readers, while also enabling teachers and therapists to motivate their students or patients towards more individual activity and independent practice.

Erik Pfeiff
Munich 2010

Guide to the pronunciation of the most frequently used Sanskrit words in this book

The vowels ā, ē, ī and ū are lengthened.
Ś and ṣ are both pronounced sh.
C is pronounced ch (like cherry).
The few other diacritical signs used here are ignored for practical reasons.

Acknowledgements

The authors thank the following:

Yogācārya Śri B.K.S. Iyengar for giving us so much knowledge about yoga, for having an open ear for my questions and for always supporting me on my way.

Dr Geeta S. Iyengar for continuing her father's unique teachings.

Professor Laurie Hartman, DO, PhD for teaching osteopathy as an art to refine the understanding of body, mind and soul, and for all his advice and encouragement.

Professor Eyal Lederman, DO, PhD for organizing seminars that formed the nucleus of this book.

Kristina Weiss and Dr. phil. Bernhard Kleinschmidt for being patient and cooperative models, Bernhard also for looking at parts of the manuscript and giving helpful advice.

Barbara Weiss for supervising the photo shoots.

Brigitte Duschek for the photograph with the real dog.

Yoga teachers Barbara Weiss, Barbara von Balluseck, Brigitte Duschek, Eva Kellermann, and Angelika Stemmer for checking the practical sections.

Karin Breitfelder, dentist, for hints concerning the head and the temporomandibular joint.

Anthony Lobo, long-time personal assistant of B.K.S. Iyengar, and Marina Alvisi for checking the preparatory practice for prāṇāyāma.

Dr. med. Heidi Hauke and Dr. med. Linnéa Roth, both also yoga teachers, for looking at the anatomy and physiology sections.

Dr. phil. Dagmar Landvogt-Aisslinger, yoga teacher, for looking at the philosophical sections.

Renate Miethge, Dipl. Psych., for giving advice on mindful exercising.

Mag. Erika Erber, yoga teacher, for correcting the Sanskrit expressions.

Wilfried Petzi for taking all the photographs.

Everyone at Elsevier, especially Claire Wilson and Sheila Black, for all their work and help.

Liz Williams for being a skilful and very helpful copyeditor.

All our patients and students for their contribution and inspiration.

Introduction to yoga

Chapter contents

A short overview of the history of yoga

Introduction

Over the last decades yoga has become very popular in the western world. Different schools, adult education centers, health centers, clinics, and private teachers are offering yoga classes and sessions. The programs for training yoga teachers are increasingly controlled by professional associations, health insurances, and other authorities. Within yoga the health aspect has become particularly relevant. An unpublished pilot study conducted by the authors of this book evaluated 200 questionnaires and 50 interviews with adult participants of yoga classes. It was found that the initial motivation to start practicing yoga was pain or discomfort, or just getting fit. Eventually yoga helped respondents to master the difficulties of life and to regain confidence or equilibrium after difficult periods of life.

When we try to describe and define yoga, we must bear in mind that yoga was developed in ancient India, in a time and a culture completely different from that of our present western world. The word "yoga" belongs to the old Indian Sanskrit language. A Sanskrit dictionary lists three pages of meanings for this term (Gode & Karve 1979). Among these interpretations, union, control, and mastery are particularly relevant (Fuchs 1990).

There follows a short history of yoga which should help readers to understand its depth. Wherever we have met teachers and students of yoga, this original Indian expression is used, not translated into any other language. Nevertheless the practice of yoga is influenced by individual and cultural factors. It is certainly not a route to the instant acquisition of knowledge and abilities. It requires the willingness to become involved in study and practice, to work with compliance and dedication. This may mean changes in lifestyle, in order to plan the time necessary for the practice of yoga.

The Vedas

Probably the oldest traces of yoga originate from the third millennium BC: stone tablets have been found dating from this epoch showing goddesses in positions reminiscent of yoga postures. The word "yoga" and the related verb "yuj" are seen for the first time in the saṃhitās. The saṃhitās are collections of texts of the Veda, that is, the holy knowledge. There are four collections: (1) the Ṛg-Veda, written in the 12th century BC or even earlier; (2) the Sāma-Veda; (3) Yajur-Veda; and (4) Atharva-Veda, probably written between 1200 and 1000 BC. The Vedas contain descriptions of methods and rituals that bring to mind the yoga techniques of mindfulness, concentration, meditation, and breathing exercises.

The Upaniṣads

The first texts on yoga are contained in the Upaniṣads. "Upa" means close to something or somebody, "ni" means down, and "ṣad" is to sit. Indeed, these texts indicate the importance of sitting close to a teacher, and of listening attentively; they emphasize the relationship between teacher and student (Bäumer 1986).

As has already been seen with the Vedas, researchers on ancient Indian texts are still unsure when these texts were written. Different authors give discrepancies of several decades for many texts. Dating seems to be particularly difficult for the Upaniṣads, some of which were contained in the Vedas, while some were written after the Vedas. Initially the Upaniṣads were only spoken and learned by heart and passed on by word of mouth from generation to generation. Eventually they were written down. In many cases the precise period is unknown and different authors and scientists give contradictory dates.

The Upaniṣads were written in the first millennium BC. The oldest ones belong to the vedic school; different schools and branches developed later on. The Upaniṣads contain descriptions of old magic rituals, mythical stories, profound philosophical thoughts, prayers, and songs. In particular the later Upaniṣads from the seventh century BC onwards begin to form the concept of yoga. These texts have been an important source for the development of yoga. The knowledge they teach is not only academic, learned by the brain; it also changes its students. They develop many ways to heighten consciousness and focus inner concentration. The concept of body and mind also originates in these texts. Overcoming obstacles to this development is called "yoga" in these texts.

Until now the Kaṭha-Upaniṣad has been considered to be the first textbook on yoga. Most authors date it to the fifth century BC, although it could be a few centuries older than that. The unknown author of this text describes yoga as inner stability and balance, both of which depend upon constant concentration (Feuerstein 2001). The highest level is reached when the five senses of perception, the thoughts, and the mind are all calm. Mastering the senses in this way and being free from distraction is yoga (Bäumer 1986).

A first description of yoga practice can be found in the Śvetāśvatara-Upaniṣad, which is usually dated to the fourth or third century BC, but also could be older. Śvetāśvatara may be the name of the author. In the second part of the text precise instructions can be found on sitting posture and breathing. The trunk, neck, and head should be held straight, and the sensory organs and the mind are focused on the heart. If the fluctuations of the mind are calmed, and the breath is controlled, the breath through the nose should be refined. Eight further Yoga Upaniṣads were written, probably after this, that are quite poetic – the Yoga Upaniṣads of the Atharva-Veda. These describe a yoga path consisting of six stages, similar to the path described in the Yoga-Sūtras of Patañjali (Michel & Deussen 2006).

The Yoga-Sūtras of Patañjali

At some point between 200 BC and AD 400 the Indian sage Patañjali collected together previous knowledge about yoga and summarized it in a concise collection of 195 aphorisms, the Yoga-Sūtras. The Yoga-Sūtras are still the primary source text on yoga.

The main pillars of the yoga path are abhyāsa and vairāgya. Abhyāsa is learning through disciplined, dedicated practice. Vairāgya is avoiding whatever is distracting from the path of learning. The core concept is the calming of the fluctuations of consciousness: "yogaś-citta-vṛtti-nirodhaḥ" (Feuerstein 1989, p. 26). "Yogaś" is the "integration from the outermost layer to the innermost self, that is, from the skin to the muscles, bones, nerves, mind, intellect, will, consciousness and self" (Iyengar 2002a, p. 49). "Citta" means consciousness, "vṛtti" fluctuations, and "nirodhaḥ" is gradual calming, becoming free from distractions.

The path of yoga practice contains eight aspects or limbs of yoga: yama, niyama, āsana, prāṇāyāma, pratyāhāra, dhāraṇā, dhyāna, and samādhi. Yama refers to the ethical, social aspects of not harming anyone, being honest, not stealing, controlling your wishes and desires, being free from envy and attachment. Niyama consists of five aspects of purifying oneself: cleanliness, contentedness, fervor for study and practice, personal immersion into the profundity of the yoga texts, and surrender to the divine source. Āsana is a firm, calm sitting posture, not being distracted. The body, mind, and soul are involved in positioning. The various āsanas that are used now and their therapeutic aspects were developed later. Prāṇāyāma is expanding the breath to control the life energy. Inhalation and exhalation are carefully elongated and refined. In the pauses between inhalation and exhalation, and exhalation and inhalation, inner stillness can be experienced. Pratyāhāra is the result of practicing the previous four stages. It is calming the senses and therefore the wandering mind, too. It is preparing for the remaining three stages. Once the senses are no longer distracted, dhāraṇā will be possible. This is concentration free of tension in all areas of the body. From the correct practice of dhāraṇā dhyāna, meditation, develops. Emotional calmness is added to the relaxed state of the body, while the mind remains fully aware and alert. The final, highest stage of this path is samādhi.

Between the first and seventh century AD Thirumoolar wrote a yoga text, Thirumandiram, in the south Indian Tamil language. There are some hints that Thirumoolar was a contemporary of Patañjali, and that both had the same teacher. The Yoga-Sūtras were originally written in Sanskrit, unlike the Thirumandiram, which was in Tamil, and it was not until 1993 that this latter text was translated into English for the first time by Govindan (Thirumoolar & Govindan 1993). It may be because the text was only in the Tamil language that many experts have been unaware that both texts share a common content.

The depth of āsana

The practice of āsana starts with a physical action. Gradually cognitive, mental, and reflective actions are integrated. The dedicated and attentive practice of āsana contains all eight stages of yoga practice. The ethical principles of yama and the aspects of purifying yourself contained in niyama are to be applied in the practice of āsana; they are also cultivated through attentive āsana practice. In a correctly practiced āsana there is no longer a duality between body and mind and mind and soul. The breath is synchronized with movement during the practice of āsanas. Inhalation is the movement from the core of the being to the skin, whereas with exhalation the body moves inwards to its source (Iyengar 2002b). In this way prāṇāyāma is connected to āsana practice.

If you are absorbed in the practice of āsana, the senses of perception and the mind are calmed, the muscles and joints are resting in their positions, and pratyāhāra is reached. The āsanas must be performed with concentration and complete attention, which is dhāraṇā. Dhyāna, meditation, is integrated into the āsana practice if there is space between receiving a message from the senses of perception and the message sent to the organs of action. This means freeing yourself from the feeling of having to act immediately. Being fully aware of the body during the practice of āsana is samādhi. "The rivers of intelligence and consciousness flow together and merge in the sea of the soul" (Iyengar 2002b, p. 76).

As mentioned above, the primary source texts on yoga are the Yoga-Sūtras. A variety of āsanas that are practiced mainly in the western world have their roots in the end of the first millennium AD. A famous text is the Haṭha-Yoga-Pradīpikā from the 14th century (Sinh 2006). This text contains a section about āsanas and one about prāṇāyāma, and describes samādhi as returning to the source of the being.

1 CHAPTER
Introduction to yoga
Yoga and health

Yoga and health

In the 20th century B K S Iyengar (born 1918) summarized and developed over 200 āsanas and prāṇāyāma techniques. Iyengar created a unique synthesis of the classical aspects of yoga from the above-mentioned sources with western medicine and science. He refined the practice to the best anatomical positioning and physiological functioning, developed the therapeutic applications of the yoga postures, and made numerous modifications for patients with ailments and disabilities. His sophisticated system of using props to support the postures is particularly relevant for therapeutic work. His own development started from experiencing serious disease at a very young age. Over 70 years of profound study and dedicated practice, Iyengar constantly refined his practice, his medical and philosophical understanding, and his teaching of yoga. In December 2008 he celebrated his 90th birthday in good health.

B K S Iyengar describes yoga as a science to free the soul through the integration of consciousness, mind, and body. Health is a side-effect of the practice, but a very important one (Iyengar 2002b).

In 1990 one of the authors of this book asked B K S Iyengar during one of his European guest seminars how to start therapeutic yoga. In a firm, enthusiastic way he answered: "Build healthy structures in your body. From there you can correct the unhealthy ones." Seeing the extent to which B K S Iyengar has succeeded in building healthy structures in his own body for his personal health, for teaching and helping students and patients, inspired us deeply. This inspiration guided our work from then on, together with the concept of healthy function. We were able to observe substantial effects on our patients' ability to heal themselves. However difficult a health condition is, there are probably still some healthy structures in the body. Working with these healthy structures activates the indidivual's self-healing power and, even in difficult situations, there is a greater likelihood of improving. Examples of healthy structures and functions include:

- centered postures in sitting, standing, walking, and many kinds of work
- symmetries
- correct alignment
- physiological positions and ranges for all joints
- balanced activity of muscles
- tissues that are well drained and well hydrated
- enough space in the body cavities.

In May 2009 Geeta Iyengar, B K S Iyengar's daughter, conducted yoga conventions in London and Cologne, with an emphasis on postural and movement patterns. During her teaching she highlighted learning to correct the posture and how to move the body, once you have found out where it is not moving or not moving properly, where it is too weak or hypermobile. To be precise, the details should be learnt correctly first, then combined to create more complex postures. This idea of learning the details first has been guiding us in our basic exercise section (see Chapter 6).

There are ways of modifying the yoga āsanas to make their beneficial effects for body, mind, and soul accessible for many people with different constitutions, health problems, and restrictions. If the therapist and teacher know the essence of the āsana, they can use different methods to adjust it for the patient. Props are used to support the patient performing the āsanas. This increases the possibility of practicing: many āsanas that cannot be done otherwise are possible with the support of props. The props allow the patient to adjust and modify the āsanas in many different ways for many different conditions. Even if patients can only manage a small change they may be able to achieve the essence of the āsana and feel a lot better.

Very stiff patients can stretch further and achieve more mobility; weak areas can be supported so as not to overwork them, and abilities that have been lost can be regained. Everybody can experience the benefits of yoga, no matter what their condition. They can go as far as they can on their own, and use support for what is not possible when unsupported. Even very ill, injured, or handicapped patients gain from practicing with props and can compensate for abilities they do not have. Without props many of them would not be able to practice any more. The props also allow patients to practice on their own what would otherwise only be possible with the help of a teacher or therapist. The performance of many āsanas can be made a lot more precise and longer with the help of props, and the student's confidence can be increased.

In a simple way props have been used by yoga practitioners from the outset. Long ago objects like stones and branches were used. In the 1970s we asked builders for a few bricks, in carpet shops we asked for remnants, we used the belts from our jeans, towels, and a lot of the furniture in our homes to support āsanas that were too difficult to perform independently. In those years we also saw B K S Iyengar refining this exercise approach for patients with different kinds of restrictions. Aging people particularly benefited from the use of props.

In the meantime a highly sophisticated system of props and the science behind them was developed (Iyengar 2001a, Steinberg & Geeta 2006, Raman 2008). In the 1980s, B K S Iyengar advised us to start with a basic amount of props, such as mats, wooden bricks, blankets, belts, and chairs. Other items such as pillows, bolsters, wooden bars, and wooden horses have been added. For this book we narrowed the props down to a sticky mat, a belt, and a cork or foam brick and improvised with things that are found in most homes, such as chairs, blankets, and pillows. Also walls, corners, windowsills, stairs, door frames, and counters may be useful.

Some authors have suggested cycles of exercises for health promotion and as a primary or adjunct therapy, using props and applying a mindful and precise exercise approach. These cycles are classified according to body systems or conditions (Mehta et al. 1990, Iyengar 2001a, b, Raman 2008). A universal underlying principle for all therapeutic yoga approaches is to improve the posture to create a sound foundation for the function of all systems. With an understanding of how to use props, an infinite variety of possibilities can be created according to individual needs.

Aims to be achieved through practice and principles underlying the exercise approach

To meet the objectives from the therapist's point of view we have compiled a set of aims that can be achieved through a healthy exercise approach. This concept can be applied to a wide range of patients. Practicing is based upon a set of principles

to improve mobility, strength, stamina, relaxation, balance, coordination, synchronization, and breathing naturally.

The basic exercises are divided according to the different areas of the body. For each area a selection of exercises is given to reach specific aims. The core aims are mobilizing stiff or hypomobile areas and strengthening or stabilizing weak or hypermobile areas. Stamina can be improved by increasing the number of repetitions or the time holding the exercise. Relaxation can be the start or the end of an exercise or an aim on its own. Balance, coordination, and synchronization play an essential role in more complex exercises. Breathing naturally is an aim for each exercise. Exercises to achieve specific aims follow the diagnosis.

There are five principles underlying this approach: mindfulness, precision, finetuning, economical practice, and a sufficient variety of approaches. The most important principle is mindful exercising – awareness, sensitivity. Therefore we have devoted a whole chapter to this principle (see Chapter 2). It is highly relevant to the health effects of practice and also to patients' education. Precision is essential and can be developed by starting slowly, learning the correct movements first. With increasing practice speed of movement can be increased, but only as long as precision is maintained. Finetuning is improving the quality of exercising. It can be used to push the boundaries of movements and ease off where necessary to avoid injury. This applies to all patients. Easing off slightly after having pushed the boundary of an exercise opens up a variety of possibilities. In this way some free play at the end of range of movement is maintained for joints and all their surrounding structures. Economical practice avoids unnecessary activity and exhaustion, and with a sufficient variety of approaches all aims can be covered.

Mindfulness, precision, finetuning and economical practice are applied to all exercises, whereas variety applies to the program selected.

Research on therapeutic yoga

Up until the mid 20th century knowledge of the effects of yoga was mainly based on empirical evidence. It was not until the 1960s that scientific research on the effects of yoga was undertaken.

There is now evidence that with regular yoga practice the immune system is strengthened, heart rate and blood pressure decrease, metabolism is better balanced, breathing becomes deeper and slower, stress hormones are reduced, and muscles are used more efficiently. Peripheral blood supply – and thus tissue nutrition – is improved. Mindful exercising and better awareness improve body posture, which helps the structures and functions. The effects start to be felt after 2 weeks of regular practice: to maintain the effects, ongoing practice is necessary.

A great deal of research about yoga has now been conducted, both on its individual effects and on its success at treating many different conditions (Raman & Suresh 2003; Kulkarni & Bera 2009; Olivo 2009). Good results have been found in stress management (Michalsen et al. 2005), cardiovascular disease (Raub 2002, Innes et al. 2005), multiple sclerosis (Oken et al. 2004), degenerative changes (Garfinkel et al. 1994, Garfinkel & Schumacher 2000, DiBenedetto et al. 2005), and carpal tunnel syndrome (Garfinkel et al. 1998). That yoga, practiced thoroughly, is an effective treatment or adjunct to medical treatment of low-back pain is supported by both empirical and scientific evidence. A comprehensive study has been conducted by Williams et al. (2005). There are few musculoskeletal and systemic conditions where a well-adjusted yoga program has failed to give improvement (Jain & Hepp 1998, Lipton 2008, Raman 2008).

What anatomy teaches for the performance of yoga exercises

Knowledge of anatomical principles aids in understanding the beneficial effects of practicing yoga. For example, cartilage is supplied with fluid by the process of diffusion, therefore pressure is important to remove waste products, and space is important so that the cartilage can fill itself like a sponge with the surrounding fluid. Yoga practice should balance loading and unloading. Cartilage that is not covered by skin cannot grow back once it has been used up. Therefore throughout practice alignment, the correct positioning of the joints, is vital to avoid degenerative changes.

Bone tissue has a strong blood supply. It is constantly being built and destroyed and changing. The shape of the bones is adapted to functional needs and bone is very hard. The building of new bone is stimulated by active exercising, particularly pressure, pulling muscles, movements against gravity, and movements that are new.

The joints need special attention in a good exercise approach. As cartilage and bones are closely related to joints, recommendations for these tissues also apply to joints. The structures and functions of the joints require precise alignment, creating enough space, and balance between loading and unloading. For the best possible supply of nutrients and to improve mobility the full range of movement should be used. For stability and to protect the joints a balanced harmony between muscles and their antagonists is important.

Anatomy explains how to work with the muscles. Tensions are released through lengthening, releasing the fibers within the muscle cells. The active contraction of the muscles works best after slight lengthening. Both in static holding and moving dynamically the balanced and coordinated activity of agonists and antagonist is important. Unnecessary movements should be avoided in order to practice economically.

Resting poses should follow practicing with effort. Breathing should be natural while working with the muscles to give a good oxygen supply. The muscles should be kept soft enough to allow good transport of fluids (Roth 2009).

Final considerations

There are many relevant and profound empirical, philosophical, and medical considerations about yoga and the effects of practicing yoga. Practicing yoga is both a science and an art.

Yehudi Menuhin, a famous 20th-century violinist, who was one of B K S Iyengar's first students, and who brought him to Europe, wrote the foreword for Iyengar's first great written text, *Light on Yoga*. There Menuhin explains: "The practice of yoga induces a primary sense of measure and proportion. Reduced to our own body, our first instrument, we learn to play it, drawing from it maximum resonance and harmony. With unflagging patience we refine and animate every cell" (Iyengar 2001b, foreword).

However profound our knowledge and experience about yoga become, there remains an unattainable secret. Krishna Raman, a medical doctor in India and a dedicated practitioner of yoga for several decades, has expressed his respect: "our body is the most marvelous piece of machinery ever made and can never be duplicated" (Raman 2008, p. 62).

References

Bäumer, B., 1986. Upanishaden: Befreiung zum Sein. Benzinger, Zürich.

DiBenedetto, M., Innes, K.E., Taylor, A.G., et al., 2005. Effect of a gentle Iyengar yoga program on gait in the elderly: an exploratory study. Arch. Phys. Med. Rehabil. 86, 1830–1837.

Feuerstein, G., 1989. The Yoga Sūtra of Patañjali. Inner Traditions, Rochester, VT.

Feuerstein, G., 2001. The Yoga Tradition: Its History, Literature, Philosophy and Practice. Hohm Press, Prescott, AZ.

Fuchs, C., 1990. Yoga in Deutschland. Rezeption, Organisation, Typologie. Kohlhammer, Stuttgart.

Garfinkel, M., Schumacher Jr., H.R., 2000. Yoga. Rheum. Dis. Clin. North Am. 26, 125–132.

Garfinkel, M.S., Schumacher Jr., H.R., Husain, A., 1994. Evaluation of a yoga based regimen for treatment of osteoarthritis of the hands. J. Rheumatol. 21, 2341–2343.

Garfinkel, M.S., Singhal, A., Katz, W.A., et al., 1998. Yoga-based intervention for carpal tunnel syndrome: a randomized trial. J. Am. Med. Assoc. 280, 1601–1603.

Gode, P.K., Karve, C.G. (eds.), 1979. Sanskrit–English Dictionary, vol. III. Prasad Prakashan, Poona.

Innes, K.E., Bourguignon, C., Taylor, A.G., 2005. Risk indices associated with the insulin resistance syndrome, cardiovascular disease, and possible protection with yoga: a systematic review. J. Am. Board Fam. Med. 18, 491–519.

Iyengar, B.K.S., 2001a. Yoga – The Path to Holistic Health. Dorling Kindersley, London.

Iyengar, B.K.S., 2001b. Light on Yoga. Thorsons, London.

Iyengar, B.K.S., 2002a. Light on the Yoga Sūtras of Patañjali. Thorsons, London.

Iyengar, B.K.S., 2002b. The Tree of Yoga. Shambhala, Boston, MA.

Jain, M.D., Hepp, H.H., 1998. Yoga als adjuvante Therapie. Hippokrates, Stuttgart.

Kulkarni, D.D., Bera, T.K., 2009. Yoga exercises and health – a psycho-neuro immunological approach. Indian J. Physiol. Pharmacol. 53, 3–15.

Lipton, L., 2008. Using yoga to treat disease: an evidence-based review. JAAPA 21, 34–41.

Mehta, S., Mehta, M., Mehta, S., 1990. Yoga the Iyengar Way. Dorling Kindersley, London.

Michalsen, A., Grossman, P., Acil, A., et al., 2005. Rapid stress reduction and anxiolysis among distressed women as a consequence of a three-month intensive yoga program. Med. Sci. Monit. 11, CR555–CR561.

Michel, P., Deussen, P. (eds.), 2006. Die Upanishaden: die Geheimlehre des Veda. Marix, Wiesbaden.

Oken, B.S., Kishiyama, S., Zajdel, D., et al., 2004. Randomized controlled trial of yoga and exercise in multiple sclerosis. Neurology 62, 2058–2064.

Olivo, E.L., 2009. Protection throughout the life span: the psychoneuroimmunologic impact of Indo-Tibetan meditative and yogic practices. Ann. N. Y. Acad. Sci. 1172, 163–171.

Raman, K., 2008. A Matter Of Health: Integration of Yoga and Western Medicine for Prevention and Cure, second ed. EastWest, Madras. Available as an e-book from www.krishnaraman.com.

Raman, K., Suresh, S., 2003. Yoga and Medical Science FAQ. EastWest, Madras.

Raub, J.A., 2002. Psychophysiologic effects of Haṭha Yoga on musculoskeletal and cardiopulmonary function: a literature review. J. Altern. Complement. Med. 8, 797–812.

Roth, L., 2009. Anatomie: Lehrbrief I. Fernlehrgang Yoga-Lehrer/in SKA. Sebastian Kneipp Akademie, Bad Wörishofen.

Sinh, P., 2006. The Haṭha Yoga Pradīpikā: Explanation of Haṭha Yoga. Pilgrims, Kathmandu.

Steinberg, L., 2006. Geeta S. Iyengar's Guide to a Woman's Yoga Practice. Parvati Productions, Urbana, IL.

Thirumoolar, Govindan, M., 1993. Thirumandiram: A Classic of Yoga and Tantra. Kriya Yoga, Quebec.

Williams, K.A., Petronis, J., Smith, D., et al., 2005. Effect of Iyengar yoga therapy for chronic low back pain. Pain 115, 107–117.

Mindful exercising

Theories of mindfulness

Introduction

Many patients start practicing yoga because of discomfort or pain. Empirical and scientific evidence has shown that a mindful state of being during exercising makes a big difference to the effect of the exercise. Mindfulness, awareness, and sensitivity, instead of an emphasis on doing, significantly increase the efficiency and effectiveness of exercising. Not without reason, mindful practice has always been used in the ancient meditation paths. The oldest known sources are found in the yoga tradition, where mindfulness is applied to physical practice, breathing, and almost all aspects of life. Different schools teaching mindfulness have developed. It is a core concept in the Buddhist tradition, and is particularly refined in Zen meditation practice, and it can also be found in martial arts such as aikido, tai chi, and other Asian training methods. Throughout the 20th century mindfulness was integrated into psychological methods. Since the 1980s aspects of physical and mental exercises, elements of yoga, and other ancient paths of meditation have been combined with mind and body therapeutic exercise and are now established in evidence-based medicine.

Mindfulness in the yoga tradition

In the yoga texts mindfulness plays a fundamental role in everyday actions, in breathing, and in particular in physical practice. The first systematic summary of this practical science was given by Patañjali (see Chapter 1). Patañjali's Yoga-Sūtras, a concise text consisting of 195 aphorisms, cover all aspects of life. The Yoga-Sūtras were written some time between 200 BC and AD 400 (Mylius 2003); they have been used since then and are still studied by yoga practitioners all over the world. The basic principles of yoga practice that are still used can be found in this ancient textbook. The sources of this work are even older, reaching back perhaps 1000–2000 years.

Patañjali describes the fluctuations which continually disturb the mind. The task of the mind is to receive information from the outside from the senses of eyes, ears, nose, tongue, and skin, and to reflect on this information in order to select or reject it. The mind is distracted and distressed if there are too many stimuli from the sense organs.

Patañjali shows various ways of stilling the organs of senses and the mind. One famous verse says: "Yoga is the cessation of movements in the consciousness" (Iyengar 2002a, p. 50). The general means of achieving this calmness are mentioned in Yoga-Sūtra I.12 (Iyengar 2002a, p. 61): constant study, practice, effort (abhyāsa in Sanskrit); detachment from desires and aspects distracting the mind (vairāgya). This includes learning what is essential for a fulfilled, healthy life.

Several practical means are described: breathing, stilling the senses, concentration, meditation. According to the Yoga-Sūtras meditation is the fruit of sustained practice of yoga. Mind and breath are closely related. Control of the breath is considered fundamental for mental stillness and peace, throughout the further development of yoga.

According to Sūtra I.34 (Iyengar 2002a, p. 87), the practice of slow inhalation and slow exhalation leads to a "state of consciousness, which is like a calm lake." This awareness of the breath brings clarity of mind, attention which is totally focused on the present moment, and is ideally applied during physical practice. In Yoga-Sūtra I.2 (Iyengar 2002a, p. 49) yoga is defined as "union or integration from the outermost layer to the innermost self, that is, from the skin to the muscles, bones, nerves, mind, intellect, will, consciousness and self."

To reach this mindful, focused attention pratyāhāra, the fifth stage of Patañjali's Yoga-Sūtras, is fundamental (see Chapter 1). Practicing pratyāhāra can calm the senses and the wandering mind. The sensory organs are withdrawn from objects that distract them and make them greedy. Therefore they are free and released. The senses are controlled and mastered (Yoga-Sūtra II.55, Iyengar 2002b, p. 170). This can be practiced with the following two exercises.

Exercise: Breathing and Listening

Sit on a chair or on the floor in a position of your choice so that your spine is upright. Close your eyes and keep them closed until the end of the exercise. Be aware of your whole body; feel the contact with the floor and your clothes. Accept everything that your senses are perceiving; be completely open to these perceptions.

Possibly sound will be the most dominant perception. Be aware of all sounds, no matter whether people are speaking, birds are singing, the telephone rings, a car is passing by, there is noisy construction work going on, or anything else.

Listen carefully without judging, without asking where the sounds are coming from, but be aware that you are listening. Remain as an observer without becoming involved. In this way your perception connects the object with your organs of the senses, while your inner observer is unaffected by it.

Focus on a particularly dominant sound, then move your awareness to a different one, and then to a few more different ones. Now listen to as many different sounds as possible at the same time. Expand your perception to the most distant sound; listen to even more subtle sounds. Expand your perception further and further: this helps to keep your thoughts calm. You perceive the sounds directly without your mind judging.

Now pull your perception inwards to your breath, just below the nostrils. Sounds from outside are excluded now. Be with your breath for some time. As long as time allows you can switch between awareness of the outer sounds and your breathing.

Partner exercise: cultivating mindfulness

Partner A is performing any exercise from this book. Before the other one, partner B, touches A's body with her hands, both talk about which area should be touched. Then, partner B feels the quantity and quality of her partner's movements. She can also feel how much pressure or support is appropriate by communicating mindfully with the partner's body tissues. This exercise leads to an even deeper experience for partner B if done with the eyes shut or with a bandage wrapped around the closed eyes.

In his book *Yoga – The Path to Holistic Health* (2001), Iyengar emphasizes the importance of being completely focused both physically and mentally during yoga practice. The effects of the exercises are mainly achieved through mindful exercising:

- reaching the different parts of the body mentally
- connecting the thoughts with the relevant part and action
- being completely aware of what you are doing.

The learning process follows four stages:

1. Beginners practice physical exercises, first learning gross movements and stability of the posture.
2. In intermediate practice the mind learns to move together with the body, and is becoming aware of the different body parts.
3. In advanced practice the mind and the body are becoming one.
4. The final stage is perfection, where the different parts of the body are reached with full awareness.

The state of mind can be influenced, too: "Through cultivation of friendliness, compassion, joy, and indifference to pleasure and pain, virtue and vice respectively, the consciousness becomes favourably disposed, serene and benevolent" (Iyengar 2002a, p. 86).

Among the classic books on yoga the Hatha-Yoga-Pradīpikā is particularly celebrated. This is the first known book where the basic yoga postures, which are still practiced today, can be found. It was written by Svātmārāma, probably around AD 1400 (Weiss 1986, Feuerstein 2001). In Chapter II.2 the connection between a steady breath and a steady mind is emphasized. According to Chapter IV, verse 29, the breath, mind, and senses are closely related; the breath is considered to be the master of the mind, and the mind the master of the senses (Sinh 2006).

In the 20th century this approach, integrating mindfulness into work with the body, was further developed by B K S Iyengar over seven decades, constantly refining awareness of the structures and functions of the body while practicing with full attention.

Iyengar (2009, p. 87) states: "The brain and the mind should be kept alert, to correct and adjust the body position and the flow of breath from moment to moment ... Complete receptivity of the mind and intellect are essential." Geeta Iyengar, his daughter, has continued and refined this work, particularly emphasizing the importance of mental and intellectual attitude. Body posture is closely connected to the mental and intellectual attitude (Iyengar 2002b).

The practice of āsanas can teach us a lot about cultivating mindfulness and intelligence throughout the body. Looking inwards, the body can constantly be adjusted and balanced. For example, if we stand with our arms spread horizontally we can look at our fingers or we can look into a mirror. We can feel the fingers and the expansion of the posture as far as the fingertips. Similarly we can look at other areas of the body or feel them, growing more and more aware of them. The awareness of the body and the intelligence of the mind and the heart should be in harmony.

While practicing the āsanas the mind should be in a calm space filled with a subtle awareness of the actions and sensations felt in performing the respective āsana. During the practice of āsanas this awareness must be renewed constantly. Practice should not become a habit and you should not be distracted. Mindfulness helps to overcome exhaustion both during practice and in everyday life (Iyengar 2005).

Over thousands of years the mindful exercise approach of yoga has been shown to be beneficial for prevention and cure or as an adjunct to curing a wide range of conditions. This knowledge is mostly based on clinical and empirical evidence. It is only during the last decades that modern research has furnished evidence for a wide range of therapeutic effects of this ancient exercise approach (see Chapter 1).

Mindfulness in the Buddhist tradition

From the Satipatthāna Sutta, one of the central teachings ascribed to Shakyamuni Buddha, we can learn a lot about the application of mindfulness to basic postures and movements. Slightly simplified, the text describes a monk's practice as follows. If the monk is walking, he knows: I am walking. If he is standing, he knows: I am standing. Sitting, he knows: I am sitting. Lying down, he knows: I am lying. He knows exactly what his posture is at every moment. By letting go of his memories and desires his mind becomes steady and focused.

Then the correct breathing method is described. The monk is sitting in a straight firm posture, maintaining his awareness. Inhaling, he knows: I am inhaling; exhaling, he knows: I am exhaling. Being fully aware of his whole body, he is inhaling; being fully aware of his whole body, he is exhaling. Stilling the actions of the body he will inhale and exhale. Through this dedicated practice he can let go of distractions and his mind becomes calm and focused. He becomes like deep water, which is not disturbed by any waves – this water reflects everything clearly and quietly (Satipatthāna Sutta 2009). From this text one of the most important meditation exercises of Theravada Buddhism has developed, called after the sutta's title, satipatthāna, or the "four foundations of mindfulness."

The same principles are practiced in the Zen tradition of China, Korea, and Japan. In order to gain a deeper understanding of the mind's actions, you learn to let go of thoughts and emotions. Then, according to Takuan Sōhō, a Japanese Zen master teaching in the early 17th century, a mental state of "no-mind" is reached (Takuan 1987). Interestingly, this state is something which cannot be seen with the eyes but only experienced with the body. Takuan states that the purpose of training is to free yourself from mental attachments. This expression refers to the regular mind which constantly attaches itself to something. No-mind, however, is free from these strings. According to the Zen tradition, our tendency to attach the mind to things around us is an enormous obstacle in training. Here again, breathing meditation is used to get rid of distracting thoughts. As Takuan explains, whenever we think of doing something, our mind is stopped by this thought. The solution is to get the mind to initiate an action without stopping in the process. The result is something called the "original mind" in Zen, a mind filling the entire body and permeating all of its parts, while our everyday state of being, the "deluded mind," is fixed at one specific point because of excessive thinking. By concentrating on breathing, even beginners can slowly learn to loosen this fixation while moving towards a more open condition.

Psychological aspects of mindfulness and movement

All therapists are aware that manual treatment and exercising can cause emotional reactions in patients. In contrast, the emotions and thoughts that patients bring with them directly influence their behavior and movements. Negative emotions such as anxiety, depression, anger, and aggression make it harder to select an exercise for the current emotional situation. They also make body and mental movements heavier. In contrast, a state of positive emotions such as joy or being in love makes movements easy and fluent.

The self-aware and self-reflective mind observes and investigates itself, including its emotions, mood, and thoughts (Kabat-Zinn 1994). Psychologists agree that the first step towards gaining control is taken with reflective self-awareness. Freud (1916) calls this "evenly hovering attention." Goleman (1996) explains that you can be angry at someone and at the same time be self-reflective and think: "I am feeling angry." This process apparently causes the brain's neural circuits to monitor the emotion, so that you gain some control. Eventually, being aware of feelings leads to emotional self-control and to emotional competence when dealing with other people. Apart from being useful in social relationships, identifying and managing emotions can also enhance cognition and task performance, as experimental research has shown.

Of special interest is the function of positive states of being. As a way to approach this function, Frederickson (2001) has developed her "broaden-and-build model" of positive emotions. This claims that the form and function of positive and negative emotions complement one another. If a negative emotion is experienced, our thought and action repertoire is narrowed to certain actions that were originally relevant for survival. Even today, these ancient survival programs are still active. Positive emotions, however, broaden our thought and action repertoire and help us build lasting personal resources. This model implies that positive emotions work to dissolve their negative counterparts.

Seen from an evolutionary perspective, positive emotions do not appear to be as important for survival value as negative emotions like fear or anger. These negative emotions trigger actions like running away or attacking, both necessary for surviving the dangers of primeval times. Feeling joy or contentment does not have such a clear survival value, but from a psychological perspective, Frederickson claims that positive emotions helped primitive humans to broaden their minds and build resources that sustained them in difficult times.

Exercises in mindfulness may help us to manage our emotions. If we are aware of our negative emotions they may be neutralized, whereas an attempt to control them may lead to suppressing them. If it is not possible to neutralize harmful emotions psychological advice should be sought and psychotherapy may be necessary. Cultivated positive emotions, however, not only counteract negative emotions but also broaden individuals' habitual ways of movement and of thinking and build their personal resources for coping.

We judge our actions. This judgment influences our future behavior. A judgment can be positive, negative, or neutral. From our past personal experience we are motivated to repeat in the future actions which we have judged positively. Through frequent repetition of the same action and the same judgment, our behavior becomes automatic. Constant avoidance also becomes automatic, although the disadvantage of avoidance is that we do not build up experience and therefore have no chance to change our behavior. This may affect other areas and functions. If we take an injured shoulder as an example, avoiding any movement within the injured area causes increasing restriction over a larger area.

This thinking is closely connected to the yoga tradition. The vṛttis, the waves or movements of consciousness, influence our actions and behavior. Remembering past events influences our behavior in the present. Yoga-Sūtra II.16 states: "The pains which are yet to come can be and are to be avoided" (Iyengar 2002a, p. 123). Yoga practice teaches us to set ourselves free from these boundaries which were created through previous painful experiences. We can learn behavior and movements that are appropriate for the present. We can do this during the practice of yoga āsanas, which are to be performed according to our individual situation – there are lots of modifications. If performed correctly the āsanas do not cause pain or negative emotions. If unpleasant emotions arise during the correct practice of āsanas, they are from remembering past events that are stored in the body. Or they can be caused by distracted senses and a distracted mind or thinking about the future. Yoga practice helps us to become calm in the present.

As we age and use habitual attitudes or body movements over a long period, it becomes increasingly difficult to discriminate between habitual movements and necessary natural movements. Often habitual movement patterns become second nature. But the constant repetition of habitual movements causes change. In the body soft tissues change and the brain loses flexibility. Restrictions in movement occur. Therefore it is important to become aware of our habits of movement.

Automatic actions save time, but the disadvantage is that we may react inappropriately in a changing context. An action which we carry out automatically because of countless previous experiences may not be suitable for a new real situation. It becomes more difficult to correct ourselves and adapt to the new situation.

Mindfulness allows us to control automatic actions: we can benefit from the advantages of automation while avoiding the disadvantages. The speed of automatic actions is useful; nevertheless mindfulness helps us to control these actions. Generally, our judgments and thoughts lead to either positive or negative emotions. In cognitive psychotherapy this is used to change behavior patterns. If we observe our automatic attitudes, judgments, thoughts, and sensations we can change them (Ellis 1994, Beck 2006). Again, this is possible using mindful awareness of these inner events.

The meaning of mindfulness for exercising

The following points are particularly relevant for mindfulness, with special emphasis on mindful exercising:

- awareness of our physical activities and sensations as posture and correcting our posture, joint positions, muscle tone, respiration, and movements against gravity

- awareness of our emotions, which can be positive, negative, or neutral

- awareness of our mental attitude, which can be positive, negative, or neutral

- the freedom to stop or change body movements, emotions, and thoughts.

In the yoga tradition the śarīras are described. These are three layers or frames that envelop the soul: (1) the gross frame, containing the anatomical structures; (2) the subtle frame, consisting of the physiological functions; and (3) the causal frame, which is described in Indian philosophy as something like a divine force (Iyengar 2009). A more refined description is given by the concept of the kośas, five layers or sheaths, interpenetrating the śarīras. These five layers include: (1) the anatomical sheath; (2) the physiological sheath, including the systems of the body, such as the respiratory system; (3) the psychological sheath, which is important for awareness, feeling, and motivation; (4) the intellectual sheath, which is important for judgment and reasoning; and (5) the spiritual sheath (Feuerstein 2001, Iyengar 2009).

To be able to move our body efficiently and without effort we need motor abilities, strength, and mobility. We also need sensory awareness to develop excellence in controlling the movement. If our sensory awareness is not well developed, we will only be able to carry out major deviations from the ideal movement. The later the finetuning happens, according to sensory feedback, the less precise the corrections will be: the movements become awkward and the risk of injury rises dramatically. This can often be observed in beginners. Therefore developing mindfulness and refining awareness quickly lead to precision and finetuning. The danger of injury is lessened, and pain can be avoided.

If we learn a new movement we refine it through repetition. The flow of movement becomes more economical, appearing more elegant. During the learning period the movements are felt more. The more we become used to the movements, the less sensory feedback we get, to a point where sensory feedback is hardly felt at all. Now the risk of injury increases again. At this point mindfulness becomes particularly important. For a better balance of movement and sensory feedback and to reduce the risk of injury, new exercises or variations can be added.

The process of refining the movements creates joy and happiness and motivates us to repeat the movements even better. Through mindful practice we improve the quality of our movements faster. Practice without mindfulness needs much longer training and is more likely to lead to injury and pain.

If we are healthy and able to move well, we are not usually aware of our movements. Pain, however, is an indication to stop or change the movement. Often pain is an emergency brake. It may indicate that the body has been overstressed, perhaps for a long time, or used in a faulty way. Greater awareness could have avoided strain and faulty use, as repeated mindful exercising refines sensory awareness.

In summary we have three modes for bodily and mental movements:

1. We move in a habitual way, without much awareness of our movement, feeling, and thinking.

2. We are aware of the kind of movement, our emotions, and our thinking. In this case change and learning will happen. This is the mindful mode.

3. Distress, pain, or too strong emotions will stop the movement.

The aim is to increase the mindful mode, our awareness of movement, emotions, and thinking, to support learning and changes.

From the 1980s new mindfulness-based methods have been developed, particularly within behavioral psychology. Jon Kabat-Zinn has developed a method called Mindfulness-Based Stress Reduction (MBSR), a training of practices based on a combination of Buddhist Vipassana and Zen traditions and on mindful yoga. Kabat-Zinn has conducted much research and published a series of studies about the effects of MBSR on chronic pain. Statistically significant reductions were observed in pain, inhibition of activity through pain, mood disturbance, anxiety, and depression. Most subjects reported that they continued their training as part of their daily lives (Kabat-Zinn et al. 1985, 1987). Later these results were confirmed and extended by Majumdar et al. (2002). These authors found improvements through mindfulness training in psychological distress, physical well-being, and quality of life.

The importance of mental practice for physical exercises has been emphasized by Lederman (2005). Based on research, Lederman shows that motor learning is improved by thinking and visualizing the movements. The thinking and visualizing have effects on the motor system, even without carrying out the movements. Clinical studies showed electromyography changes. Mental practice also improves physical activities, both endurance and muscle strength.

Summary

We have considered mindfulness in:
- yoga
- Buddhism
- Zen meditation
- modern psychology and medicine (supported by evidence-based medicine).

From the publications on these topics we selected those that were particularly relevant for mindful physical practice. We came to the conclusion that mindfulness in exercising increases the efficiency (a minimum of effort, economical exercising) and effectiveness of exercises and reduces the risk of injury.

Teaching mindfulness and mindful exercising

General considerations

The points given below are not meant to be applied all at once for every patient or student; rather, select and adjust them to the individual with whom you are working. The teaching steps should be small enough so that students or patients can be aware of what they have learned. Mindfulness and awareness are developed for the body and its activities, for the emotions, and for mental attitude. The student and teacher observe how far movements, emotions, and thoughts can be controlled and calmed. The emotions during āsana practice are positive and calm: all other emotions are vṛttis, memories.

The practical aspects of mindful exercising

Awareness of the body can be trained in the following ways:
- touching and feeling the relevant area
- moving the area passively with the hand
- moving the area actively, feeling the movement with the hands

(avoiding eye contact in these three types of exercise increases tactile awareness)
- performing the movements with resistance and/or weight-bearing.

These exercises should be performed first without looking at the area that is worked on. After the exercises have been completed you can look at the area.

Reducing visual feedback during movement can also enhance proprioception [perception and control of the body position in space]... if vision is reduced early in the learning process, it increases the reliance of the subject on proprioception for correcting and learning the movement.
(Lederman 2005, pp. 155–156)

The following points are important for awareness and control of emotions and mental attitude:
- Ask yourself: what is your mental attitude and your emotion at the beginning of the exercise?
- Develop an attitude of curiosity, as when small children explore their body.
- Develop an innocent attitude totally detached from any expectations and memories.
- Experience each exercise like the first breath of a newborn baby.

- Modify and combine the exercises to make them pleasant.
- Make the steps of practicing and learning small enough that you can follow them mindfully.
- Give yourself or the patient the chance to stop or change to a different exercise.
- Adjust the exercises so that you are looking forward to practicing them again.

Exercise to develop awareness and to refine the approach to the barrier of movement

Example for developing mindfulness through stretching and activating muscles:

1. Begin any stretch that you wish and go to the point where you feel the muscles lengthening.
2. It may help to close the eyes and feel the sensation of stretching.
3. Ease off a tiny bit. If you still feel the stretch, your first movement was too strong.
4. Repeat the process of backing off a tiny bit until the sensation of stretching disappears.
5. Now you have the right point and you can return to the most recent position where you can feel the stretch comfortably.
6. Within 10–20 seconds the stretching sensation will disappear.
7. Now you can activate the muscle with full awareness.

Relevant for all exercises

Mindfulness is the fundamental and most important principle. It should be integrated into each exercise and āsana. The practice approach, speed, and length should be such that mindful exercising is possible.

References

Beck, A.T., 2006. Cognitive Therapy and the Emotional Disorders, second ed. Guilford, New York.

Ellis, A., 1994. Reason and Emotion in Psychotherapy. Citadel, New York.

Feuerstein, G., 2001. The Yoga Tradition. Hohm, Prescott, AZ.

Frederickson, B.L., 2001. The role of positive emotions in positive psychology: the broaden-and-build theory of positive emotions. Am. Psychol. 56, 218–226.

Freud, S., 1916. Vorlesungen zur Einführung in die Psychoanalyse. Gesammelte Werke, Studienausgabe Bd. 1, Vienna.

Goleman, D., 1996. Emotional Intelligence. Bloomsbury, London.

Iyengar, B.K.S., 2001. Yoga – The Path to Holistic Health. Dorling Kindersley, London.

Iyengar, B.K.S., 2002a. Light on the Yoga Sūtras of Patañjali. Thorsons, London.

Iyengar, G.S., 2002b. Yoga: a Gem for Women. Timeless, Spokane, WA.

Iyengar, B.K.S., 2005. Light on Life. Rodale, Emmaus, PA.

Iyengar, B.K.S., 2009. Light on Prāṇāyāma. Crossroad, New York, NY.

Kabat-Zinn, J., 1994. Wherever you Go, There you Are. Hyperion, New York.

Kabat-Zinn, J., Lipworth, L., Burney, R., 1985. The clinical use of mindfulness meditation for the self-regulation of chronic pain. J. Behav. Med. 8, 163–190.

Kabat-Zinn, J., Lipworth, L., Burney, R., 1987. Four-year follow up of a meditation-based program for the self-regulation of chronic pain: treatment outcomes and compliance. Clin. J. Pain 2, 159–173.

Lederman, E., 2005. The Science and Practice of Manual Therapy. Elsevier, Edinburgh.

Majumdar, M., Grossman, P., Ditz-Waschkowski, B., et al., 2002. Does mindfulness meditation contribute to health? Outcome evaluation of a German sample. J. Altern. Complement. Med. 8, 719–730.

Mylius, K., 2003. Geschichte der altindischen Literatur. Harrassowitz, Wiesbaden.

Satipatthāna Sutta: frames of reference (MN 10), transl. Thanissaro Bhikkhu. Access to Insight, June 7, 2009 Available online at: http://www.accesstoinsight.org/tipitaka/mn/mn.010.than.html.

Sinh, P., 2006. Haṭha Yoga Pradīpikā: Explanation of Haṭha Yoga. Pilgrims, Kathmandu.

Takuan, S., 1987. The Unfettered Mind: Writings of the Zen Master to the Sword Master. Kodansha, Tokyo.

Weiss, H., 1986. Quellen des Yoga. Scherz, Bern.

CHAPTER 3

Diagnosis

Chapter contents

General considerations for diagnosis and testing

Diagnosis and examination are fundamental to all medical and therapeutic interventions:

- to design the treatment plan
- to see the improvement, how the patient is responding to treatment
- to adjust and modify the treatment accordingly.

Manual therapists have a special responsibility for diagnosis. During treatment patients seem to become more aware and remember their problems more. Often they tell their therapist what they should have told their doctor or counselor. The manual therapist must be able to guide the patient towards the appropriate diagnostic steps. It is also important to recognize red flags indicating when the patient has to be referred for medical investigation. This is the case if any of the following applies:

abdominal pain, anorexia, bilateral symptoms, bowel/bladder changes, chills, constipation, diaphoresis, diarrhea, dizziness, dysesthesia, dysphagia, dyspnea, early satiety, fatigue, fever, headaches, heartburn, hemoptysis, hoarseness, indigestion, jaundice, nausea, night pain, night sweats, palpitations, paresthesia, persistent cough, skin rash, vision changes, vomiting, weakness, weight loss/gain.

(Goodman & Snyder 2000, pp. 492–493)

Particular care is necessary when there is:

- severe feeling of sickness

- severe night pains

- spasms

- psychological problems

- no history of trauma or injury

- no known etiology

- conspicuous recent changes

- case history which indicates that exercise could cause tissue damage; for example, with fractured ribs be careful not to cause a pneumothorax with exercise

- pain that does not improve with medication, treatment, position, movement, or rest

- any doubt or the feeling that something is not right.

We are not dealing with systemic diseases in this book; nevertheless we should be aware that systemic diseases could mimic neuromusculoskeletal problems due to viscerosomatic reflexes or referral patterns of viscera. Particular care is necessary if the case history shows related signs and symptoms (Goodman & Snyder 2000).

Sammut & Searle-Barnes (1998, p. 136) summarize the important principles of examination:

- *understanding what has happened to the various tissues that cause the symptoms*
- *understanding how the body has reacted locally and globally to these changes, particularly how these have affected the functions*
- *considering the predisposing and maintaining factors for these tissues and functional changes.*

These aspects are helpful for developing appropriate exercises, and changing harmful habits and everyday activities.

Tests of our aims of exercising

From the vast array of tests available we are giving a brief introduction of those that relate particularly to our aims of exercising. The tests indicate which

therapeutic aims should be developed, maintained, or reduced. The diagnostic outcome will lead to the appropriate exercise prescription and help patients to understand why these exercises were chosen, how to perform them, and see the improvements for themselves. Many tests are exercises as well, and most exercises can also be considered as tests. Therefore we will give suggestions for tests and refer to suitable basic exercises or āsanas. As soon as patients have developed mindfulness in their approach to exercise, they will be able to see and feel the changes more clearly.

For details of musculoskeletal examination there are many publications to refer to, such as Magee (1997), Sammut & Searle-Barnes (1998), and Goodman & Snyder (2000). For tests referring to motor abilities, see Lederman (2005, 2010).

We will mainly focus on active tests that are most relevant for showing improvement through exercise and can be understood, performed, and evaluated by patients themselves, once the therapist has taught them.

The baseline is the patient's ability at the start of the exercise treatment. All improvement is measured in relation to this baseline. This individual approach is consistent with the traditional view of yoga, meeting patients where they are. A sensible objective is to tailor the exercise aims to the patient's needs and expectations, as far as possible. This subjective approach has been useful in the authors' exercise approach.

A non-specific but highly relevant factor indicating general health and stamina is the overall quality of movement and willingness to move. Experience has shown that any change in range of movement, however small, can improve the patient's function and well-being. To judge this, mindfulness is fundamental. In itself mindful exercising is an important basis for testing that patients can do themselves.

We have mentioned the importance of testing in the initial diagnosis and observation of improvement through exercising. Particularly important for the patient is the motivation to continue exercising. Therefore tests that enable patients to judge their own improvement for themselves are particularly relevant. With continued practice, mindfulness and the ability to self-test will be increasingly refined.

The following sections suggest a selection of tests, with an emphasis on the close relation between testing and exercising. Results can be documented in different ways according to individual preference. For example, measurements can be taken, or drawings, photographs, verbal descriptions, or a combination of any of these can be used. In this way the patient's success rate can be observed over a period of time. The baseline indicates where the patient was at the beginning.

The meaning of mindfulness

As explained in Chapter 2, mindfulness is a fundamental aspect of the ancient eastern paths of meditation. Applying this principle to the physical practice of the yoga path leads to the following reflective aspects:

- observing the body's signals
- cultivating inner awareness from the center to the periphery of the body
- observing and feeling: where awareness can go, which parts of the body can be penetrated with the mind, how long this awareness can last, how long you can be calm in a posture.

In mindfulness the exercise path is entered from both directions. It is a basis for measuring the improvement in all objectives as well as the quality of exercise and the boundary of movements. It is enhanced through continued practice. Improving mindfulness is not restricted by most conditions, nor by aging. Iyengar (2005) emphasizes that we have the capacity to refine our awareness as we get older. It is worth cultivating this. Mindfulness is a strong diagnostic tool that can be applied to all exercises and can constantly be honed.

Mobility and stability

For a successful exercise prescription it is important to consider hypomobility as well as hypermobility and the possible relationship between the two. It is particularly important to understand hypermobility in order to protect the relevant areas and avoid injury through overexercising. We need to distinguish between pathological instability and hypermobility (Magee 1997).

Pathological instability is an excess of the small accessory movements in the joints, such as translation or anterior/posterior shift. A small amount of this joint play is important for painless, good joint function; it is not under voluntary control. Pathological hypermobility is an excess of gross anatomical movements, such as flexion, extension, side-bending, rotation, and circumduction. It is very individual, and is dependent on age, gender, and many other factors. Hypomobility and hypermobility can be generalized or local. Hypermobility is often adjacent to a restricted area and a consequence of it.

Clinical instability of the lumbar spine is frequently discussed (Richardson et al. 1999, Panjabi 2003). When the practitioner can see more pronounced deviations from natural curves during active examination, showing hypermobile segments, the patient often experiences pain. This is an important connection between the testing done by the therapist and the patient. These hypermobile segments also need special care during exercise. If movements at these segments are causing pain, this area may be overworked. The movements should remain in the pain-free range or come back to this range if performed too far.

Patients and yoga students who are generally hypermobile are often admired and envied for their abilities and impressive performance of yoga āsanas. Nevertheless, they tend to have pain that does not improve, and sometimes is even worsening despite their regular, beautiful practice. Their muscles, tendons, and ligaments are often overstretched and irritated. They should not go to the limit of their mobility; rather they need to adjust their postures so that the muscles are strengthened and work together in a balanced way. For hypermobile individuals precise alignment is very important. The muscles should be used sufficiently to finetune the movements of the joints and to protect the vulnerable joints. The instructions for both the āsanas and the basic exercises are designed to fulfill this. Very mobile people may need to come away from their limits of movement and use props to support stability first. Details need to be decided on a case-by-case basis.

Standing active examination for hip and spinal mobility

Stand with your feet as close together as possible. Keep the knees straight throughout the movement test. Perform side-bending, rotation, bending backwards, and bending forwards. Find and document the painfree range of movement.

To test yourself you can slide your hands down the sides of your legs for side-bending, and down the backs of your legs when bending backwards. When you bend forwards you can measure the distance from your fingertips to the floor. You may like to use a stick lined up beside your legs: make a mark on this stick to indicate how far you get down, and observe your development over a period of time.

Rotation can also be tested sitting on a chair, turning to either side, and observing the angle of rotation (see Chapter 6, exercise 2.8).

Note that hip mobility and thigh muscle tone influence the result. When testing forward bending in particular it is useful to decide the main limit at the outset. If short hamstrings restrict hip flexion the lumbar spine will be more curved. If the lumbar spine itself is restricted it will show less curve from the side (Sammut & Searle-Barnes 1998).

To test the hamstrings lie on your back and raise one leg, keeping that knee straight (see Chapter 7, āsana Supta Pādāṅguṣṭhāsana). Check the angle of hip flexion.

Tests for the feet

It is essential to observe the transverse and longitudinal arches of the feet during standing and how they change with exercising (see Chapter 6, exercises 10.4 and 10.6).

Active mobility without weight-bearing can be tested sitting with straight legs. Move the feet into plantar- and dorsiflexion, inversion and eversion, and circumduction. Move the toes in all possible directions. Extension of the big toe is particularly important for gait (see Chapter 6, exercise 10.3).

To test these abilities with weight-bearing, stand and invert and evert your feet, then raise the heels and stand on the heels, raising the forefoot (see Chapter 6, exercise 10.9). Toe extension can be tested in squatting with the heels raised. The hands can be supported on a couch.

While wear and tear of the soles of the shoes may not help to judge improvement over just a few weeks, it is a useful diagnostic tool at the outset or over a longer period.

Tests for the knees

Look into the mirror for:

- valgus or varus

- swelling around the joints

- shape and position of the kneecap

- shape of the quadriceps muscle, which is very important for good function of the knee joint. Tighten both thighs simultaneously. Observe whether the kneecaps move evenly upwards.

To test flexion and extension without weight-bearing:

- Stand on one foot. Support yourself against a table or wall using the hand on the same side. Bend and stretch the other knee.

- Sit on a chair. Bend and stretch one knee at a time; when you are stretching the knee the leg is horizontal.

- Test flexion in the knee hug position, lying on your back (see Chapter 6, exercise 1.4, Figure 6.4).

To test flexion and extension on weight-bearing, look in the mirror:

- Stand on both feet. Stretch both knees; observe whether they can stretch equally.

- Raising your heels, squat down as far as possible. Look for deviations and stability.

Tests for the hips

Here we have chosen positions in which it is easy to test movement. Some movements can also be performed in different positions.

Standing

To test extension of the hip, stand on one foot. Support yourself with the hand of this same side against a wall or table. Keep your pelvis stable (you can control this with your free hand) and move your leg backwards.

If the pelvis tilts downwards on the side of the lifted leg, this is called a positive Trendelenburg's sign (Magee 1997). If there is no serious pathology this is a reliable test for hip stability, particularly strength of the hip abductors. This stability is essential for all exercises on one leg. When these exercises are performed correctly they build up this stability (see Chapter 6, exercises 8.4 and 8.6, and Chapter 7, Vṛkṣāsana).

Sitting on a chair or on the floor

- To test adduction cross one leg over, so that one thigh is resting on the other one.
- To test abduction spread the legs apart.
- To test external rotation bend the knee and rest the foot on the other thigh (see Chapter 6, exercise 8.5, variation c).

Internal and external rotation can also be tested with straight legs (see Chapter 6, exercise 8.1).

Lying on the back

With bent knees, hip flexion and circumduction can be tested (see Chapter 6, exercise 8.2).

Lying on your back and bending one hip and knee can also give important information (see Chapter 6, exercise 7.1). If the straight leg comes off the floor or the knee bends, a flexion contracture is indicated; frequently there will be hypertonia of the psoas on that side. A deviation of that leg to the side indicates hypertonic lateral muscles.

Tests for the iliosacral joints

Of the many possibilities for testing the iliosacral joints we select the following:

Lie on your back with one hip and knee bent (see Chapter 6, exercise 7.1).

There are three different positions of movement:

1. Keep bending only as long as the hip is not moving off the floor at all. This mainly shows movement in the hip joint.

2. Bend further so that the hip moves away from the floor or couch but the curve of the lumbar spine does not change. This is iliosacral movement: by changing the direction of the knee you can reach different joint planes. In most

cases it is sufficient to move the knee towards the same shoulder and towards the opposite shoulder.

3. If you bend even further the lumbar spine will flatten more.

In hypermobile iliosacral joints precise alignment is extremely important and pelvic torsion should be avoided in all exercises and postures.

Tests for the shoulders

Full examination of the shoulder may be extensive and also includes examination of the cervical spine.

To make it easier for the patient to do the movement in the shoulders and not the lumbar spine and to avoid tilting the pelvis, self-testing of flexion and abduction lying on the back is recommended:

Keep the contact of the back of the pelvis and the middle back unchanged. Keep your arms parallel, and move them above your head. Then bring your arms beside your body. Keeping them on the floor, slide them sideways and over your head. Find the painfree range of movement and compare left and right.

Extension of the shoulders, moving the arms backwards, can be tested in sitting. Again it is important to be aware of the stability of the pelvis and the lumbar spine (see Chapter 6, exercise 4.9, part 4). The back of a chair or wall may be a useful measure of this backwards movement of the arms.

External rotation and abduction and internal rotation and adduction can be tested at the same time with the Apley scratch test (Magee 1997):

1. Sit or stand. Again, be aware of the stability of the pelvis and lumbar spine.

2. Internally rotate the left arm. Move it backwards; bend the elbow and touch the back with the back of the hand, as high as possible towards the head.

3. Externally rotate and raise the right arm. Bend the elbow, touch the neck with the palm, and slide it down between the shoulder blades as far as possible.

4. Feel whether the fingers can touch or overlap. If not, use a belt to measure the distance between the hands.

5. Ask your partner or a friend to take this measurement.

6. Repeat for the other side.

The Apley scratch test covers an important part of the functional capacity of the shoulder and is also an exercise (see Chapter 6, exercise 4.11).

Tests for elbows, wrists, and hands

A quick examination of the elbow observes the shape of the stretched elbow for valgus. Then bending, extending, and hyperextending can be observed. For combinations with supination and pronation, see Chapter 6, exercise 6.6. To test the different aspects of the wrist, see Chapter 6, exercises 6.2–6.4 and 6.7.

Tests for the atlanto-occipital area and the cervical spine

Lie on your back with your head supported comfortably. The direction you are looking now indicates the tilting of your head, and a possible tightness of the atlanto-occipital or cervical area on the side where your head is tilting.

When sitting or standing the head movements bending forwards, backwards, side-bending and rotation can be tested (see Chapter 6, exercises 5.3–5.5). Stability of this area is as important as good mobility, as the cervical area contains vulnerable parts. The muscles moving the cervical spine should be strong enough and cooperate in a balanced way to protect these vulnerable areas (see Chapter 6, exercises 5.2 and 5.6).

Tests for the temporomandibular joint

When there are problems in this area dental and orthodontic investigation is necessary. Meanwhile patients can check a few simple changes for themselves:

- Look in the mirror for deviations of the chin on opening and closing the mouth.
- Feel the joint with the finger pads when opening the mouth. Feel which side moves

first, and feel whether the movement is smooth (see Chapter 6, exercise 5.7).

- Feel the chewing muscles while clenching the teeth.

Testing strength

As a taxonomy of muscular strength, the categories of static, dynamic, and yielding strength have proved to be a useful tool in practical work (Zatsiorsky & Kraemer 2006). In real life and yoga practice no sharp distinction between these types of strength is made. In our therapeutic yoga approach we mainly use static and yielding strength. We suggest that you use some of the basic exercises and āsanas and count how long or how often you can perform them.

Some examples are found in Chapter 6, exercises 1.2, 1.15, and 4.9. All āsanas are suitable as well.

Testing stamina

For the musculoskeletal system it is firstly relevant to measure the improvement in how long you can hold a contraction and how many times you can repeat certain movements without becoming tired and breathless. An everyday test is the distance you can walk or go up the stairs you have to use regularly.

In general systemic diseases are not considered here. However, as the cardiovascular system is closely related to the musculoskeletal system, it is stressed with every activity of the musculoskeletal system. Therefore we will include the following basic evaluation of the cardiovascular system:

Patients can note their increase in heart rate compared to their resting pulse after aerobic activities they do regularly for the same length of time, and observe how the heart rate changes over time.

Testing relaxation

From the physiological relaxation responses, such as reducing heart rate, metabolism, rate of breathing, blood pressure, and brain waves (Lasater 1995, p. 5), we choose the breath and heart rate as indicators of relaxation.

The breath rate and heart rate can be counted. In addition the following qualities can be observed:

- quality and smoothness of the flow of breath

- relaxing thoughts with exhalation: how many breaths can you count without becoming distracted?

- quietness in the eyes. Feel it with exhalation: can you maintain it with inhalation? This aspect is very subjective, but as we include mindfulness in exercising it is sensible to consider this aspect.

Testing balance

The gait is a non-specific balance test that can be used regularly. More specific balance tests include:

- Romberg test (Magee 1997): stand with your feet together and your arms down the sides of your body. Keep your eyes open at first. If you do not have a balance problem, close your eyes for at least 20 seconds. Where there are serious balance problems, medical investigation is necessary.

- Stand on one foot with the eyes open, then with the eyes closed.

- Four-point kneeling position: raise one arm so that it is parallel to the floor and stretch the opposite leg also parallel to the floor (see Chapter 6, exercise 1.14).

Compare left and right in all asymmetrical tests.

Testing coordination

Finger coordination

1. Touch the tip of the thumb and fingertips of one hand together quickly, one finger after the other.

2. Touch the thumb and fingertips of the left and right hand together, one after the other. Start with the right index finger on the left thumb, then the right thumb on the left index finger. Continue with the right middle finger and the left thumb, right thumb and left middle finger, right ring finger and left thumb, right thumb and left ring finger, right little finger and left thumb, right thumb and left little finger.

Then return until the right index finger is on the left thumb again. Repeat this several times for a brilliant exercise.

For a test of coordination in hip circumduction, see Chapter 6, exercise 8.2.

Testing synchronization

Synchronization can be observed within your own body during different movements. The āsanas test and teach how to synchronize the movements of the legs and arms, trunk and head, trunk, legs, and arms, or integrate all areas and all layers of the body (see the explanations from the Yoga-Sūtras in Chapters 1 and 2).

Synchronization with your surroundings is also relevant, such as exercising in a group, with a partner, moving to music, and dancing.

Testing breathing

As we place a lot of emphasis on mindful exercising, it is sensible to observe and feel the quality of the breath.

The breathing movements can be observed in a mirror, looking at the upper chest, the costal arches, and the abdomen. If you have the equipment to see your back in a mirror, also look at the breathing movement in the upper lumbar area and between the shoulder blades. With your hands, feel the sternum, the upper ribs, the costal arches, the abdomen, the upper lumbar area, and, if possible, one shoulder blade at a time for the breathing movements. Expansion with inhalation can be measured with a belt around the chest. Counting the number of breaths per minute also gives information.

Summary

Most of the exercises and āsanas described in the practical sections are diagnostic tools for one or more aims. Testing and exercising are closely related, and become one in mindful exercising. Various methods of measuring and documenting improvements can be applied. The more yoga practitioners cultivate mindfulness and awareness, the more they can refine their own diagnosis. Observation of the posture is an important diagnostic aspect as well, as many musculoskeletal and systemic diseases affect not only the quantity and quality of movement, but also the posture. Likewise posture affects the functions. In a compressed trunk fluid transport and nerve supply to all tissues and organs are compromised. A poorly lifted spine also affects the functions of the central and autonomous nervous system. Good posture improves the functions of all connected tissues and organs.

Exercise and pain

Pain during and after exercising is a frequently debated topic. First you need to find out whether the pain is caused by the exercise being performed wrongly, or whether it indicates disease. If the pain persists after the exercise has been adjusted correctly and to the intensity appropriate for the patient, a thorough investigation is necessary.

Pain is an important warning signal to prevent danger to health. It is a complex perception of different qualities: it can be an ache or a sharp or burning pain. Individuals perceive and rate pain differently; it cannot be measured objectively.

According to Pschyrembel (2007), there are several categories of pain:

- excitation of sensory nerve fibers and conduction to the central nervous system

- neuropathic pain caused by damage to the peripheral or central nervous system

- pain from disturbed function, such as muscle pain caused by wrong posture or emotional stress.

Pain syndromes, conditions associated with chronic pain and lasting longer than 6 months, are categorized as:

- pain caused by inflammation, such as arthritis, myositis, or inflammation caused by injury

- spastic pain caused by excessive contractions of the smooth muscles in organs

- neuropathic pain or neuralgia, caused by direct irritation of or damage to the nerves or directly from the central nervous system without the pain receptors being involved

- headache

- pain caused by dysfunction or bad posture

- psychosomatic pain, e.g., muscle hypertonia from emotional stress.

The myofascial pain syndrome frequently occurs in muscles or muscle groups and can be caused by overwork or strain of muscles, trauma, cold temperature, degenerative or inflammatory conditions, systemic diseases, or emotional stress (Pschyrembel 2007).

In referred pain the cause is remote from the area of pain sensation. The most common cause is the convergence of pain-sensitive nerve fibers from organs and skin areas, the so-called Head zones. Excitation of nerve fibers from organs is felt in corresponding areas of the skin. The area for the heart is in the chest, frequently spreading into the left arm or the upper abdomen (Silbernagl 2007).

We shall now consider pain in connection with the practice of yoga. First of all you should abandon the idea that exercising only helps if it is painful. Exercising should not be painful, particularly afterwards. There are very few exceptions to this rule. Pain should ease after a while; it can be released with exhalation or sustained sensitive stretching. As mentioned above, where there are serious signs and symptoms a medical investigation is necessary before using yoga as a therapy or adjunct to a medical treatment. This also applies to serious pain.

Pain during exercise

If stretching muscles or scars causes pain, it is sensible to tolerate the discomfort to a certain degree, as long as there is no irritation and the structures are not overstretched or torn. This intensity must be felt and handled very carefully. For muscles to lengthen takes 3–5 breaths. During stretching the pain should be relieved, there should be a feeling of give. If the barrier felt is too hard, painful, and not releasing, ease off slightly and continue the stretching more gently. Often it helps to let a stretch go as you breathe out.

With the same sensitive awareness, scars older than 6 months and shortened connective tissue fibers can be stretched, except that it takes 2–4 minutes to get a release and needs many repetitions (Pullig Schatz 1992). The pain of both muscle and scar stretching must not cause any radiating pain and must stop after the stretching is finished.

In any other type of pain, such as joint pain or radiating pain or in paresthesia, such as tingling or numbness, check how the exercise is being performed. If the pain or tingling or numbness persists despite the exercise being performed correctly and adjusted to what the patient can tolerate, an investigation is necessary. Exercising despite the feeling of pain may be dangerous. If pain-sensitive nerve fibers are stimulated, they release chemical substances that may cause inflammation of the adjacent vessels (Silbernagl 2007).

Pain after exercise

If pain occurs after exercising, thorough observation, and possibly investigation, is necessary.

Pain after exercising often indicates an inflammatory process such as arthritis. You need to check how the exercise was being performed – its quantity, quality, and intensity. In particular, hypermobile patients may overwork themselves during exercise. If they are not very aware, they may not feel the effects of the overwork until afterwards.

Muscle soreness or stiffness after unfamiliar or intensive use of muscles is probably caused by multiple microruptures of muscle fibers (Pschyrembel 2007).

In summary, where there is pain after exercise the main pillars are the medical investigation and the style of exercise. If the medical investigation is clear, the exercise approach should be checked. In the beginning the help and correction of a well-trained yoga teacher should be sought. With increasing practice, mindfulness and awareness are progressively cultivated. Natural biofeedback can help you to be aware of the very first signals that something is not right (Pullig Schatz 1992). Yoga practice is a good training for learning to feel and interpret these first warning signals. With increasing practice this learning can be applied to everyday life to improve posture and movement patterns, to be more aware of them, and to learn to avoid unhealthy postures, movements, and habits.

Contraindications

As for any other therapeutic and medical treatment there are contraindications for prescribing certain yoga āsanas for certain conditions. Some very experienced yoga teachers may succeed in their work by intuition based on profound knowledge and long experience. However, a thorough consideration is necessary.

Where there is acute disease, a life-threatening condition, or a condition needing surgery or special medication yoga therapy is not indicated.

The variety of approaches and modifications is rich in yoga. Once the necessary medical measures have been applied, at the very least a gentle resting pose with appropriate support or sensitive breathing can make the patient feel better. There are contraindications to performing full āsanas (Iyengar 2001). Inversions should not be practiced in cases of high blood pressure, glaucoma, or during menstruation.

Much of the knowledge about indications and contraindications for certain āsanas is based on empirical evidence. There is plenty of scope for further research on therapeutic yoga (Raman 2008a).

One remarkable recent finding relates to intraocular pressure. Measuring the pressure in 75 subjects during headstand showed that in all cases the intraocular pressure was twice as high as before starting headstand. Therefore according to present knowledge glaucoma patients should avoid standing on their head, even if they are well controlled with medication. Another observation has shown that intraocular pressure in a resting pose has been lower in subjects regularly practicing headstand than in a group who were not practicing inversions. More research is necessary into the preventive evaluation of headstand for glaucoma (Baskaran et al. 2006, Raman 2008b).

As mindfulness is an essential principle for performing yoga, students and patients should refine their awareness during their practice. In this way they will improve their ability to feel what they can do and what it is best to avoid. This also depends on their constitution and state of mind, which changes from day to day.

Mindfulness, awareness, and clear observation are also very important for the teacher and therapist.

During practice some signs indicate either exhaustion or health problems. These are change of skin color, red eyes, perspiration, change in breathing, trembling, or any other unusual reaction. It is important to keep an eye open for these signs as students and patients may have undiagnosed disease. Also if someone is afraid of certain exercises or refuses to do them, this may give an important diagnostic clue. In his work *A Matter of Health*, Raman (2008a, p. 3) states: "as an eminent doctor has put it: With all our varied instruments, useful as they are, nothing can replace the watchful eye, the alert ear, the tactful finger and the logical mind."

In summary, if there is any doubt, seek advice from an experienced colleague and a medical expert. A synthesis between modern medicine and the traditional art and science of yoga will be a good approach to the patient.

References

Baskaran, M., Raman, K., Ramani, K.K., et al., 2006. Intraocular pressure changes and ocular biometry during Śīrṣāsana (headstand posture) in yoga practitioners. Ophthalmology 113(8), 1327–1332.

Goodman, C.C., Snyder, T.E.K., 2000. Differential Diagnosis in Physical Therapy, third ed. Saunders, Philadelphia.

Iyengar, B.K.S., 2001. Yoga – The Path to Holistic Health. Dorling Kindersley, London.

Iyengar, B.K.S., 2005. Light on Life. Rodale, Emmaus, PA.

Lasater, J., 1995. Relax and Renew. Rodmell, Berkeley, CA.

Lederman, E., 2005. The Science and Practice of Manual Therapy. Elsevier, Edinburgh.

Lederman, E., 2010. Neuromuscular Rehabilitation in Manual and Physical Therapies: Principles to Practice. Churchill Livingstone, Edinburgh.

Magee, D.J., 1997. Orthopaedic Physical Assessment, third ed. Saunders, Philadelphia.

Panjabi, M.M., 2003. Clinical spinal instability and low back pain. J. Electromyogr. Kinesiol. 13, 371–379.

Pschyrembel, W., 2007. Klinisches Wörterbuch, 261st ed. Walter de Gruyter, Berlin.

Pullig Schatz, M., 1992. Back Care Basics: A Doctor's Gentle Yoga Program for Back and Neck Pain Relief. Rodmell, Berkeley, CA.

Raman, K., 2008a. A Matter of Health: Integration of Yoga and Western Medicine for Prevention and Cure, third ed. EastWest, Madras.

Raman, K., 2008b. Augeninnendruck in Śīrṣāsana. Abhyāsa 1, 23–27.

Richardson, C., Jull, G., Hodges, P., et al., 1999. Therapeutic Exercise for Spinal Segmental Stabilization in Low Back Pain. Churchill Livingstone, Edinburgh.

Sammut, E., Searle-Barnes, P., 1998. Osteopathic Diagnosis. Stanley Thornes, Cheltenham.

Silbernagl, S., 2007. Taschenatlas der Physiologie, seventh ed. Thieme, Stuttgart.

Zatsiorsky, V.M., Kraemer, W.J., 2006. Science and Practice of Strength Training, second ed. Human Kinetics, Champaign, IL.

Motivation and cognitive-behavioral intervention strategies

General considerations

Health care practitioners frequently find that patients react skeptically to advice. Sometimes we need to persuade patients into behavioral change, such as taking more exercise. Patients seem not to like being told what to do. Despite this, public health campaigns often try to increase individual risk perception through emotional messages based on fear appeal theory, for example, the graphic warnings on cigarette packs. Such warnings are rarely successful – although fear is an important factor in human perception, we need strategies to deal with this fear. Practical research has demonstrated that, although some patients react favorably when given advice, success rates are not very high, according to brief intervention studies (Mason & Butler 1999; Marcus et al. 2000; Lawlor & Hanratty 2001).

This leads to the question: which type of intervention would be successful in therapeutic practice? A word of warning: studies researching the effectiveness of different interventions have found inconsistent results. For instance, in their review Lewis et al. (2002) state that definitive conclusions could not be reached, because of measurement error, lack of importance of a particular variable, or unsuccessful interventions with changing variables.

We can still ask: how it is possible to enhance our patients' motivation and guide them to self-motivated, responsible behavior? In this ideal state, patients act autonomously, changing their unhealthy habits into healthy ones.

Useful strategies for motivational counseling were originally developed to treat addiction (Prochaska & DiClemente 1983, Rollnick et al. 2008). These tactics can be applied to change other forms of behavior.

As shown by everyday experience as well as empirical research, it is difficult to develop the ability to suppress strong habitual or situational impulses in favor of new needs that have been rationally recognized. For instance, your intention to diet stalls when you are faced with your favorite food. By the same token, patients may accept rationally their therapist's advice for daily practice of certain exercises but be unable to carry it out. One reason for this is because we prefer small short-term gains over greater long-term rewards (Ainsli 2005).

This impulsive, unwholesome behavior can be explained by the existence of multiple competing evaluation and control systems (McClure et al. 2004). Because of their attitudes and subjective norms, people do not always do what they intend to do. In social psychology this is called the intention–behavior gap (Bandura 1986, 2000; Sniehotta et al. 2005). Therefore, we need special self-control strategies in order to achieve long-term objectives in the face of passing emotions or proven habitual reactions.

One self-control strategy recommends you to arrange your environment so that it is less likely that you will yield to temptation. As an example, a woman who wishes to change her activity pattern may arrange to meet a friend so that they can perform the new activity together. This gives her an additional motivation because of her social commitment. In the same way, if there is a good team spirit within an exercising group, the individual participants are more motivated to participate regularly.

Self-control techniques recommend learning to influence your individual motivation level. This means selectively focusing your attention on information that will help you achieve your goal while ignoring stimuli that distract you from that goal (Kuhl 1985). For example, if an eagerly awaited vacation starts with a dawn flight, a traveler will motivate himself to get up in time by imagining the expected pleasures of the trip. Rising early then becomes the lesser evil compared with missing the plane.

A factor that is important in achieving a desired behavior is the difference between goal intentions (i.e., "I want to go on vacation") and implementation intentions ("Tomorrow at 5 a.m. I will take a taxi to the airport") (Gollwitzer 1999). Studies have shown that participants who try to smoke less, achieve healthier eating habits, or follow an exercise program are more successful if they have set out their specific intentions (Abraham & Sheeran 2000).

It has been repeatedly demonstrated that patients' physical activity patterns can improve through short, one-off cognitive-behavioral interventions. In a review of studies published between 1966 and 2006, Smitherman et al. (2007) give the following general recommendations:

- Give patients time to make their decisions.
- Present several options instead of a single course of action.
- Describe how other patients have acted in a similar situation.
- Tell patients that they can judge best what is good for them.
- Provide information in a neutral, impersonal way.

These ideas are similar to a technique called motivational interviewing, presented by Rollnick & Miller (1995). According to the authors, this method is determined by its "spirit" and its "interpersonal style." Here, different cognitive and personality variables are taken into account, and there is a conscious attempt to avoid reactance (the strengthening of a contrary attitude).

Practical measures

Let us now explore a number of attitudes, measures, and techniques that can be used to minimize possible resistance against intended behavioral changes while allowing for patients' cognitive and personal differences.

Small steps

Changing your lifestyle is always difficult because an old, tried and tested position has to be given up. Depending on our own personal experience with changes, this triggers fears. The bigger these steps towards change, the more likely it is that fear will be aroused. Thus any change is hampered. As Maurer (2004, p. 21) notes, "fear of change is rooted in the brain's psychology, and when fear takes hold it can prevent creativity and change. The brain is designed that any new challenge triggers some degree of fear." As a result, it is best to suggest that patients take small, individually appropriate steps, to help them reach their goal. These steps should be so small that they avoid triggering the fight or flight response. Of course, everyone's reaction will be different. The therapist and patient should work together to define the patient's goals, the steps needed to reach these goals, and an appropriate exercise program. In the process, the therapist asks about previous changes that the patient has achieved. From the starting point of these personal experiences, the exercise program is planned.

Bear in mind that excessive demands lead to frustration and fear while not enough challenge incites boredom. Although the exercises must be constructed in small steps, they can be adapted to each patient's capacities by increasing the speed of an exercise and progressing to more difficult ones. In this way boredom is avoided. Ultimately, the speed of progress is determined by patients, in line with their ability and aspirations.

Every exercise should be a small challenge that leads to a personal sense of achievement once it has been performed for a set number of repetitions. Avoid strain and failure. You can adapt each step by varying the difficulty of the exercise, the number of repetitions, and the speed of execution. The patient's individual needs govern the program.

Asking questions

You may find it helpful to guide patients towards accessing their own resources by asking questions. Even if patients cannot immediately answer, if you repeat the question, it will have an ongoing effect, and take root in the patient's memory. At some later point patients will find a solution because they are mentally prepared. Through repeated questioning the patients' attention is focused selectively on essential information that will help them achieve their exercise aims. Patients are able to find a solution for themselves, and their motivation to act is greater than if you yourself give them the solution. In this way their self-reliance is improved.

The first step is the decision to change something, and patients will already have taken this decision before they choose a therapist. They really want to change their state of health. In other words, they already have some risk awareness, even if this does not effectively predict future health behavior change by itself (Weinstein 2003). In addition patients need appropriate strategies. You can reinforce patients' decisions to change by asking what resources they used to solve other problems and talking about role models in similar situations.

Even when patients have decided to change, they may not be prepared to carry out exercise programs on their own. First you should help patients accept the need for exercise and then point the way to self-help. Patients' decisions depend on their outcome expectancies – their beliefs about the positive and negative results of different forms of behavior. Every patient knows: "If I exercise I will gain mobility and be able to control my weight, but exercising is demanding and exhausting." Only if the positive outcome expectancies (the "pros") outweigh the negative ones (the "cons") is there the chance to change behavior. Here you could recount how other patients have acted in similar situations and direct patients' attention to the pros by asking appropriate questions.

Once patients have made a conscious decision to exercise, the time is right to inquire about their personal experiences. It is vital to bolster their confidence in their own efficacy since they must believe that they are able to practice regularly in spite of everyday obstacles. For instance, their resolve could be strengthened by the sentence: "In spite of my heavy workload, I am certain that I can exercise daily."

The next step is to identify the setting and the specific exercises. Ask questions about realistic times and places and discuss how long the patient is willing to practice and how success can be measured. This kind of exchange supports the decision to exercise (Gollwitzer 1999). Through the questioning process, patients visualize a context for exercise and become familiar with it.

By repeating such questions, the patient is guided towards the conditions of practicing regularly in the future. Patients can decide on their individual exercise options because they now have a realistic idea of what is involved. Their outcome expectancies boost their belief in their own effectiveness, and this belief helps them to complete a realistic plan. Behavior change begins.

If patients want to keep up their changed behavior, they must be able to see the success of their exercise practice. Here again, asking questions guides them towards noticing perceptible changes. You should help them to accept even small changes as positive steps. Physical activity must be joy if it is to be sustained, so success should be assessed appropriately. It is the patient's evaluation system that is crucial, not the therapist's.

Appropriate questions could be:

- Can you think of small things that will tell you something has changed?

- What would you like to achieve? What would show you that there is hope that you will reach that aim?

- When would you be proud of yourself?

If you ask open questions (such as what, how, when, where), patients have the freedom to weigh their options and decide for themselves. Give information in the form of different options rather than ordering patients to follow a single course of action: avoid closed questions that only allow a "yes" or "no" response. When patients feel they can decide freely, they are able to develop the self-motivation to change their behavior.

Immediate or delayed reward

If there is a choice between a proven immediate reward and a not yet proven and therefore theoretical delayed reward, we usually decide in favor of the short-term gain. As a result familiar behavior patterns often persist and change does not take place. In order to adopt a good new habit it is necessary to minimize the influence of the "now" and to remind ourselves of the "later." In this way patients' attention is directed towards future success.

During an exercise session we need to put in an immediate extra effort while at the same time abstaining from momentary relaxation or other pleasurable activities. In the long term the profit is clear: improved circulation, reduced risk of disease, weight loss, increased energy and mobility, greater self-esteem. Through questions the therapist again points to this delayed reward. Additionally, questions about the choice of the exercise context (time, length, place) help patients to focus on their practice instead of succumbing to their habits and to fleeting emotions.

In a skillfully constructed exercise sequence, the last exercises are chosen so that patients see some success. Then, at the end of a sequence it is easy to point out an immediate improvement (for instance of mobility) or to demonstrate it during the coordination phase. The patient's attention is directed by questions like: What has changed? How does … feel now?

At the end of a sequence, most patients experience relaxation as a form of reward. This is because relaxation is perceived more clearly compared to the time before and during an exercise. It is even more important that this relaxation lasts for some time after the sequence so that it can be experienced positively in everyday life.

The known and the unknown

The main problem in relearning movements is that a well-known movement that has become unhealthy must be replaced by a similar movement that meets current demands. In this way a new movement pattern is created that is not a health hazard or is more beneficial. While learning this pattern there is the risk that patients try only to modify something they already know instead of giving up their old pattern and developing the desired movement from scratch (Hotz & Weineck 1988, p. 46).

It is sensible to start with simple but usually unknown movements, referred to in this book as "basic exercises." Here patients' perception is guided by questions about different types of sensory information (verbal, visual, kinesthetic). With the help of sensory perception, patients are able to repeat and hone the exercise on their own and to form a correct pattern of movement. From these simple new movements the more complex forms of the āsanas are later developed. If those more complex forms are practiced regularly, they will then be transferred into simple everyday movements.

As soon as a basic exercise has been mastered and can be executed independently, correctly and easily, patients are encouraged to try out variations. In doing this they will be able to find out which movements feel more pleasant or more effective. Patients can do this on their own or under your direction. Patients' creativity should always be welcomed and reinforced.

Patients should become so attentive that they are able to recognize, and stop, unhealthy movement patterns quickly. At the same time they learn to recognize which movements are more economic and efficient, and where the body works too hard because of unnecessary muscle activity. Again, these insights are openly hailed as a success.

The patient's regular good habits can be used to establish new habits faster. A useful suggestion would be to schedule the exercise cycle before something the patient does automatically. For instance, if a patient always takes a shower in the morning, advise her to exercise beforehand. Or if one specific exercise is already practiced regularly, an extra new one can be added before it. Thus a new habit can be added to an old one (Premack 1970).

"Just do it!"

Often we tend to boycott something we had resolved to do. This happens along these lines: at the very moment when you intended to carry out your plan, you think about how you are feeling at this precise moment – you simply don't feel like doing something new and would rather keep your familiar habits. At this point, even tedious activities can seem much more attractive than the new, unfamiliar activity. This is why most students start preparing for exams only when they are under pressure or why people repeatedly postpone unpleasant phone calls by taking care of something else instead.

In large companies it is frequent practice to collect information about specific problems. Based on this information management then decides on a course of action, and this decision is relayed to employees in the form of a directive, with which staff inevitably comply. This is partly because of the hierarchical structure of the company, although it is best if employees are convinced that the directive is based on a correct decision. In any case, the directive is executed without going back over the decision process.

Patients should apply the same principle. After they have made their decision to exercise they should decide on the exercise, its start, and its length. Then they should simply start without questioning whether they feel like doing the exercise at that time. Often patients will go back on their intention to exercise if they think too much about whether they have the time and energy to exercise.

It is easy to explain this pattern of behavior to patients, and in so doing, you are increasing their chance of starting to exercise at their chosen time. It is also helpful for patients to visualize in advance carrying out their intention, including all the variables such as type, place, length, and success of the exercise.

Memory tools

If a new type of behavior is to be established in daily life there is always the chance that the patient will simply forget it. This is because ingrained habits override new and unknown ones. With the help of memory tools patients can overcome their forgetfulness. Small stumbling blocks are used to remember the intention and to trigger an exercise. Examples include:

- Putting a towel on the floor where the patient will see it in the morning prompts the patient to pick it up and start an exercise linked with this action.

- The habit of stepping on the scales can be a prompt to burn some calories first, i.e., by starting a specific exercise.

- A towel hanging over the bathroom mirror can act as a prompt to do something to improve your posture before looking in the mirror. Again, this should be linked to a certain exercise.

There are countless possibilities for creating associative stumbling blocks. These blocks should always be placed in relation to a predictable daily routine; then the patient is forced to see the reminder at the desired moment.

When placing a stumbling block, it is advisable first to connect it to a conscious visual and verbal instruction. Later on this link will then call up the desired memory.

Consolidating new habits and transferring them to daily life

As soon as exercises are practiced regularly, the skills that have been developed should be transferred to everyday life. Once patients have established their exercise routines, encourage them to practice in different situations and in new sequences, varying the place, time, length, and procedure. It is a good idea to vary just one thing first, e.g., practicing in another room, outside, or while traveling. After that all the other variables can be changed one at a time or all together.

To transfer basic exercises into everyday movements, patients should choose any frequently performed movement from their daily routine. The patient then carries out this movement in slow motion, at significantly lower speed than normal. If the exercise is not performed optimally, this will be difficult. If that is the case, patients can start to refine the movement in accordance with the principles and aims they have been taught (for example, precision, mindfulness, finetuning, coordination, and synchronization).

In addition, patients are asked to integrate parts of their basic exercises into their everyday movements, i.e., to modify that familiar movement slightly. The movement is at its optimum level when it can be stopped and varied at any point. Only then does it become possible to execute the movement easily in slow motion. Patients should explore their problematic everyday movements – and their improvement – on their own.

Positive attitude

Behavior that generates less aversion and fear tends to occur increasingly often, and it is easy for such avoidance behavior to take root. If, however, unpleasant feelings are stopped by solution-oriented measures (like setting appropriate positive goals, planning a realistic exercise schedule, and taking small steps if pain arises), a constructive momentum develops in the course of time (Ludwig 2000).

In a spirit of mindfulness patients are told about the importance of their inner dialogue and positive imagery. By observing themselves mindfully, they will become aware of this internal conversation. Then they can create positive statements in the form of an inner dialogue or visualize a realistic image of future success.

A positive inner attitude and positive images lead to a readiness to change our behavior in a goal-oriented way. While an inner dialogue can express itself as bitter self-criticism ("I can't do that; it's impossible!"), it can also be phrased positively ("I'm curious how many days I'll need to learn this" or "At present this doesn't work yet but if I persist it will get better").

Usually a feeling manifests itself as a facial expression, which can also be used the other way round (Ekman et al. 1983). In other words, a relaxed, friendly face can change our emotional state and ease tensions within the body. Patients should be encouraged to use this method because exercising should be joy.

Here, the therapist acts as a role model by presenting a positive attitude that is transferred to patients. For that reason explanations as well as demonstrations of exercises should always be given very carefully. It is vital to use positive phrases like "Breathe naturally!" instead of negative ones like "Don't stop breathing!"

Correcting mistakes

If you correct mistakes, some patients may feel offended, which will reduce their motivation to exercise. To avoid this, it is advisable not to insist on what is "right" and "wrong." Instead, give extra advice. Encourage patients to try out variations and compare them by asking questions like "Which movement feels good?" or "Which movement is easier, more pleasant, or more effective?"

If the patient makes a mistake during a sequence of movements, don't always stop the sequence but wait until the patient finishes, unless there is a danger of injury. Then explain the correct movement as a variation so that the patient can make a comparison before repeating that movement. Explain that it is good to enlarge the exercise routine (Hotz & Weineck 1988).

You can also correct mistakes by pointing out even the smallest changes that lead in the desired direction, and affirming the patient's progress. Through a large number of small steps the patient improves slowly but surely, and the feeling of success persists.

Control of therapeutic behavior

Of course, you should be able to explain why an exercise is performed. This rational explanation helps patients strengthen their motivation.

You also need to ask patients whether they understand an exercise to make sure they will practice the exercise correctly. It is even more important to let patients demonstrate all exercises while you are watching. If patients are to work on their own, write down the exercises or make a simple drawing of them to help them remember.

Finally it is essential to inquire how patients have got on while they were exercising on their own, before asking them to demonstrate the exercises once more. Then you can affirm the exercise behavior by pointing out success and correcting mistakes that have crept in. If a patient has failed to exercise, ask what the obstacles were and what would help. For some patients it is useful to keep a list of their successes.

References

Abraham, C., Sheeran, P., 2000. Understanding and changing health behaviour: from health beliefs to self-regulation. In: Norman, P., Abraham, C., Conner, M. (eds.), Understanding and Changing Health Behaviour. Harwood, Amsterdam, pp. 3–24.

Ainsli, G., 2005. Precis of breakdown of will. Behav. Brain Sci. 28, 635–673.

Bandura, A., 1986. Social Foundations of Thought and Action: A Social Cognitive Theory. Englewood Cliffs, New York.

Bandura, A., 2000. Cultivate self-efficacy for personal and organizational effectiveness. In: Locke, E.A. (ed.), Handbook of Principles of Organizational Behaviour. Blackwell, Oxford.

Ekman, P., Levenson, R.W., Friesen, W.V., 1983. Autonomic nervous system activity distinguishes among emotions. Science 21, 1208–1210.

Gollwitzer, P.M., 1999. Implementation intentions: strong effects of simple plans. Am. Psychol. 54, 493–503.

Hotz, A., Weineck, J., 1988. Optimales Bewegungslernen: Anatomisch-physiologische und bewegungspsychologische Grundlagenaspekte des Techniktrainings. Perimed, Erlangen, pp. 46.

Kuhl, J., 1985. Volitional mediators of cognitive-behavior consistency: self-regulatory processes and actions versus state of orientation. In: Kuhl, J., Beckmann, J. (eds.), Action Control: From Cognition to Behavior. Springer, Berlin, pp. 101–128.

Lawlor, D.A., Hanratty, B., 2001. The effect of physical activity advice given in routine primary care consultations: a systematic review. J. Public Health Med. 23, 219–226.

Lewis, B.A., Marcus, B.H., Pate, R.R., et al., 2002. Psychosocial mediators of physical activity behavior among adults and children. Am. J. Prev. Med. 23, 409–418.

Ludwig, P.H., 2000. Imagination. Leske+Budrich, Opladen.

McClure, S.M., Laibson, D.I., Loewenstein, G., et al., 2004. Separate neural systems value immediate and delayed monetary rewards. Science 306, 503–507.

Marcus, B.H., Dubbert, P.M., Forsyth, L.H., et al., 2000. Physical activity behavior change: issues in adoption and maintenance. Health Psychol. 19, 32–41.

Mason, S., Butler, C., 1999. Health Behavior Change: A Guide for Practitioners. Churchill Livingstone, London.

Maurer, R., 2004. One Small Step can Change your Life: the Kaizen Way. Workman, New York.

Premack, D., 1970. Mechanisms of self-control. In: Hunt, W.A. (ed.), Learning Mechanisms in Smoking. Aldine, Chicago, pp. 107–123.

Prochaska, J.O., DiClemente, C.C., 1983. Stages and processes of self-change of smoking: toward an integrative model of change. J. Consult. Clin. Psychol. 51, 390–395.

Rollnick, S., Miller, W., 1995. What is motivational interviewing? Behav. Cogn. Psychother. 23, 325–334.

Rollnick, S., Miller, W.R., Butler, C.C., 2008. Motivational Interviewing in Health Care: Helping Patients Change Behavior. Guilford Press, New York.

Smitherman, T., Kendzor, D.E., Grothe, K.B., et al., 2007. State of the art review: promoting physical activity in primary care settings: a review of cognitive and behavioral strategies. Am. J. Lifestyle Med. 1, 397–409.

Sniehotta, F., Scholz, U., Schwarzer, R., et al., 2005. Bridging the intention–behaviour gap: planning, self-efficacy, and action control in the adoption and maintenance of physical exercise. Psychology and Health 20, 143–160.

Weinstein, N.D., 2003. Exploring the links between risk perceptions and preventive health behavior. In: Suls, J., Wallston, K. (eds.), Social Psychological Foundations of Health and Illness. Blackwell, Oxford, pp. 22–53.

CHAPTER 5

Preparatory practice for the yoga art of breathing

General introduction

Breathing is the source of our life energy. Inspiration has a much wider meaning than just taking in air: it also means being creative, in a very deep, complex sense. Expiration not only means exhaling air; it is relaxation, letting go, finally also letting go of life. This link between life, death, and breath has been considered by many religions and philosophical systems. In the Bible we read that God made man from the dust of the earth and breathed into his nostrils the breath of life, and man became a living being. In those ancient Indian texts that are particularly relevant to yoga, such as the Vedas, Upaniṣads, Yoga-Sūtras, and Haṭha-Yoga-Pradīpikā, breathing is described as the essential process related to life.

Our life starts with our first inhalation and ends with our last exhalation. We can survive without taking fluids for about 4 days, without solid food for about 4 weeks, but without breathing for only 2–3 minutes. Breathing also connects our inner body with the environment. Philosophically speaking it connects the individual with the universe. It also connects physical and psychological aspects and is related to all bodily systems. Therefore we need to ensure that our breathing and all related structures and functions work as well as possible. As breathing is fundamental for life and all structures and functions of our body, we will give a short introduction to the anatomy and physiology of respiration, as a preparation for the practical parts of this chapter.

Basic anatomy and physiology of respiration

External and internal respiration

Respiration consists of two processes: external and internal respiration. External respiration consists of all processes involved in the intake of oxygen and the elimination of carbon dioxide through the lungs. Internal or cellular respiration is the absorption of oxygen, metabolic processes that produce energy, and the elimination of carbon dioxide through the body cells. This acts to regenerate the cells. External respiration also serves other functions, such as smelling and producing sounds such as speaking and singing, laughing, and coughing (Hauke 1980).

The passage of air

Air enters the system through first the nostrils, then the nasal cavity and the paranasal sinuses. After this comes the pharynx, which consists of three parts: (1) the upper pharynx, behind the nose and connected to the ears via the eustachian tube; (2) the middle pharynx, where food and respiratory pathways cross; and (3) the lower part, connecting to the larynx (Figure 5.1). The structures from the nostrils to the lower pharynx form the upper respiratory system, whereas the larynx is the beginning of the lower respiratory system. The epiglottis covers the larynx during swallowing, interrupting the passage of air. The larynx produces the voice and also the cough reflex to protect the lower structures – the trachea, bronchi, bronchioli, and alveoli of the lungs. The lungs contain about 300 million alveoli, surrounded by pulmonary capillaries (Figure 5.2). Oxygen and carbon dioxide are exchanged between the alveoli and the pulmonary capillaries by diffusion through the respiratory membrane.

The pleura covers the lungs and connects them to the thoracic wall. There are two layers in the pleura: the visceral and the parietal pleura. These layers cannot be separated, as they adhere together; however, they slide over each other. In this way the lungs passively follow the movement of the thorax.

Normally we inhale and exhale through the nose. The warm air of exhalation helps to dilate the blood vessels, improving blood supply. Air inhaled through the nose is moistened, warmed, cleaned, and examined through the sense of smell.

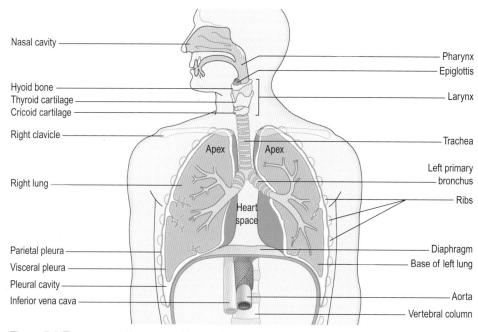

Figure 5.1 The upper and lower respiratory system.

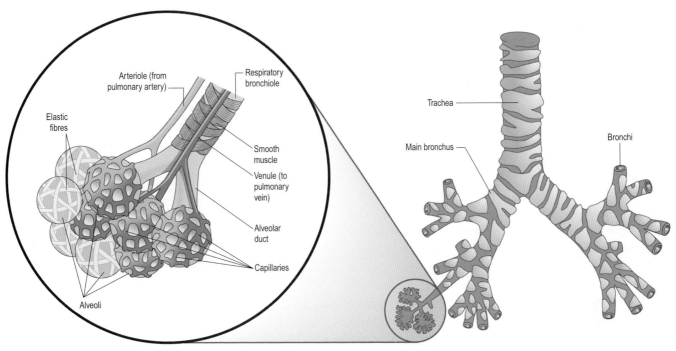

Figure 5.2 The alveoli.

The muscles of respiration

The muscles of inspiration

The main muscles of inspiration are the diaphragm and the external intercostal muscles. Parts of the internal intercostal muscles are also involved (Netter 2006).

The diaphragm is a dome-shaped, musculotendinous structure, separating the thoracic from the abdominal cavity (Figure 5.3). It is attached to the upper three lumbar vertebral bodies via the crurae, which are tendinous pillars. It is also attached to psoas and quadratus lumborum muscles through the arcuate ligaments, the lower six ribs and their cartilages, and the xiphoid process of the sternum. Good diaphragmatic function assists other structures, and vice versa.

With inhalation the diaphragm contracts and its central tendon moves downwards a few centimeters. The vertical diameter of the thorax is increased. The lower ribs are elevated and therefore the diameter of the lower thorax also increases. The upper ribs are elevated and the anteroposterior diameter of the chest increases. The organs underneath the diaphragm influence the mobility of the diaphragm and the experience of respiration. The

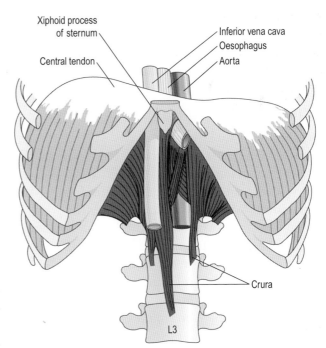

Figure 5.3 The diaphragm.

dome of the diaphragm above the liver on the right side is higher than above the stomach and spleen on the left side. The liver is more solid and less compressible than the stomach and the spleen. Mindful awareness of the breathing movement in the area of the diaphragm allows us to feel more resistance on the right side during inhalation. Due to the mobility of the liver this difference can be balanced with practice. During normal exhalation the diaphragm relaxes; the dome moves upwards a few centimeters, and the lungs go into passive rebound.

The accessory muscles of inspiration are the sternocleidomastoid, scalenus anterior, medius, and posterior (some fibers of which are attached to the fascia covering the top of the lungs), serratus anterior, pectoralis minor, and erector spinae.

In inspiration the air is drawn into the lungs through active expansion of the thoracic cavity. The diaphragm is contracted and moved downwards a few centimeters. This causes 75% of air intake in normal breathing. Raising the side ribs at the beginning of inhalation can enhance movement of the diaphragm. The intercostal muscles raise the ribs, resulting in the remaining 25% of the air intake. Combining both actions, normal breathing can become quite deep yet still be very subtle. The breathing techniques we explain later in this chapter are based on this. This subtle, conscious, deep breathing is different from forced breathing using the accessory muscles of respiration. These accessory muscles are not very active in normal, quiet respiration.

The muscles of expiration

Normal, quiet exhalation is passive. The diaphragm relaxes and moves a few centimeters towards the head. The costal cartilages and the ribs are depressed through the transversus thoracis muscle and the internal intercostal muscles. In this way the space is reduced and air moves out of the lungs. The activity of all the abdominal muscles and the latissimus dorsi muscle causes forced exhalation. As forced inhalation, this is not relevant to our approach to breathing techniques. These accessory muscles are rather used in a balanced, mindful way to improve and stabilize the sitting postures for the breathing techniques.

The thoracic cage

The thoracic vertebrae, the ribs, and the sternum form the thoracic cage, the skeleton of the chest (Figure 5.4). This protects the thoracic organs; the respiratory muscles are also attached to the thoracic cage.

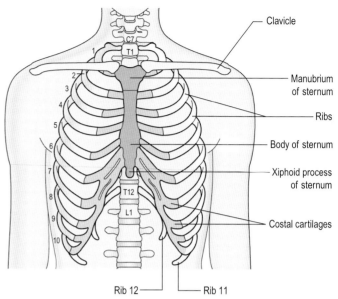

Figure 5.4 The thoracic cage.

The ribs and their movements with inhalation and exhalation

There are 12 pairs of ribs. The upper seven ribs, the true ribs, are directly connected to the sternum by separate costal cartilages. The eighth to twelfth ribs are the false ribs. The costal cartilages of the eighth, ninth, and tenth ribs are fused, forming the costal arch and connected to the costal cartilage of the seventh rib. Ribs 11 and 12, the floating ribs, are connected just to the thoracic vertebrae, but not the sternum. All other ribs are also connected to the thoracic vertebrae. The costovertebral joints are between the head of the rib, the vertebral body, and the intervertebral disc. The costotransverse joint is between the costal tubercle and the tip of the transverse process. The many different joint planes throughout the different segments of the thoracic spine and the corresponding ribs lead to rib movements in different planes around different axes and therefore to a very complex movement pattern of the ribs during inhalation and exhalation. The three main movement directions can be summarized as follows: (1) elevation of the lower ribs increases the transverse diameter of the thorax; (2) elevation of the upper ribs increases the anteroposterior diameter of the thorax and raises it; (3) elevation of the middle ribs increases both diameters. Ribs 11 and 12 move like callipers to create more space in the lower thorax (Kapandji 2008).

Due to adhesion between the visceral and parietal pleura, this expansion of the thoracic cage leads to an expansion of the thoracic space that is filled by the lungs. Through this expansion the pressure in the thoracic cavity is decreased in relation to the abdominal cavity and the outside. This increases venous return to the right atrium of the heart. Therefore more blood is supplied to the lungs for gas exchange. More air is sucked into the lungs, to supply oxygen for gas exchange. In normal exhalation these movements are reversed passively; during forced exhalation they are enhanced using the accessory respiratory muscles. Due to the attachments of the serratus anterior muscles the shoulder blades are closely related to the ribs as well. Therefore good mobility of the shoulder blades is important for breathing.

The spine

The spine needs a good balance between stability and flexibility. Activating the abdominal muscles sufficiently during inhalation stabilizes the lumbar spine. Due to contraction of the pelvic floor muscles the sacrum moves into counternutation, which lengthens the spine.

The thoracic spine bends backwards slightly. B K S Iyengar (2009) gives an elegant description that the ninth thoracic vertebra and the sternum move slightly towards the chin. As a result the physiological curves of the spine become flatter (Hartman 2001). Good mobility of the costovertebral joints is important for breathing. Good mobility of this area also improves the blood supply and drainage of the sympathetic chain that is close to the costovertebral joints.

The sternum

During inhalation the sternum moves forwards and upwards. Anterior movement of the upper sternum is more than that of the lower sternum (Kapandji 2008). This also involves various movements of the costal cartilages, the sternocostal joints, and the costochondral junction and is important for rib movement. In connection with sternal mobility the transverse thoracic muscle is particularly relevant and should be stretched and mobilized.

The exchange of oxygen and carbon dioxide between the alveoli and the blood vessels

The alveoli are the terminal air saccules of the lungs. Fine pulmonary capillaries surround them. Both are lined by layers of extremely thin epithelium and separated by membranes. In the alveoli the concentration of oxygen is higher than in the capillaries. Therefore oxygen moves passively by diffusion into the capillaries. In contrast the concentration of carbon dioxide is higher in the capillaries and moves passively by diffusion into the alveoli. Air containing less oxygen and more carbon dioxide is removed by exhalation. The fresh oxygen diffused into the capillaries is carried into all tissues and organs of the body by red blood cells for absorption by the cells of the body.

In conclusion, a basic understanding of these processes shows how important a good pattern of respiration is for sufficient oxygen supply, to maintain the acid/alkaline balance, and to support the functioning of all systems of the body. Breathing is also important for the musculoskeletal system and its functions, including exercise. By the same token, practicing breathing techniques contributes to good lung function. The supply of the alveoli with air and the capillaries with blood can be significantly improved through good posture and practicing.

The rhythm and volume of respiration

There is a significant difference between the normal respiratory volume of 500 ml and the maximum capacity of respiration of up to 5 litres (Martini & Nath 2008). In quiet breathing the main respiratory muscles are used for inhalation; exhalation is passive, by elastic rebound. The emphasis can either be on the contraction of the diaphragm or on raising the ribs through contraction of the external intercostal muscles to increase thoracic volume so that air can be drawn into the lungs. Normally diaphragmatic breathing is deeper – 75% of total volume – whereas costal breathing is shallower – 25% of total volume. It can be further differentiated between high, clavicular breathing, intercostal mid breathing, and diaphragmatic breathing (Iyengar 2009). In full breathing in yoga all areas can be integrated. Capacity is greatest if the ribs are raised when the diaphragm is pulled down. In forced breathing the accessory muscles of inhalation and exhalation are used. In general, quiet deep breathing moves more air than forced, noisy breathing. The normal respiratory rate is 12–18 breaths per minute, slightly higher in children. It is directed by the breathing center in the medulla oblongata, influenced by the concentration of oxygen and carbon dioxide in the blood, the autonomous nervous system, and emotions. It is also adapted to movement (Hauke 1980).

Connection of respiration with the other systems of the body

Through oxygenization and elimination of carbon dioxide, respiration is connected with all tissues of the body which receive a blood supply. There are a number of special connections of the respiratory system with other systems of the body. The axial skeleton protects and surrounds the lungs; rib movements are important for inhalation and exhalation. The sternum is important for the production of red blood cells. Movement stimulates this production, too. Muscles actively control and generate the flow and movements of breath and the sounds connected with breathing. The nervous system controls the rhythm and volumes of respiration, and blood gas levels. Epinephrine and norepinephrine stimulate respiration. The cardiovascular system is particularly related to the respiratory system. The heart and lungs are connected through their veins and arteries. Red blood cells carry oxygen and carbon dioxide between the lungs and the tissues. In the alveolar capillaries converting enzymes, important for the regulation of blood pressure, are produced (Martini & Nath 2008). The rhythmic movements of the diaphragm stimulate fluid movements in the arteries, veins, and lymphatic vessels by a change in pressure between the abdominal and thoracic cavities. The support of the venous flow back to the heart increases the volume of the heart and the blood supply to the coronary arteries, and decreases the heart rate (Roth 2008). This fluid movement improves the immune system and the health of the tissues in general. It also improves mobility and therefore the functions of the abdominal and thoracic organs. Respiration is both a conscious and an unconscious process, connecting these two areas.

In conclusion, an understanding of these anatomical and physiological connections shows that breathing well and exercising connected with good respiration are beneficial for health, both in prevention and therapy. It is important not to force these processes, rather to communicate with them in a sensitive, mindful way.

Preparation for prāṇāyāma, the yoga art of breathing

Introduction

In the classical yoga texts prāṇa is defined as the basic life energy for all living beings and the whole universe. There is a close connection between prāṇa, breath, and mind. Āyāma is expansion, extension of this energy, controlling, distributing, and storing it. Prāṇāyāma is the aspect of yoga concerned with breathing. It fits well with the anatomy and physiology described above. Patañjali (see Chapter 1) describes prāṇāyāma in his Yoga-Sūtras 49–51, part II. Verse II.49 teaches: "Prāṇāyāma is the regulation of the incoming and outgoing flow of breath with retention" (Iyengar 2002, p. 161). Verse II.50 explains: "Prāṇāyāma has three movements: prolonged and fine inhalation, exhalation and retention; all regulated with precision according to duration and place" (Iyengar 2002, p. 165). From verse II.51 we learn: "The fourth type of prāṇāyāma transcends the external and internal prāṇāyāmas, and appears effortless and non-deliberate" (Iyengar 2002, p. 166).

From a consideration of the anatomy and physiology of respiration as well as the classical yoga textbooks we can see that precision, mindfulness, and dedicated practice are essential for prāṇāyāma. The basic breathing movements can be understood from the anatomy; deep understanding comes through practice. As we have seen in Chapter 2, the sensory organs play an important role in concentrated, mindful, quiet practice. So an awareness of eyes, ears, nose, tongue, and skin will be fundamental to the practice of prāṇāyāma, in addition to softness of the base of the skull and pharynx. Calming the senses is essential for mindful exercising, and for prāṇāyāma, as well. The practice of prāṇāyāma is very fine and subtle.

The aim of prāṇāyāma is to improve the capacity of respiration and the functions of the respiratory system, related to all other systems of the body. It is very important for health – it is a "medicine of health." Changes in frequency, depth, and quality improve the efficiency and effectiveness of respiration. Prāṇāyāma improves mindfulness, and calms the mind, heart, nerves, and senses. In this way our constant stimulation is reduced, and the body and mind can recover much better. The ancient yoga masters have taught that we are born with a finite number of breaths. We should not use them up rapidly (Roth 2008).

Modern research on prāṇāyāma

As with general yoga practice, numerous studies on prāṇāyāma can be found. The long tradition of prāṇāyāma as an adjunct to the medical management of asthma has been confirmed in studies (Vedanthan et al. 1998, Singh et al. 1990). It is certainly worthwhile to conduct more research on this matter.

Breathing through the right nostril has stimulated the sympathetic nervous system (Telles et al. 1996). The observation of a group practicing slow breathing over a period of 3 months showed increased parasympathetic and decreased sympathetic activity (Pal et al. 2004). So prāṇāyāma seems to have an effect on the autonomous nervous system, and by implication on a large variety of conditions caused by autonomous dysfunction. In one study it had a beneficial effect in irritable bowel syndrome (Taneja et al. 2004). Metabolic effects could also be measured. Following yoga āsana, prāṇāyāma, and meditation practice over 9 days, there was a significant improvement in blood glucose and cholesterol levels (Bijlani et al. 2005). The positive effect that practicing breathing techniques has on mental and physical energy and on mood almost goes without saying.

The practical experience of inhalation and exhalation

Introduction

The instructions for these supine and sitting breathing techniques are consistent with the anatomic and physiologic explanations given above. These techniques are suitable as introductory steps for prāṇāyāma, both for beginners and for advanced students. For a deeper insight into prāṇāyāma see the textbook *Light on Prāṇāyāma* (Iyengar 2009).

If you are short of time, you can practice one or other of these techniques. If you have more time, you can combine them together or with other, more complex techniques, as described in *Light on Prāṇāyāma*. You may also find the principles of these techniques useful building blocks to integrate into a variety of techniques if you are experienced.

Special attention should be paid to mindful exercising and the penetration of all layers of the body, as described in Chapter 2. Expanding the breathing space through special positions considered later in this chapter will allow more alveoli to be filled with air, and the area for gas exchange will be increased. The breaths will be longer and slower and more blood will move in the capillaries surrounding the alveoli during one breath. More oxygen can be absorbed and more carbon dioxide can be expelled during one breath (Roth 2008).

All prāṇāyāma techniques start with an exhalation to free the lungs. They end with an inhalation to support the heart. Inhalation is felt more in the inner, lower part of the sinuses, exhalation in the outer, upper part (Iyengar 2009). If you listen carefully to your breath, inhalation is more an sss sound, exhalation more like hhh. Normally the eyes are closed, soft, looking towards the heart while practicing prāṇāyāma. Occasionally they can be slightly opened to control the posture without disturbing the inner stillness. The middle of the forehead stays relaxed. The ears are relaxed, listening to the sound of the breath.

First we will consider suitable positions for breathing. Even normal breathing will be different, more conscious and deeper in these positions. Then specific areas of the body that are particularly relevant for breathing will be considered in detail. The integration of these details into one breath will gradually lead towards deep breathing, which should not be forced. Long experience has shown that subtle breathing gives many beneficial effects. It also gives a better oxygen supply than forced breathing.

The supine, supported position (Figure 5.5)

For a detailed description, see Supta Sukhāsana, a variation of āsana Sukhāsana (see Chapter 7).

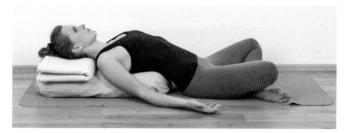

Figure 5.5

Adjust the height of the support so that it is right for you. You can use folded blankets instead of the bolster if you need a lower support. In particular the back of the head, the neck, and throat should be relaxed, the thorax expanded, the lumbar area relaxed, and the lower abdomen should sink slightly towards your back.

Instead of Supta Sukhāsana, Supta Vīrāsana or Supta Baddha Koṇāsana (see Chapter 7) can be practiced. If you practice with straight legs you may like to support the knees or lower legs with a roll or a bolster.

The correct sitting position (Figure 5.6)

Sit in a firm and comfortable position on the floor with the legs in a simple cross-legged position. Find the balance for your pelvis between tilting it forwards and backwards, so that your spine is lifting without effort. Rest your hands on your thighs, palms facing upwards, so that your elbows and shoulders move slightly backwards and downwards. Keeping your chest lifted and the throat relaxed, bend your head, and lengthen the back of your neck. If this causes stress in the neck or throat, keep your head upright. Keep your pelvis slightly tilted forwards when you pull your lower abdomen towards the lumbar spine and the diaphragm. Maintaining this stable pelvic position, lift your side ribs, sternum, and upper ribs. All these adjustments of the posture prepare you for correct breathing. Alternatively you can sit in Vīrāsana (see Chapter 7) or on a chair.

Experiencing detailed areas that are relevant for breathing

Applying anatomical principles to the practical experience of breathing movements, the following preparatory practice is suggested. To improve awareness of the area and movement, the hands are

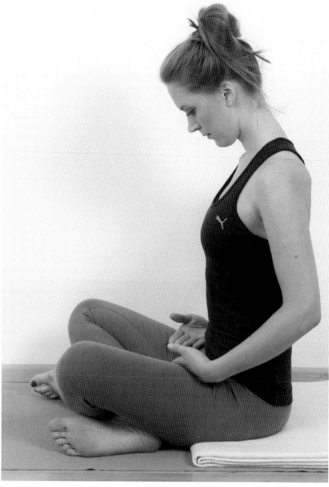

Figure 5.6

placed on specific areas, feeling the movement with inhalation and exhalation. Keep the hands on each area for 1–3 minutes. Start the contact from the little finger side, then gradually put the whole hand on the area. Gently release your hands with the end of an inhalation. Practice lying on your back or sitting. Work on the following areas:

* costal arches

* upper lumbar area

* sternum and middle ribs

* upper ribs and clavicle

* area below the navel.

The gentle movement of the area below the navel towards the lumbar spine and the diaphragm during exhalation can be maintained during inhalation by gently pulling the skin of this area towards the underlying muscles, the lumbar spine, and the diaphragm.

Once you have mastered these preparatory techniques with sufficient awareness you can practice them without using your hands. Gradually more and more of these details can be integrated into one breath.

Deep inhalation supine

Start with normal fine, subtle inhalation. Maintain the softness in your eyes, ears, nose, tongue, and skin of the face; gradually integrate the following sensations into one breath:

- slight contraction of the anterior lower abdominal wall, as if you were moving gently from this abdominal wall through the underlying muscles and organs towards the lumbar spine and the diaphragm. This movement can be seen and felt on the lower abdominal wall
- expansion of the upper lumbar area and the area of the floating ribs
- elevation and expansion of the lower ribcage
- elevation and expansion of the middle and upper ribcage
- gentle stretching sensation of the skin over the clavicles.

In summary the inhalation goes from the lower abdomen through all layers of the body to the skin over the clavicles.

Deep exhalation supine

The exhalation is mainly a passive rebound. In prāṇāyāma special emphasis is placed on slow and smooth exhalation to calm the mind. This slow, controlled exhalation is achieved by keeping the upper chest lifted at the start of exhalation, only slowly releasing the intercostal muscles in this area. To slow down the recoil of the floating ribs, control the lumbar area. At the end of exhalation let the lower abdomen be relaxed to finish the exhalation smoothly and prepare for the movement starting at the lower abdomen with the beginning of inhalation. Even if you are not able to keep the upper chest lifted while breathing out, just feeling the area soft and listening to the inner sound of breath helps to slow down exhalation.

In summary the exhalation can be felt from the upper chest to the lower abdomen through all layers of the body.

Deep inhalation sitting

Sit as explained above for the correct sitting posture. Slightly lift yourself from the lower abdomen or from your center of gravity deep inside the pelvis. Start inhalation by widening the lumbar area and the costal arches, then lift the lower and middle ribs, the sternum, the upper ribs, and the clavicles. Move your shoulder blades apart slightly. An important source for lifting the sternum is the slight back-bending of the thoracic spine. The distance between the thoracic spine and the sternum is increased.

As an alternative to bending the head towards the throat, it can be kept upright. A subtle adjustment of the head on the cervical spine, slightly lengthening the head away from the neck, keeping the chin on the same level, helps to correct the posture if the head is kept upright. This adjustment frees the area of the medulla oblongata where the center for respiratory control is located. Furthermore this head movement supports the lifting of the sternum and upper chest, so it is a useful correction at the end of inhalation and the beginning of exhalation.

Integrating these fine adjustments and sensations into normal quiet breathing leads towards deeper inhalation. Practice for 5–10 minutes. If this causes any irritation, just continue normal breathing. If you are exhausted, continue normal breathing in the supine, supported position.

Deep exhalation sitting

As mentioned before, exhalation starts with holding the upper chest lifted, supported by upwards movement of the back of the head, if you practice with your head straight. The final effect is that the downward movement of the ribs becomes slower; exhalation itself becomes slower and smoother. Avoiding or slowing down the downward movement with exhalation corresponds to the movement of the diaphragm towards the head. This movement can be followed mentally in the inner chest. Moving the center of the diaphragm upwards creates a length between this center and the center of the pelvic floor.

This can be perceived as a column between these two areas supporting the whole posture, which prevents you collapsing with exhalation, and prepares you to lift for inhalation. Integrating these fine adjustments and sensations into normal quiet breathing leads to deeper exhalation. Practice for 5–10 minutes. If this causes any irritation, just continue normal breathing. If you are exhausted, continue normal breathing in the supine, supported position.

Combining these techniques and experiencing inner stillness

Depending on your constitution choose the supine supported position or the correct sitting position or a combination of both. Combine deep inhalation and deep exhalation as described above. Learn to practice so gently that no irritation is created. First pay particular attention to the end of inhalation and the end of exhalation. Then become aware of the tiny pause between inhalation and exhalation. Do not force these pauses, just observe them carefully. Even if they are ever so tiny, they lead towards the experience of inner stillness and calmness of mind.

Summarizing considerations for the preparatory practice for prāṇāyāma

Even when this approach leads towards deep, full breathing, it is not forced breathing. The accessory muscles of respiration are not used for the breathing movements; they are only used to stabilize and finetune the posture. In particular the muscles of the shoulders, neck, and throat are relaxed. The facial muscles are also relaxed. As a result there is no pull on the eyes, ears, nose, skin, or tongue. This helps to calm the brain and mind. A sensation of free space between tongue and palate is important. This can be supported by slightly lifting the upper teeth away from the lower teeth. Combine this with slightly lengthening the back of the head away from the neck. All these corrections, as well as the breathing itself, have to be practiced in a subtle and mindful way. They should only be practiced once you have developed good awareness of posture and movements of the body.

Resting poses and exercises for preparing prāṇāyāma

As we have seen, all bodily systems are interrelated with the respiratory system. Therefore each function and each movement will influence respiration, and vice versa.

It is particularly important to develop the following abilities before practicing the preparations for prāṇāyāma. A well-balanced practice of the different groups of āsanas helps develop these abilities:

1. posture: we have seen the importance of good posture from anatomical and physiological considerations
2. lifting of the spine: the diaphragm, the ribs, and many respiratory muscles are connected to the spine
3. mobility of the joints between the bony structures of respiration and the "functional joints" between related soft tissues
4. good function, ability to contract and relax the muscles of respiration
5. increasing the "respiratory space"
6. balance between lung ventilation and perfusion
7. calming the mind.

If you are practicing breathing techniques after a sequence of āsanas calm down first. It is best to practice Śavāsana (see Chapter 7) for 10 minutes. Also finish the sequence of breathing techniques with Śavāsana.

Below is listed a summary of relevant resting poses that are described in detail in Chapters 6 and 7. A sequence of passive exercises useful for teaching and private practice is described by Zugck (2008):

1. Forward-bent Vīrāsana (see Chapter 7). Alternatively forward-bent Sukhāsana can be practiced (see Chapter 7). Stay in the position up to 5 minutes.
2. Supported supine resting position (see Chapter 6, exercise 2.4). Alternatively Supta Baddha Koṇāsana or Supta Vīrāsana (see Chapter 7) can be practiced or the legs can be kept straight. Stay in the position for up to 5 minutes.

3. Viparīta Karaṇī (see Chapter 7): instead of straight legs pointing upwards, the lower legs can be rested on a chair or the knees can be bent and the soles of the feet placed on the floor (see Chapter 6, exercise 2.5). Stay in the position for 5 minutes.

4. Śavāsana (see Chapter 7): use sufficient support for your head and legs, if necessary. Make sure you are warm: this significantly improves relaxation. Stay in the position for 10 minutes.

This is a well-balanced sequence of resting poses in preparation for breathing techniques. If you are short of time you can practice a selection from this cycle; even just one part is helpful. Always finish with Śavāsana (see Chapter 7).

The following basic exercises can be combined in a similar manner:

1. side-lying rotation (see Chapter 6, exercise 3.2)

2. side-bending over a bolster (see Chapter 6, exercise 2.6)

3. supported forward-bending (see Chapter 6, exercise 2.7). Adho Mukha Śvānāsana in a rope and supported Halāsana (see Chapter 7) are good preparations for breathing techniques and to calm the mind.

Further relevant preparations for good breathing include:

- To stabilize the posture and lift the spine: exercises 1.1 and 1.2 (see Chapter 6) and all standing poses (see Chapter 7) are particularly relevant.

- The mobility of the thoracic joints is improved by bending in all directions; rotations are very important (see Chapter 6, exercise 2.8, and āsanas Marīcyāsana III, Utthita Marīcyāsana, and Bharadvājāsana I, in Chapter 7).

- Hypomobile spinal segments or ribs can be mobilized lying over a rolled towel, adding specific movements (see Chapter 6, exercise 2.2).

- Scapular mobility is improved by all-embracing shoulder work (see Chapter 6, exercise 4.11).

- The respiratory muscles are strengthened in all exercises which include arm and trunk movements.

- The respiratory space is expanded through forward bends posteriorly (see Chapter 6, exercise 2.7), supported supine positions anteriorly (see Chapter 6, exercise 2.4), and through side-bending on the opposite side (see Chapter 6, exercise 2.6). Due to gravity ventilation and perfusion are greatly affected by inversions and side-bending exercises. In supine positions the effect on ventilation and perfusion is balanced.

References

Bijlani, R.L., Vempati, R.P., Yadav, R.K., et al., 2005. A brief but comprehensive lifestyle education program based on yoga reduces risk factors for cardiovascular disease and diabetes mellitus. J. Altern. Complement. Med. 11, 267–274.

Hartman, L., 2001. Handbook of Osteopathic Technique, third ed. Nelson Thornes, Cheltenham.

Hauke, H., 1980. Lehrbrief IX, Fernlehrgang Yoga-Lehrer/in SKA. Sebastian-Kneipp-Akademie, Bad Wörishofen.

Iyengar, B.K.S., 2002. Light on the Yoga Sūtras of Patañjali. Thorsons, London.

Iyengar, B.K.S., 2009. Light on Prāṇāyāma, Crossroad, New York, NY.

Kapandji, I.A., 2008. The Physiology of Joints, vol. 3, sixth ed. Churchill Livingstone, Edinburgh.

Martini, F.H., Nath, J.L., 2008. Fundamentals of Anatomy and Physiology, eighth ed. Pearson, London.

Netter, F.H., 2006. Atlas of Human Anatomy, fourth ed. Saunders, Edinburgh.

Pal, G.K., Velkumary, S., Madanmohan, 2004. Effect of short term practice of breathing exercises on autonomic functions in normal human volunteers. Indian J. Med. Res. 120, 115–121.

Roth, L., 2008. Die Anatomie von Raum und Zeit. Vylk-aktuell 2, 18–21.

Singh, V., Wisniewski, A., Britton, J., et al., 1990. Effect of yoga breathing exercises (Prāṇāyāma) on airway reactivity in subjects with asthma. Lancet 335, 1381–1383.

Taneja, I., Deepak, K.K., Poojary, G., et al., 2004. Yogic versus conventional treatment in diarrhea-predominant irritable bowel syndrome: a randomized control study. Appl. Psychophysiol. Biofeedback 29, 19–33.

Telles, S., Nagarathna, R., Nagendra, H.R., 1996. Physiological measures of right nostril breathing. J. Altern. Complement. Med. 2, 479–484.

Vedanthan, P.K., Kesavalu, L.N., Murthy, K.C., et al., 1998. Clinical study of yoga techniques in university students with asthma: a controlled study. Allergy Asthma Proc. 19, 3–9.

Zugck, K., 2008. Vorbereitende Āsanas zum Einstimmen auf Prāṇāyāma. Vylk-aktuell 2, 10–13.

ॐ 6

The basic exercises

General introduction: basic exercises

How to use the basic exercise section

In the section on yoga and health in Chapter 1, we emphasized finding and developing healthy structures in the body as a fundamental approach for therapeutic yoga. To learn how to use these structures in a sensible way to improve their function we have applied the principles of mindfulness, variety of exercise approaches, economical practice, precision, and finetuning to the exercise approach. Specific aims for improving bodily structure and function are mobility, strength, stamina, relaxation, balance, coordination, synchronization, and breathing naturally.

The instructions are designed in order to achieve healthy postures and movements. Nevertheless students and patients will need guidance to stay within this healthy range or to move back a level by using appropriate props.

Our experience with patients' motivation has shown (see also Chapter 4):

- The learning steps must be small enough so that patients can improve in line with their ability.

- However, they should be challenged as far as possible, so that they do not become bored.

- They should see success early onto motivate them to continue. This experience of success should come from their performance of the exercises and be confirmed by the therapist.

- They should understand why they are practicing the chosen exercises.
- They should enjoy the exercises and look forward to continuing to practice them. The therapist or instructor who is teaching the exercises should also enjoy the process.

The therapist's own posture and movement patterns should set a good example. This is important for patients and also to protect therapists and teachers, who should themselves be in good condition, and only teach from their own experience and understanding.

We have collected together this set of basic exercises as a tool for therapists, instructors, and patients. The exercises are divided according to the areas of the body. This is not a strict division; rather it is a focus. Some exercises are similar for different areas, focusing on different areas, sensations, or movements. A different emphasis or applying a prop in a different way brings the focus to another area. For example, in supported forward bending, placing a rolled blanket underneath the lower abdomen targets the lumbar spine (exercise 1.7, Figure 6.13), whereas placing the rolled blanket underneath the costal arches targets the dorsolumbar junction and the lower ribs (exercise 2.7, Figure 6.49). For each area there are exercises emphasizing one or more aims. These aims are stated at the start of the exercise. In each and every exercise you should aim for a good quality of breathing. The rib exercises are particularly helpful to improve breathing.

These basic exercises are modified from more complex yoga āsanas or their preparation. Most of these basic exercises are teaching details of āsanas and help us to understand fine adjustments of the āsanas. Even if the exercises are small and subtle it is important to integrate them into a good all-over posture while working with the whole body in a sensible way. An important example is to maintain a stable position of the pelvis and keep the spine lifted while practicing exercises for the thorax, shoulders, cervical spine, or head. Therefore these basic exercises are yoga exercises, too, particularly as we put a great deal of emphasis on applying the principles of mindfulness, variety of exercise approaches, economical practice, precision, and finetuning

during exercising. All the principles are relevant for all exercises, and should be applied during practice. Mindfulness is paramount among the principles (see Chapter 2) and particularly connects to the spirit of yoga. It underlies all the other principles: variety, economical practice, precision, and finetuning.

The exercises are not meant to be carried out one by one as presented here. They can be selected and combined for each patient according to the diagnosis. The sequences should gradually increase in intensity and finish with a quiet exercise or Śavāsana (see Chapter 7). Some of the basic exercises have several variations. This was designed to cater for the great variety of anatomical shapes and movement possibilities, to meet individual needs.

As emphasized in Chapter 3, it is essential to carry out a thorough case history and examination, including contraindications in certain conditions. Keeping in mind your patient's particular aims and selecting and applying the exercises accordingly, this approach can be applied to many conditions. In particular it is useful to help target restricted areas and protect hypermobile ones, which is fundamental in many musculoskeletal problems. Patients who have many symptoms will probably already have had a lot of therapy. Do not add more; rather start the patient on exercises he can still do to encourage him. Other exercises can gradually be added to help the body correct itself and improve the patient's chance of self-healing.

It is important to respect patients' abilities and restrictions. Many of the exercises can be modified to meet the needs of different patients. If, for example, patients find it impossible to lie down or get up from the floor, they can practice the exercises on a bed or couch or table. It is also worth thinking about exercises that improve getting up. If patients cannot lie flat, particularly older patients or those with circulatory problems, many of the supine postures can be modified with the head or thorax raised. Many modifications for positioning patients on the treatment table can also be applied to exercise positions, and throughout the practical sections we have given suggestions for using props. There are countless variations to modify and adjust exercises to individual needs. As mindful exercising is one of our fundamental exercise principles, awareness and feeling are important guides when building up and modifying the exercises. Considering these possibilities of modification, this exercise approach is suitable for patients with many different kinds of restrictions and for all age groups.

The recommended timings and number of repetitions are based on long-term observations, what feels right for many patients, and on research results (Pullig Schatz 1992, Tanzberger et al 2004, Lederman 2005). However, the results vary within a range of possibilities: again, careful observation and mindful exercising will be a helpful guide. Frequently used timing for holding stretches or strengthening is 3–5 breaths, for repetitions of basic exercises 3–5 times. Unless directed otherwise, by breath we mean one inhalation and one exhalation. For beginners the time may be shorter, gradually increasing with practice. Within a sensible range it also depends on the desired effect. The lengthening of a muscle in a relaxed position may take much longer, depending on the individual situation. It usually takes several minutes to get into deep relaxation. So it is important that the therapist and the patient are clear about the aims of the exercises and understand the principles.

Exercises should not be held so long or repeated so often that the patient becomes exhausted or uncomfortable. Ask patients how they feel, and then adjust the intensity, timing, and way of performing the exercises according to the feedback. If a stretch is painful, modify the challenge so that it becomes tolerable. After exercising patients should feel comfortable. If they feel continuing pain after exercising, they should be referred for medical investigation (see Chapter 3). If the results are negative, check again that the patient is carrying out the exercises correctly, and perhaps make the practice shorter or less intense.

Many basic exercises are suitable for beginners. There are refined or stronger versions for experienced practitioners, indicated at the start of the exercise. However, advanced practitioners may not need harder exercises than beginners. Each exercise can be performed and experienced very differently depending on the level of practice. To begin with the exercise approach will be less detailed, more like building a frame. With increasing practice you come closer to the inner work, refining the movements and sensations, connecting more and more layers of the body. This can all be done within one exercise. Different patients have different needs and wishes. Some only practice basic exercises for a long time and make good progress. Others need different exercises to move ahead. Even without any variations the beginners' exercises will be experienced differently and understood in greater depth by more experienced practitioners, who can create their own combinations according to their level of awareness. With increasing practice mindfulness is further refined, and more variety is added. Economical practice is also learned in more complex āsanas. Finetuning develops into excellence. The speed at which you perform the exercises as well as how long you hold them can be increased to improve stamina.

These basic exercises are like building blocks for more complex ones. They emphasize a specific area of the body and show in detail how to work according to the principles and reach your aims. Once you have mastered the relevant basic exercises they can be combined into more complex tasks, further developing the aims. This leads towards the classical āsanas. The basic exercises place greater emphasis on mobilizing, stretching, strengthening, and relaxation. Coordination and balance are also practiced in basic exercises, but even more so in the more complex tasks, the āsanas. Synchronization is particularly developed in partner or group work. Synchronizing movements of different parts of the body also plays an important role in āsana practice.

Yoga teachers will also find the basic exercises helpful to lead step by step towards the more complex āsanas.

In summary the basic exercises are modified from classical āsanas:

- teaching important details of the āsanas; the details can be combined and integrated into more complex tasks
- helping to understand the essence of the āsanas
- leading to a mindful, precise exercise approach.

There are many more possibilities to move and correct different areas of the body than can be presented here. Once you have learned and understood some of these exercises you may wish to create variations or design your own exercises according to your patients' diagnosis and needs.

Most exercises are illustrated with photographs. Some of the fine movements cannot be seen very easily on the pictures, but can be followed from the description.

Frequently used positions and movements

In the exercise instructions we prefer to refer to individual measures like the patient's foot length or hand width, as body measurements are individual. Knees hip width apart is particularly used for parallel alignment of the thighs: this corresponds to the knees one fist width apart.

For the position of the feet we sometimes use dorsiflexion and plantar flexion (exercise 10.3, Figure 6.194). Dorsiflexion is the movement at the ankle towards the superior surface of the foot. When wearing flat shoes the foot is mainly in dorsiflexion. Plantar flexion is the movement at the ankle towards the sole of the foot: the higher the heels, the more the foot is in plantar flexion. In dorsiflexion the foot has more stability, whereas in plantar flexion it its more vulnerable. Inversion is the movement of the foot inwards (exercise 10.3, Figure 6.195), while eversion is an outwards movement (Figure 6.196), both without rotation at the hip or knee joints (Kingston 2001).

Supination and pronation in the elbow joint are the rotation of the radius on the ulna. Supination is the rotation of the forearm so that the palm is facing forwards, with the thumb outwards, whereas pronation is the rotation of the forearm so that the palm is facing backwards, with the thumb inwards. The joint surfaces of the carpal bones also allow some complex supination and pronation movements (Kingston 2001).

The neutral position is a fundamental position for many exercises. "Lumbar neutral position is midway between full flexion and full extension as brought about by posterior and anterior tilting of the pelvis … the neutral position places minimal stress on the body tissues. Also, because postural alignment is optimal, the neutral position is generally the most effective position from which trunk muscles can work" (Norris 2000, p. 10). In this neutral position the joints and their soft tissues are least stressed. The neutral position must be distinguished from the concept of neutral zone. This is "the zone in which movement occurs at the beginning of the range of motion before any effective resistance is offered from either the muscular system or the spinal column" (Norris 2000, p. 9). The less stable a spinal segment is, the larger the neutral zone.

The concept of the neutral position can be applied to the whole musculoskeletal system. For the neutral lumbopelvic position the neutral zone between the sacrum and the fifth lumbar vertebra is relevant. Feel your way towards it by tilting the pelvis forwards and backwards within the comfortable range. Make the movements smaller and smaller, until you reach the midrange position. When you are lying on your back, this is often the most relaxed position for the abdomen and the lumbar area. Sitting and standing, the neutral position is the basis for the upright position with the minimum stress. In neutral position the spine is stable during all movements, including movements of the legs and arms. It is a good foundation for lifting and lengthening the spine to support the nutrition of the discs and create enough space for the nerve roots. The neutral position will be applied in many of our exercises and āsanas. Depending on the context it is described in different ways, for example tilting or stabilizing the pelvis, lifting from the lower abdomen, or adjusting the costal arches.

Supine means lying on your back. To achieve the optimum neutral, relaxed position you may need support. To support from the bottom, place a rolled blanket or bolster underneath the knees or a chair under the lower legs. To support from the top, put a pillow underneath the neck and head (see Śavāsana, Chapter 7). There are various methods to support lying supine (Lasater 1995). You may need to experiment to find the best for individual patients. To come up from the supine position, stretch your right arm over your head and turn on your right side, with the right arm supporting the head. Bend both knees, keeping your left hand on the floor in front. Stay lying comfortably on this side for a few breaths in a neutral lumbopelvic position. To push yourself up to sitting, set your left leg slightly free from the bent position. If you prefer to finish on the left side, turn onto your left side in the same way. Moshe Feldenkrais has written a very detailed description of this and other transitions between different positions (Feldenkrais 1984).

Prone means lying on your front. As with the supine position, this may need a variety of supports for patient comfort. We are not using this as a relaxation position, rather as a starting and finishing position for some exercises. There are different ways to come up from the prone position. We prefer a gentle method: stretch one arm besides the head, turn on this side and push yourself up to sit as described for coming back from the supine position.

We have described several basic exercises and āsanas sitting on the floor. As sitting on the floor is not suitable for all patients, there are modifications. If the patient cannot sit on a support like a brick or pillow, many of the sitting exercises can be done sitting on a chair or on the treatment couch. If the patient finds it difficult to get up from the floor, it can be helpful to hold onto a chair or table for support.

The knee hug position (exercise 1.4, Figure 6.4) is the starting and finishing position for lumbar mobilizing and abdominal strengthening exercises. It is a relaxing pose on its own.

Four-point kneeling (exercise 1.14, Figure 6.28) and variations is used in several chapters, with different emphasis. Patients may find it comfortable to kneel on a soft support like a folded blanket. This also increases the height of the pelvis so that the back is closer to the horizontal line.

Forward-bent kneeling (exercise 1.9, Figure 6.16) is a suitable position to finish four-point kneeling variations as well as the dog pose. It is a relaxing pose on its own, particularly if performed with props, as shown in exercise 1.9 (Figure 6.16). In addition to the supported relaxation poses we have given a few examples of oscillations. These gentle rhythmic movements are particularly inspiring fluid movements (Lederman 2001). To refine the exercises and sink into deeper relaxation it is important to feel softness in the eyes, ears, palate, tongue, and larynx, and to be receptive and mindful during practice (see Chapter 2).

Many of the exercises get easier and more accessible by using props. The questions of what patients can do and which exercises should be avoided are replaced by the question of how to modify the exercises. We describe important basics for this exercise approach, as this is an important factor in therapeutic exercising. Most of the props we suggest can be found at home. We recommend buying a sticky mat, a foam brick, and a belt (see Chapter 1).

Breathing during exercising

Breathing during exercising should be natural and light. The natural breathing movements and patterns should not be disturbed. In this way it is possible to take deeper breaths in harmony with activity. Some movements, particularly downwards movements and stretches, are frequently done while exhaling. Moving with exhalation helps you to relax in the exercise. Some movements, particularly upwards movements, are frequently done while inhaling. If the movement matches the upwards movement of the side and frontal ribs it is sensible to perform it while inhaling, whereas if it is closer to a downwards movement of the ribs, perform it while exhaling. But this is not a dogma. For some individuals it may be better to coordinate this differently, so it is often useful to play with matching the movements and the breath. In particular very mobile, loose patients may prefer to perform more movements while inhaling. Mindful, attentive practice often gives the best answer. Breathing during exercising should only be through the nose.

1. Basic exercises for the lumbar spine

With reference to the lumbar spine, low-back pain should be mentioned as this is the most common condition for which patients present to manual therapists or start exercising.

As many different pathologies can cause low-back pain, a thorough diagnosis is necessary. Particular caution is necessary if the low-back pain is associated with neurological signs and symptoms, bowel and bladder problems, or the patient has lost weight or is feeling ill. If, after thorough medical investigation, exercise therapy is appropriate, you need to bear in mind the general function of the lumbar spine as a weight-bearing structure that needs to be able to lift against gravity and change direction, in addition to being well balanced. Strengthening and mobilizing exercises are required.

Mobilizing exercises may cause a problem if they reach hypermobile areas instead of restricted ones. We have seen patients' conditions worsening, particularly after intensive, ambitious practice. In many cases we could see that the hypermobile segments were vulnerable to being overstretched or overmobilized. For these patients two things were helpful:

* easing off slightly from the boundary, the limit of movement
* combining mobilization with muscle strengthening.

Muscle strengthening is performed with only part, about one-third, of full strength and repeated several times. These exercises should be performed within the painfree range.

Mobilization exercises should give a feeling of ease and relaxation. This experience of easy, painfree exercises can help eliminate conditioned pain reactions.

To integrate these abilities into more complex and everyday actions we recommend the balance, coordination, and synchronization exercises. For healthy movement patterns of the lumbar spine a wider context is important, particularly targeting the pelvis, iliosacral joints, and the hips, as well as the feet and knees. The functions in the middle and lower thoracic spine can also influence the lumbar spine. All these connections contribute to a healthy balance of stability and mobility of the lumbar spine. In this way the cooperation between the muscles, the nutrition of the discs, and the nerve roots can improve and be kept at a healthy level. All the bony and soft tissues and fluids can function in a healthy way.

Exercise 1.1: Lumbopelvic stability

Aims: strengthening the lower abdomen, pelvic floor, and lumbar area.

1. Lie on your back with your hips and knees bent, the soles of the feet resting on the floor, the heels one foot length away from the buttocks. Use a pillow for your head if necessary.

2. Gently tilt your pelvis until you find the neutral lumbopelvic position. Maintain this neutral position throughout the following series of exercises.

3. Put your fingertips on the central line of your lower abdomen about 5 fingers below your navel. Keeping your throat and your shoulders relaxed, slightly pull this area of the lower abdomen inwards and towards your lumbar spine as you exhale; feel the slight contraction of the lower abdomen beneath your fingertips. Then inhale normally, keeping your abdomen relaxed.

4. Perform point 3 3–5 times, with 1–2 normal breaths in between if necessary. You may feel the associated activity of the pelvic floor and the lumbar area as well.

5. With an exhalation repeat the contraction, hold it for up to 3 breaths, and release it while exhaling.

6. Relax for a few breaths.

7. Keeping your throat and shoulders relaxed, practice the gentle contracting action of point 3 while inhaling; relax as you exhale; feel the slight contraction with your fingertips on the central line of the lower abdomen.

8. Perform point 7 3–5 times.

9. Again hold the contraction for 3 breaths, and release it while exhaling, hands comfortable.

10. Stay calm for a few breaths; feel the softness in your abdomen and pelvic floor.

Refined work

Resting your arms besides your body on the floor, follow points 2–10 without controlling the lower abdomen with the fingertips.

Exercise 1.2: Abdominal strength

Aims: gentle strengthening of the abdominal muscles, stabilizing the lumbar spine.

1. Lie on your back with your hips and knees bent; rest your head so that your neck is relaxed, if necessary on a pillow; hold the knees close towards the chest so that the back is comfortable on the floor; feel your lumbar area long and broad (Figure 6.1).
2. Without changing the position of your pelvis, lower your right leg as you exhale until the sole of the foot touches the floor (Figure 6.2); you can feel the position of your lower back with your hands, while you lower your leg.
3. Keep the foot on the floor while you inhale; if necessary you can keep it there for 1–2 breaths.
4. With another inhalation bring the leg back to the starting position, without changing the position of the pelvis.
5. Perform points 2–4 3–5 times.
6. Repeat points 2–5 for the left leg.
7. Lower your right leg towards the floor in three sections: breathing out, lower one-third, breathing in, pause; breathing out, lower the second third, breathing in, pause; breathing out, lower the last third, put the foot on the floor, then pause for 1–2 breaths. Control the position of your lower back with your hands.
8. With an inhalation bring the leg back to the starting position.
9. Perform points 7 and 8 twice.
10. Repeat points 7–9 for your left leg.
11. Finish in the knee hug position (Figure 6.4) for a few breaths. Feel the softness in the abdomen and lumbar area.

Variation

You can also move the leg in three sections while lifting it from the floor.

Stronger variations

Variation a

1. Lie on your back with your hips and knees bent; hold the knees close towards the chest so that the back rests comfortably on the floor (Figure 6.1). Maintain this contact of the pelvis with the floor throughout the exercise.
2. Keeping the pelvic position stable and the throat and shoulders relaxed, lower both legs as you exhale until the soles of your feet touch the floor. Stay there while you inhale; if necessary wait for 1–2 breaths. If the pelvis starts tilting while you lower your legs, stop and reverse the movement.

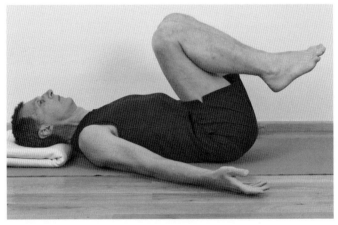

Figure 6.1

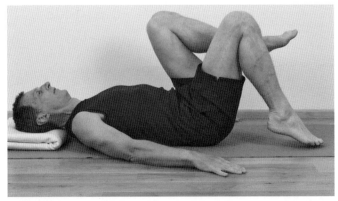

Figure 6.2

3. With another inhalation bring both legs back to the starting position (point 1).

4. Perform points 2 and 3 3–5 times.

5. Lower both legs towards the floor in three sections: breathing out, keep your pelvis stable, lower one third; breathing in, pause, breathing out, keep your pelvis stable and lower the second third; breathing in, pause, breathing out, keep your pelvis stable and lower the last third, feet on the floor; then pause for 1–2 breaths.

6. With an inhalation bring the legs back to the starting position.

7. Perform points 5 and 6 twice.

8. To finish stay in the starting position (point 1) for a few breaths.

Variation b

Lie on your back with your hips and knees bent; hold the knees close towards the chest so that the back rests comfortably on the floor (Figure 6.1). Maintain this contact of the pelvis with the floor throughout the exercise. Practice as described in variation a, except that you move the legs in three sections while lifting them off the floor.

Variation c

Perform the movements described with knees and feet slightly apart; do the exercise 3–5 times, each time slightly changing the distance of the knees and feet, within a sensible range for your hips.

Variation d

1. Lie on your back with your hips and knees bent; hold the knees close towards the chest so that the back rests comfortably on the floor. Maintain this throughout the exercise.

2. Without changing the position of the pelvis lower both legs as you exhale until the soles of your feet touch the floor. Stay there while you inhale; if necessary wait for 1–2 breaths.

3. Maintaining the position of the pelvis slide your heels along the floor away from your hips with another exhalation, until your legs are straight.

4. Inhaling again, slide your heels towards the hips, and bring your legs back to the starting position (point 1).

5. Perform points 2–4 3–5 times.

6. To finish lie on your back with relaxed legs for a few breaths; be aware of the position of the back of your pelvis and your lumbar spine; adjust your abdomen and lumbar area so that they are soft.

Exercise 1.3: Rhythmic relaxation

Aim: gentle mobilization of the lumbar spine.

1. Lie on your back, with your hips and knees bent and the soles of your feet on the floor and the heels one foot length away from the sitting bones.

2. Bring your pelvis into a comfortable, neutral position on the floor.

3. With an exhalation slightly slide away one hip in the direction of the same foot, then the other one, about 3 times during this exhalation, to oscillate the lumbar spine into rhythmic side-bending (Figure 6.3). Finish with your pelvis in symmetry.

4. While breathing in, stay calm.

5. Perform points 3 and 4 3–5 times.

6. Stay relaxed for a few breaths and feel the change in your lumbar spine.

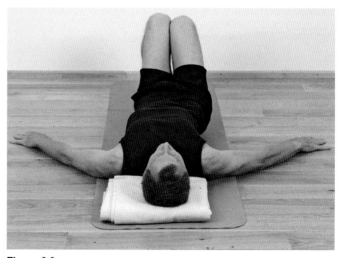

Figure 6.3

7. Lie on your back with your hips and knees bent; hold the knees close towards the chest so that the back is comfortable on the floor (Figure 6.1).

8. Gently rock your legs from side to side, about 20°, slightly lifting the opposite hip, to oscillate the lumbar spine into rotation, up to 3 times within one exhalation; finish in the starting position (point 7).

9. While breathing in, stay calm and feel the relaxation of your abdomen and lumbar area.

10. Perform points 8 and 9 3–5 times.

11. Stay relaxed for a few breaths in the knee hug position (Figure 6.4).

Refined work

Play with the scope and frequency of the oscillation to find the easiest and most comfortable rhythm.

Exercise 1.4: Knee hug rotation variation

Aims: mobilizing the lumbar spine into rotation, balancing the trunk muscles.

1. Start with the knee hug position (Figure 6.4); hold the knees close towards your chest so that the back is comfortable on the floor; holding a brick or pad between your knees may be useful to help position the hips and knees (Figure 6.5).

2. Bring your arms down in line with your shoulder girdle, with the palms facing the ceiling; you may like to also try it with the palms facing the floor, as shown in Figure 6.7, below.

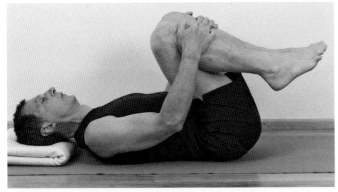

Figure 6.4

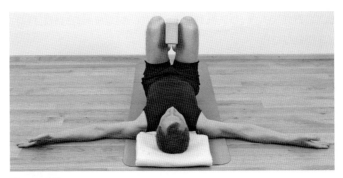

Figure 6.5

3. Without shifting the knees move your legs to the right side as you exhale; the left hip comes off the floor; the left shoulder and arm should remain on the floor, so only go this far and as long as you can control the rotation (Figure 6.6); keep your head in line with your spine.

4. Hold this position for 1–2 breaths.

5. Bring your legs back to the center as you inhale.

6. Repeat points 3–5 for the left side, keeping the right shoulder and arm on the floor.

7. Perform points 3–6 3–5 times.

8. Relax in the knee hug position (Figure 6.4) for a few breaths; feel the softness in your abdomen.

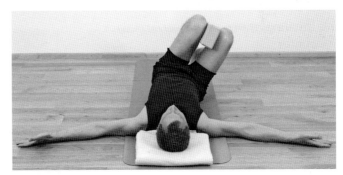

Figure 6.6

Refined work

Try different angles for your hips and knees, but no more than 90°. Hold up to 3 breaths at the end of range of rotation.

Hint

If you are very mobile you may prefer to perform the rotation movements during inhalation instead of exhalation.

Exercise 1.5: Knee hug side-bending variation

Aims: mobilizing the lumbar spine into side-bending, balancing the trunk muscles.

1. Start with the knee hug position; hold the knees close towards your chest so that the back is comfortable on the floor; a brick or pad between your knees may be useful to position the hips and knees (Figure 6.4).

2. Bring your arms down in line with your shoulder girdle, with the palms facing the floor. You may also like to try this with your palms facing the ceiling, as shown in exercise 1.4 (Figure 6.5).

3. Keep your lower legs horizontal while moving your knees away from the chest as long as you can keep your pelvis stable; only go as far as the thighs are perpendicular to the floor.

4. Exhaling, slowly swing your lower legs towards the right, so that the left hip slides away from the lower ribs; this is side-bending the lumbar spine (Figure 6.7).

5. Inhaling, move the lower legs back to the center.

6. Repeat points 4 and 5 to the left.

7. Perform points 4–6 5–10 times.

8. Relax in the knee hug position for a few breaths; let your abdomen be soft.

Exercise 1.6: Roll the back

Aims: mobilizing the lumbar spine into flexion, strengthening the front aspects.

1. Sit with your hips and knees bent, the soles of your feet on the floor (Figure 6.8).

2. Lean back on your hands (Figure 6.9), then on your elbows.

3. Tilting your pelvis backwards, lower the back of your pelvis onto the floor as you exhale.

4. Lower your lumbar spine to the floor, one segment at a time.

5. To finish the exercise lie on your back with the pelvis and lumbar spine in neutral position; rest for a few breaths (Figure 6.10).

6. Turn to one side (whichever is more comfortable) and sit; repeat points 1–6 once.

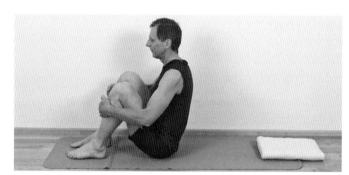

Figure 6.8

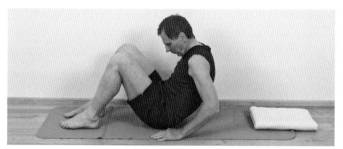

Figure 6.9

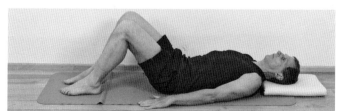

Figure 6.10

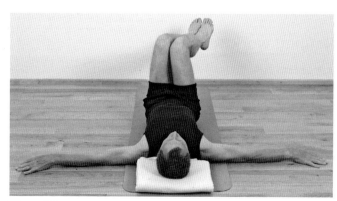

Figure 6.7

Refined work

This following exercise gives a more detailed segmental mobilization of the lumbar spine by slightly reversing the movement described above. This movement is repeated, and 1–2 further lumbar segments are lowered in addition.

1. Sit with your hips and knees bent, with the soles of your feet on the floor.

2. Lean back on your hands, then on your elbows; stay on your elbows until point 9.

3. Tilting your pelvis backwards, lower the back of your pelvis onto the floor as you exhale.

4. Slightly tilt your pelvis forwards to lift the back of your pelvis off the floor as you inhale.

5. Exhaling again, bring the back of your pelvis and the lower 1–2 segments of your lumbar spine on the floor, elbows sliding apart if necessary to stay comfortable in the shoulders.

6. Inhaling, bring these segments and the back of the pelvis slightly off the floor; the buttocks stay on the floor.

7. Exhaling, bring these areas and 1–2 further lumbar segments down to the floor again, one by one.

8. Inhaling, reverse this movement to the neutral lumbopelvic position.

9. With another exhalation, bring the back of your pelvis and the whole lumbar spine down to the floor using this segmental movement.

10. To finish lie on your back with your abdomen and lumbar area soft and rest for a few breaths.

11. Perform points 1–10 once or twice.

Exercise 1.7: Roll the back on a chair

Aim: mobilizing the lumbar spine into flexion.

1. Sit on a chair with a straight back rest, with the soles of your feet firmly on the floor (Figure 6.11).

2. As far as possible your back is in contact with the back of the chair or a wall.

3. Breathe in and lengthen your spine.

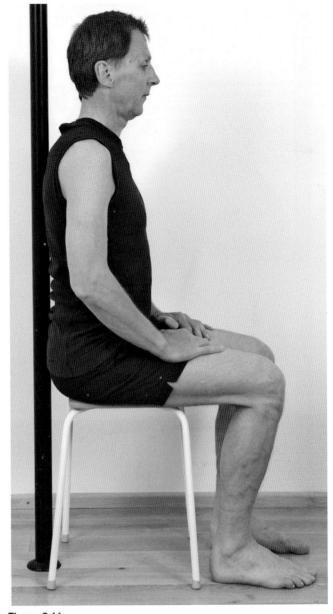

Figure 6.11

4. Breathing out, bend your head forward, then one segment of your spine after the other; this will need a few breaths (Figure 6.12).

5. Pay particular attention to removing one lumbar segment after the other from the back of the chair or the wall.

6. Rest on your thighs for a few breaths; use a pillow or rolled blanket on your thighs if necessary. Breathing in, lengthen your spine (Figure 6.13).

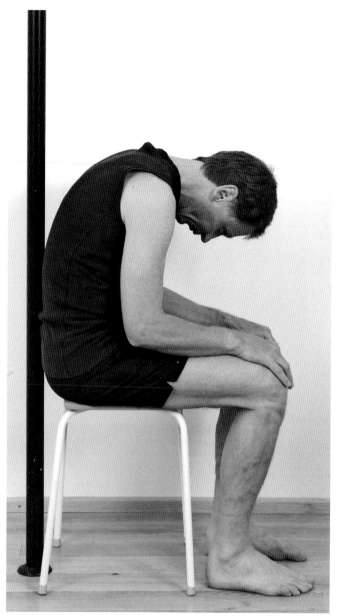

Figure 6.12

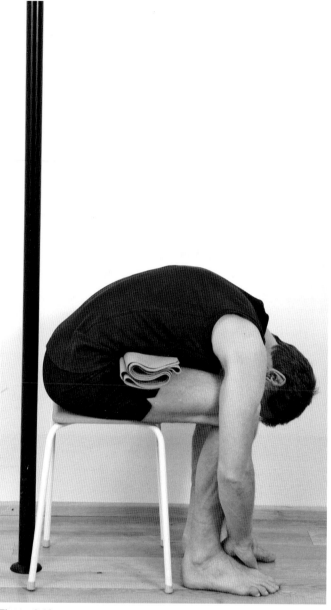

Figure 6.13

7. Bring the back of your pelvis to the back of the chair or the wall.

8. Move your lumbar spine to the back of the chair, one segment at a time.

9. Sit upright for one or two breaths.

10. Perform points 2–9 once or twice.

Exercise 1.8: Coachman relaxation

Aim: relaxing the lumbar spine.

1. Sit on a chair or stool, with the soles of your feet on the floor and feet and knees hip width apart.

2. Put your elbows on your knees (Figure 6.14).

3. Feel the lengthening of your spine during an inhalation.

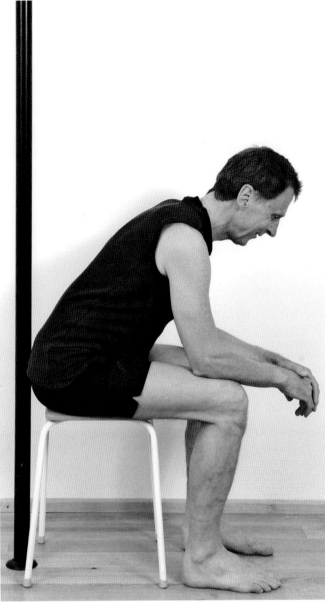

Figure 6.14

4. Maintain this length while you exhale.

5. When you inhale feel the lumbar area getting longer and wider.

6. Let the lumbar area be relaxed and soft while you exhale.

7. Keep the position described in points 1 and 2 for 3–5 breaths or longer.

8. To finish come back to sit straight as you inhale.

Variation

1. Sit on a chair or stool, with the soles of your feet on the floor and feet and knees hip width apart. Put a folded blanket or a thin pillow on your thighs, close to the groin.

2. Feel the lengthening of your spine during an inhalation.

3. Maintaining this length, bend forward to rest your abdomen on the blanket or pillow.

4. Let your head and arms hang naturally (Figure 6.13).

5. When you inhale feel the lumbar area getting longer and wider. Let this area be soft as you exhale.

6. Hold for 5–10 breaths; with practice you can gradually increase the time.

7. To come back place your palms on your thighs or the edges of the chair. Press your palms down to lift your trunk as you inhale.

8. To finish remain seated on the chair for a few breaths.

Exercise 1.9: Arched and hollow back with side-bending

Aims: mobilizing the lumbar spine, coordination.

Preparation: arched and hollow back

1. Kneel on a folded blanket to have a soft support for your knees and enough height so that the back is horizontal; the knees and feet are hip width apart and the thighs are perpendicular to the floor; the hands are on the floor, with the wrists underneath your shoulder joints.

2. Adjust the neutral lumbopelvic position.

3. With an exhalation, round your back like a cat; you may like to stay there for 1–2 breaths (Figure 6.15).

4. With an inhalation hollow your back.

5. Perform points 3 and 4 3–5 times.

6. To finish come back to the neutral lumbopelvic position.

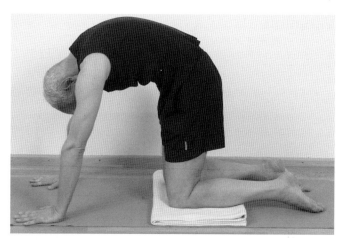

Figure 6.15

7. Bring your buttocks close to your heels and bend forwards; stay calm for a few breaths (Figure 6.16); if necessary use a pillow or rolled blanket between your buttocks and heels.

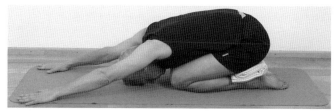

Figure 6.16

Refined work: arched back and hollowing with side-bending

1. Kneel on a folded blanket to have a soft support for your knees and enough height so that the back is horizontal; the knees and feet are hip width apart and the thighs are perpendicular; the hands are on the floor with the wrists underneath your shoulder joints.

2. Adjust the neutral lumbopelvic position.

3. With an exhalation round your back like a cat; you may like to stay there for 1–2 breaths (Figure 6.15).

4. With an inhalation hollow your back and side-bend to the left, looking towards your left hip; shift your right hip backwards (Figure 6.17).

5. Bring your head and pelvis back to the center and again round your back as you exhale.

6. With another inhalation hollow your back and side-bend to the right, looking towards your right hip; shift your left hip backwards.

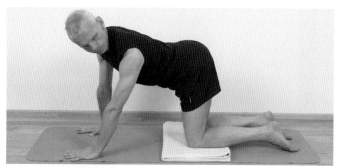

Figure 6.17

7. Bring your head and pelvis back to the center.

8. Perform points 3–7 3–5 times.

9. To finish come back to the neutral lumbopelvic position.

10. Bring your buttocks close to the heels and bend forwards; stay calm for a few breaths (Figure 6.16); if necessary use a pillow or rolled blanket between your buttocks and heels.

Hint for points 3 and 4

If you find that one or more segments bend too much when you round your back, which may be uncomfortable, ease off by slightly lengthening the corresponding front aspect of your trunk. If you have a weak, hypermobile segment in your spine, ease off from hollowing slightly in this area.

To begin with these finetuning corrections need to be carefully supervised.

General hint for this exercise

To develop awareness for the correct side-bending action and the coordination to get it right, a partner can guide the movement with one hand on the sacrum and the other hand between the shoulder blades.

Exercise 1.10: Side-bending strength

Aims: mobilizing the lumbar spine into side-bending, strengthening the lumbar spine, balance.

1. Lie on your right side with your trunk in line with your outstretched legs. Use a folded blanket as a soft support for your hip and thigh.

Lean on your right elbow and support your head with your right hand. Your left hand on the floor helps keep your balance.

2. With an exhalation lift both legs together (Figure 6.18); bring them down with an inhalation.

3. Perform point 2 3–5 times.

4. After lifting the legs the last time, hold them for 3–5 breaths, then slowly put them back on the floor.

5. Adjust your right arm on the floor, so that your head can rest on it.

6. Bend both hips and knees; stay there for a few breaths and feel the softness in your left hip.

7. Turn on your left side and repeat points 1–6.

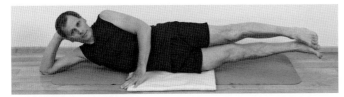

Figure 6.18

Refined work, particularly emphasizing balance

1. Lie on your right side; your outstretched right arm supports your head; your right hip and thigh are supported by a folded blanket; the left arm rests on the side of your trunk; if necessary, use a small pillow underneath your head.

2. With an exhalation lift both legs together (Figure 6.19); bring them down with an inhalation.

3. Perform point 2 3–5 times.

4. After lifting the legs for the last time, hold them for 3–5 breaths, then slowly put them back on the floor.

5. Adjust your right arm so that your head can rest on it.

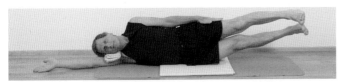

Figure 6.19

6. Bend both hips and knees; stay there for a few breaths and feel the softness in your left hip.

7. Turn on your left side and repeat points 1–6.

Exercise 1.11: Balance on the side

Aims: strengthening the lumbar spine, balance.

1. Prepare a blanket or soft mat for support for your elbow and knee.

2. Lie on your right side; with the help of your left hand, raise your upper trunk to bring your right elbow underneath your shoulder, with the right palm facing the floor, fingers pointing forwards; the left arm lies on the left side of the trunk.

3. Bend your right knee 90° so that it remains underneath the left knee and the lower leg is pointing backwards.

4. With an exhalation lift your pelvis so that the left leg, left hip, and left side of the trunk are in a line (Figure 6.20).

5. Hold for 3–5 breaths.

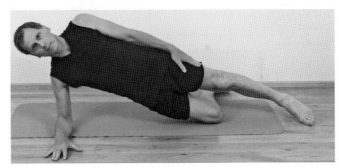

Figure 6.20

6. With an exhalation bring the right hip back onto the floor; stay there for 1–2 breaths.

7. Perform points 4–6 once or twice.

8. Lie on your right side; adjust your right arm so that the head can rest on it.

9. Turn on your left side and repeat points 2–8.

10. To finish bend both knees, push yourself up with your hands from the floor and sit cross-legged or with straight legs for a few breaths.

Stronger variation

For more strength and balance work, you can add the variation shown in Figure 6.21:

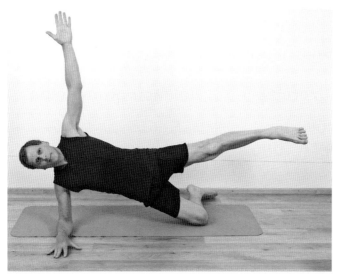

Figure 6.21

1. Prepare a blanket or soft mat for support for your elbow and knee.

2. Lie on your right side; with the help of your left hand raise your upper trunk to bring your right elbow underneath your shoulder, with the right palm facing the floor, fingers pointing forwards; the left arm lies on the left side of the trunk.

3. Bend your right knee 90° so that it remains underneath the left knee and the lower leg is pointing backwards.

4. With an exhalation lift your pelvis so that the left leg, left hip, and left side of the trunk are in one line.

5. Stretch your left arm perpendicular in line with the shoulder girdle.

6. Abduct your left leg rhythmically 3–5 times; before abducting the leg, the foot touches the floor; after the last go, hold the left abducted leg for a few breaths.

7. With an exhalation bring the left foot and the hip back onto the floor; stay there for 1–2 breaths.

8. Perform points 4–7 once or twice.

9. Lie on your right side; adjust your right arm so that the head can rest on it.

10. Turn on your left side and repeat points 2–8.

11. Lie on your left side; adjust your left arm so that your head can rest on it.

12. To finish bend both knees, push yourself up with your right hand from the floor and sit cross-legged or with straight legs for a few breaths.

Exercise 1.12: Baby back-bends

Aims: mobilizing the lumbar spine into back-bending, strengthening and relaxing the lumbar area.

1. Lie comfortably on your stomach, with your arms besides your trunk and palms facing the ceiling; if you need a soft support for your hip bones, use a folded blanket underneath your abdomen; support your forehead with a small pillow or folded towel so that your nose is free and your neck is relaxed.

2. Slightly pull your lower abdomen inwards, so gently that you can continue normal breathing.

3. Feel your groins moving towards the floor.

4. Maintaining the slight contraction of your lower abdomen, lift your right leg with an exhalation; the knee is straight and the foot is in dorsiflexion (Figure 6.22).

5. Hold for 2–3 breaths; as soon as you loosen the slight contraction of the lower abdomen, lower the leg so that you can get this action again.

6. With an exhalation bring the leg down; feel the relaxation in your lumbar area and relax your abdomen.

7. Stay relaxed for 1–2 breaths.

8. Repeat points 2–7 for the left leg.

9. Perform the whole cycle up to 5 times, but only as long as you can breathe naturally.

10. After the last go stretch your right arm besides your head; supporting yourself with your left hand, turn on your right side with your right arm under your head; bend both knees; stay comfortably lying on this side for a few breaths. While pushing yourself up to a sitting position with the left hand, let your left foot move away from you freely. If you prefer finishing on the left side, turn on your left side in the same way.

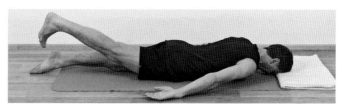

Figure 6.22

Stronger variations

a. Repeat points 1–7, except lifting both legs at the same time (Figure 6.23). You can put your hands flat underneath your front hip bones (Figure 6.24).

b. Bend both knees, feet in dorsiflexion; repeat points 2–7, lifting both bent legs at the same time (Figure 6.25). If this exercise is performed correctly, the knees do not move far from the floor.

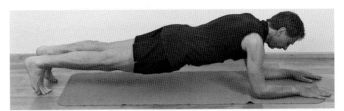

Figure 6.26

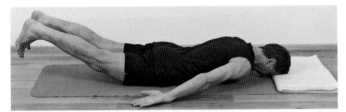

Figure 6.23

2. Stretch one leg backwards at a time, knees away from the floor; only the toes touch the floor; your legs, trunk, and head are in a line (Figure 6.26).

3. Keep your buttocks firm and slightly suck your lower abdomen in.

4. Hold for 1–3 breaths.

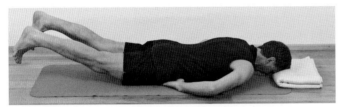

Figure 6.24

5. Keeping your elbows and shoulders the same, lower your knees to the floor, one at a time. If your hands are moving closer together, use a brick or book in between them.

6. Perform points 2–5 3–5 times; for the repetitions change the order in which you stretch the left and right leg backwards, and the order in which you lower your knees at the end.

7. To finish stay in the modified four-point kneeling position for a few breaths; bring your buttocks onto your heels or a folded blanket (exercise 1.9, Figure 6.16), relax for a few breaths.

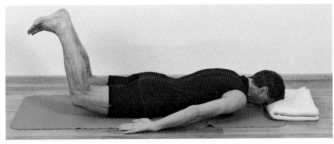

Figure 6.25

Stronger variation

1. Start as described in points 1–3, shown in Figure 6.26.

2. Maintaining the neutral lumbopelvic position, through a balanced activity of buttock and abdominal muscles, lift your right leg only as long as the hips stay on the same level and there is no rotation (Figure 6.27).

Exercise 1.13: Stick on four roots

Aims: strengthening the lumbar spine, balance.

1. Start with a modified four-point kneeling position; knees and feet are together, elbows bent, elbows underneath your shoulder joints and lower arms parallel. If necessary, rest your elbows on a folded blanket.

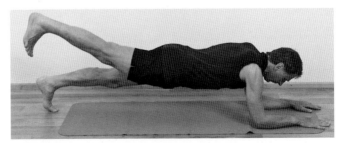

Figure 6.27

3. Hold for 1–3 breaths.

4. Come back to the starting position (point 1).

5. Lift your left leg as described in points 2 and 3, then come back to the modified four-point kneeling starting position.

6. Perform points 2–5 3–5 times.

7. To finish come back to the modified four-point kneeling position; bring your buttocks onto your heels or on a folded blanket (exercise 1.9, Figure 6.16) and relax for a few breaths.

Exercise 1.14: Four-point kneeling – variations

Aims: integrating lumbar stability and balance, coordinating and synchronizing arm and leg movements.

1. Kneel on a folded blanket to have a soft support for your knees and enough height so that the back is nearly horizontal; the knees are hip width apart and the thighs are perpendicular; the lower legs are parallel and the tops of the feet are on the floor with the toes pointing backwards; put your hands on the floor with the wrists underneath your shoulder joints (Figure 6.28).

2. Adjust the neutral lumbopelvic position.

3. Maintaining this neutral position, with the left thigh perpendicular to the floor and the arms unchanged, stretch your right leg backwards, with the foot in dorsiflexion; the toes are pointing towards the floor; the height of the leg does not matter, but the stability of the lumbar spine and the position of the left thigh and the

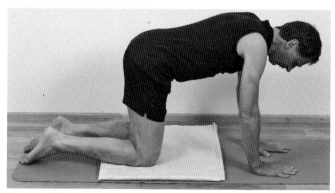

Figure 6.28

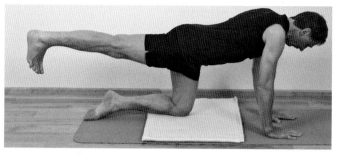

Figure 6.29

arms are important; particularly watch that your left elbow does not bend (Figure 6.29).

4. Hold the position up to 3 breaths, as long as you can maintain the neutral lumbopelvic position and breathe normally.

5. Come back to the starting position (point 1).

6. Repeat points 2–5 for the left leg.

7. Perform both sides 2–3 times.

8. To finish bring your buttocks onto your heels or on a folded blanket (exercise 1.9, Figure 6.16) and relax for a few breaths.

Hint

To improve awareness of the lumbopelvic position a partner can put her hands on the iliac crests or a sandbag can be placed on the lumbar area (Figure 6.30). Your partner can give you verbal feedback. You will feel whether the sandbag changes position and its weight distribution. Keep the pelvis stable so that the sandbag does not move.

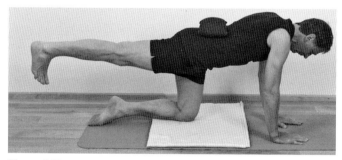

Figure 6.30

Refined work

1. Kneel on a folded blanket to have a soft support for your knees and enough height so that your back is nearly horizontal; the knees are hip

width apart and the thighs are perpendicular; the lower legs are parallel; the tops of the feet are on the floor and the toes are pointing backwards; put your hands on the floor, with the wrists underneath your shoulder joints.

2. Adjust the neutral lumbopelvic position.

3. Maintaining the neutral position, with the left leg perpendicular and the right arm unchanged, stretch your right leg backwards, with the foot in dorsiflexion, and stretch your left arm forwards in line with the side of your trunk (Figure 6.31).

4. Hold for 2–3 breaths, constantly feeling the balance between the abdomen and the lower back.

5. Repeat for the other side.

6. Perform both sides 2–3 times.

7. To finish bring your buttocks onto your heels or on a folded blanket (exercise 1.9, Figure 6.16) and relax for a few breaths.

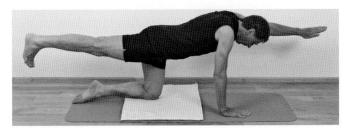

Figure 6.31

Variation

Lifting one arm and the opposite leg several times quickly builds coordination; a sensible rhythm is lifting the arm and leg with the inhalation, and bringing them down with the exhalation. With more experience you can try different rhythms; be aware of synchronizing the arm and leg movements.

Exercise 1.15: Shoulder bridge and variations

Aims: strengthening and mobilizing the lumbar spine.

1. Lie on your back.

2. Keep your throat relaxed throughout the following sequence.

3. Keep your pelvis in a neutral position; bend your knees, keeping the feet parallel and one foot length away from the buttocks; knees and feet are hip width apart; the arms are beside your trunk, the palms are facing the ceiling.

4. While exhaling lift your pelvis, maintaining it in a neutral position and contracting the buttock muscles.

5. While coming down during one or two breaths, feel your spine coming to the floor like a necklace, one pearl after another.

6. Perform points 4 and 5 3–5 times as a slow, rhythmic motion.

7. Then hold the lifted pelvis for 3–5 breaths, balancing the action of the buttock and abdominal muscles, and coming down as described in point 5.

8. Lie on your back for several breaths, feeling the relaxation in your lumbar and abdominal area; knees either bent or straight.

Hint

To work more precisely put a brick or pad between your knees (Figure 6.32) and keep the knees and feet at the same distance; then follow points 2–8. With increasing practice you may perform this exercise without a brick and reduce the distance of the knees and feet.

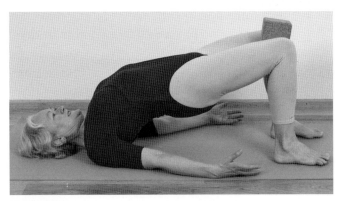

Figure 6.32

Variation a

Additional aim: balance.

1. Lie on your back.

2. Keep your throat relaxed throughout the following sequence.

3. Bend your knees, keeping the feet parallel and one foot length away from the buttocks; knees and feet are at the same distance; the arms are beside your trunk, the palms are facing the ceiling; the pelvis is lying in a neutral position.

4. Maintaining the pelvis in a neutral position, lift it with an exhalation, contracting the buttock muscles.

5. Maintaining the alignment of your hips (you may like to control them with your hands), lift your right leg as you exhale, bringing the knee towards your chest (Figure 6.33).

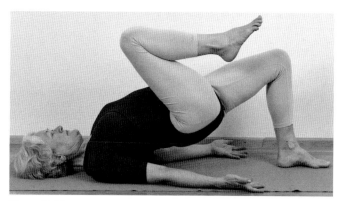

Figure 6.33

6. Hold for 1–3 breaths, then bring the right leg back to the starting position.

7. Repeat points 5 and 6 for the left leg.

8. While coming down with an exhalation, feel your lumbar spine like a necklace coming to the floor one pearl after another.

9. Perform points 4–8 3–5 times.

10. After the last go lie on your back for a few breaths and feel the relaxation in your lumbar and abdominal area; knees either bent or straight.

Variation to train coordination, synchronization, and stamina

Lift alternately the right and left leg rhythmically, gradually increasing speed.

Variation b

1. Lie on your back.

2. Keep your throat relaxed throughout the following sequence.

3. Bend your knees, keeping the feet parallel and one foot length away from the buttocks; hold a brick between your knees; knees and feet are at the same distance; the arms are beside your trunk, the palms are facing the ceiling; the pelvis is lying in a neutral position.

4. Maintaining the neutral lumbopelvic position, lift your pelvis, contracting the buttock muscles.

5. With an exhalation lift your right leg straight, nearly horizontally; the foot is in dorsiflexion, slightly relaxed (Figure 6.34).

6. Hold for 1–3 breaths, then bring the leg back to the starting position.

7. Repeat points 5 and 6 for the left leg.

8. While coming down, feel your lumbar spine like a necklace coming to the floor one pearl after another.

9. Perform points 4–8 3–5 times.

10. After the last go lie on your back for a few breaths and feel the relaxation in your lumbar and abdominal area; knees either bent or straight.

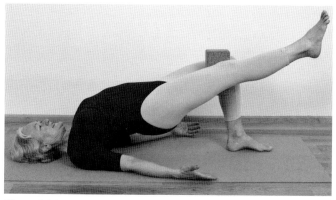

Figure 6.34

Variation c

1. Lie on your back.

2. Keep your throat relaxed throughout the following sequence.

3. Bend your knees, keeping the feet parallel and one foot length away from the buttocks; knees and feet are at the same distance; the arms are beside your trunk, the palms are facing the ceiling; the pelvis is lying in a neutral position.

4. Maintaining the neutral lumbopelvic position, lift your pelvis as you exhale, contracting the buttock muscles.

5. With an exhalation bring your right knee towards your chest, then straighten the leg vertically; the foot is in dorsiflexion, slightly relaxed (Figure 6.35).

6. Hold for 1–3 breaths, then bring the right leg back to the starting position (point 4).

7. Repeat points 5 and 6 for the left leg.

8. While coming down with an exhalation, feel your lumbar spine coming to the floor like a necklace one pearl after another.

9. Perform points 4–8 3–5 times.

10. After the last go lie on your back for a few breaths and feel the relaxation in your lumbar and abdominal area; knees either bent or straight.

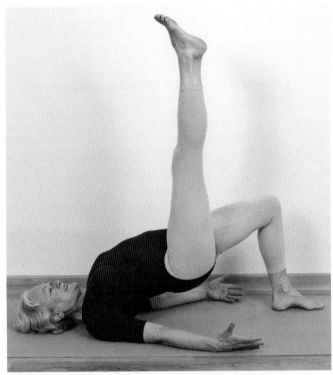

Figure 6.35

2. Basic exercises for the thoracic cage and ribs

There are 12 pairs of ribs: the upper seven ribs are the true ribs, whereas the eighth, ninth, and tenth rib are the false ribs, and the 11th and 12th ribs are the floating ribs. All ribs articulate with the thoracic vertebrae. The cartilage parts of the true ribs articulate with the sternum. The cartilage parts of the false ribs are connected together and to the cartilage part of the seventh rib, therefore they are indirectly connected to the sternum. There is no connection with the floating ribs. The cartilage parts of the ribs are important for elasticity of the thorax, and so it is important to stretch the transverse thoracic muscle connecting the sternum and the ribs.

The ribs move specifically with the breath. With inhalation the upper two ribs move forward and up, whereas the lower ribs flare outwards, and the middle ribs combine these movements. The upper sternum moves upwards and forwards, and the lower sternum mainly upwards. During exhalation these movements are passively reversed.

The basic exercises have been selected to mobilize all these structures. The supported bending exercises forwards, backwards, and to the sides in particular stretch the intercostal muscles and improve the mobility of the joints with the ribs. Stretching of the front of the upper thorax is also important, as it is too short in many patients (Roth 2009). To target the movements specifically at the ribs it is essential to maintain a neutral lumbopelvic position. The elasticity of the thorax and the quality of breathing can be maintained or even improved with age. When the thorax is expanded more alveoli in the lungs can also expand. This increases the surface for the exchange of oxygen and carbon dioxide, with the result that all the bodily systems receive a better oxygen supply.

Rib restrictions may be a cause of shoulder problems. To make the rib exercises more effective, it is important to maintain a neutral lumbopelvic position, so that the movements do not dissipate into the lumbar spine. Many rib exercises can be slightly modified to work on the thoracic spine. The rib exercises also work on the diaphragm, particularly if combined with breathing well. One of the best diaphragmatic exercises is laughing. Positive effects of laughing include:

- releasing muscle tension
- stimulating brain activity
- improving blood circulation
- long-term decrease in heart rate, after a short-term increase
- deeper breathing with an associated improvement in oxygen exchange (Titze & Eschenröder 2003).

If the patient has chest pains, think of heart problems; if the pain is in the costovertebral joints, think of lung problems. The thorax is particularly vulnerable to emotional stress. If the exercise therapy is generating an emotional reaction, the patient should be referred to a counselor for psychotherapeutic investigation and treatment if necessary.

Exercise 2.1: Communicating with your breath

Aims: training awareness of the breathing movement; mobilizing the costovertebral and costosternal joints.

1. Lie on your back in a comfortable position.
2. Use support for your legs if necessary, so that your abdomen and lumbar area are relaxed; use support for your head so that the throat and neck are relaxed.
3. Place your hands on the costal arches (Figure 6.36).
4. Breathing should be very subtle and fine, with no resistance; feel the movement with inhalation and exhalation for 3–5 breaths; the hands are only feeling, not guiding, the movements.

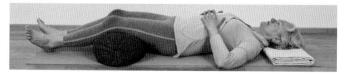

Figure 6.36

5. Release your hands at the end of an inhalation.

6. Place your hands on the upper lumbar area, so that the back of your hands or fingers are touching the lumbar area (Figure 6.37).

7. Repeat points 4 and 5 for this hand hold.

8. Place your hands on your upper ribs underneath your clavicles (Figure 6.38).

9. Repeat points 4 and 5 for this hand hold.

10. Place your arms comfortably on the sides of your trunk and be aware of the areas you have been feeling; stay calm for a few breaths.

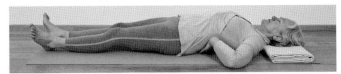

Figure 6.37

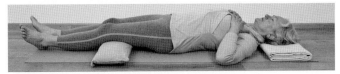

Figure 6.38

Exercise 2.2: The rib wave

Aims: mobilizing the costovertebral joints, relaxing the intercostal muscles.

1. Sit in a comfortable position and, while inhaling and exhaling, feel your thoracic movement with your hands on different areas to discover the restricted area. (Beginners should be instructed on this.)

2. Lie on your back, using a rolled towel underneath the restricted level of your ribcage; the hips and knees are bent; feet are hip width apart and knees together.

3. If necessary use a suitable pillow for your head.

4. Cross your arms over your chest, the right arm is on top, the elbows are together, and the hands are close to the opposite shoulder blade (Figure 6.39).

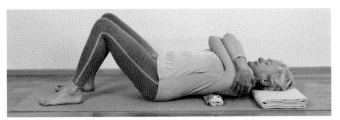

Figure 6.39

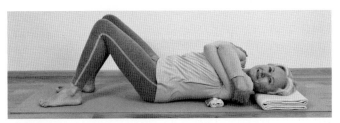

Figure 6.40

5. Move your elbows from side to side in a slow rhythmic movement, for 3–5 breaths; the ribcage is rotating slightly, and the head goes comfortably with the movement; the pelvis and knees are stable (Figure 6.40).

6. Change the arms; put the left arm on top and repeat point 5.

7. Let your arms release beside your trunk and feel the breath in your chest.

8. If you want to work on one particular rib or one pair of ribs, repeat points 4–6 2–3 times, placing the rolled towel under these ribs.

9. For more general mobilization change to different segments, performing points 4–6 once for each segment.

Hints

This exercise can be done for all ribs, but works best for ribs 5–9. If you are stiff, try to do this rhythmic movement only during exhalation; if you are hypermobile, then it may help to move during inhalation. Otherwise this exercise can be done during inhalation and exhalation. If you cannot cross the arms, they can be folded instead. Carefully adjust the diameter of the rolled towel until it feels right.

Refined work

To focus even more on a particular segment you can slightly side-bend to one side and maintain this side-bending while performing the movement with the elbows. Maintaining this slightly rotated and side-bent position for a few breaths, you can hold your elbows and position the arms over your head instead having crossed arms.

Exercise 2.3: Caterpillar movement

Aims: mobilizing the costovertebral and sternocostal joints, relaxing the intercostal muscles.

1. Prepare a board to lie on, either a foam board or folded blankets, of 3–5 cm height, which is large enough for your whole back.

2. Lie on this board with your whole back; the knees are bent and hip width apart; the head is off the board; support the back of your head with both hands, with fingers interlocked (Figure 6.41).

3. Constantly support your head and apply a slight traction with the thumbs under the lower ridge of the back of the head.

4. Keeping your knees stable, perform a slow, rhythmic side-bending; the elbows move away from the armpits, as if paddling with your elbows; slide down from the board, in the direction of the head, one rib at a time, alternating left and right; take up to one breath for each rib movement (Figure 6.42).

5. If you find an area that does not move well, stay in this passive back-bending over the edge of the board for a few breaths; place your arms loosely to the sides, beside the head and shoulders. If you cannot get any release after 3–5 breaths, try again on a thinner board.

6. After you have moved your whole thorax down from the board, move a little further; stay with your pelvis on the board; adjust yourself into a symmetrical position; feel the breathing movement in your ribs. Lift your pelvis to remove the board; gently lower your thorax, lumbar area, and pelvis onto the floor; bring your knees together; stay calm for a few breaths.

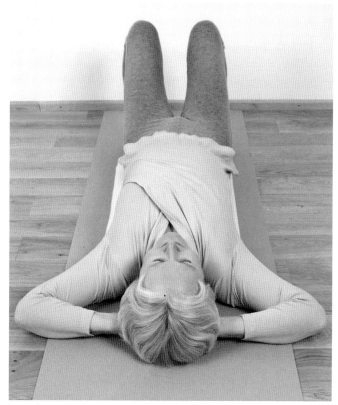

Figure 6.41

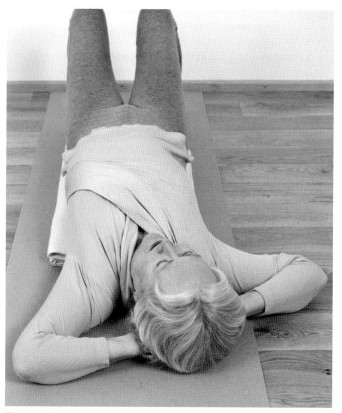

Figure 6.42

Exercise 2.4: Supported supine resting position

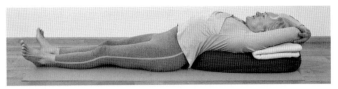

Figure 6.44

Aims: releasing the sternocostal and sternoclavicular joints, relaxing the area between the ribs and the first rib and clavicles.

1. Prepare a bolster for your back and a folded blanket for your head, as shown in Figure 6.43.

2. Sit in front of the bolster with bent knees; the soles of the feet are on the floor.

3. Supporting yourself on your hands, slowly bending your elbows lie down on the bolster; adjust the distance of your pelvis from the bolster so that you can maintain a neutral lumbopelvic position and relax your abdomen; slightly pull the thorax away from the abdomen.

4. Lie on the bolster, supporting your head so that the neck and throat are relaxed; if you can maintain a neutral lumbopelvic position and the abdomen relaxed, you can straighten the legs; otherwise keep the knees bent.

5. For the first part rest your arms sideways on the floor, so that you can feel the space from your sternum into the clavicles and upper ribs widening (Figure 6.43).

6. If you cannot relax your arms this way, rest them on pillows or folded blankets, or put your hands on your costal arches.

7. Feel the widening with inhalation, and the softness with exhalation; the inhalation is so subtle that there is no resistance in the widening and the throat stays relaxed.

8. For the second part bring your folded arms over your head, or alternatively straighten your arms; while moving the arms up, take

particular care to maintain the neutral lumbopelvic position; while resting the arms over your head, feel the lengthening from your side ribs through the armpits into your arms while you inhale; feel the area soft during exhalation. If you are holding the elbows, change your grip in between (Figure 6.44).

9. In the beginning a suitable timing is 5–10 breaths for each arm position; with increasing practice you can gradually increase to several minutes, whatever feels right for you.

10. To come back turn on one side to come down from the bolster; then remove the bolster and finish lying flat on your back for a few breaths.

Hint

If you cannot relax your back and abdomen with this support, put a folded blanket underneath your buttocks or use a thinner bolster.

Exercise 2.5: Supported shoulder bridge (Figure 6.45)

Aim: relaxing the areas between the lower and middle ribs.

1. Sit on a bolster placed across a mat; the knees are bent and the soles of the feet are on the floor; the knees and feet are hip width apart.

2. Put your hands on the floor behind the bolster; slide your pelvis towards the feet till the back of your pelvis is on the bolster; slowly bend

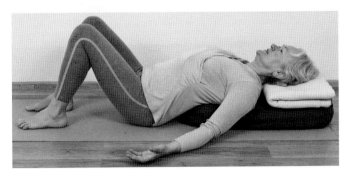

Figure 6.43

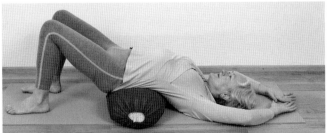

Figure 6.45

your elbows to lower your trunk, then bring your shoulders and head down onto the floor, keeping your throat relaxed.

3. Adjust yourself so that the pelvis is in a neutral position on the bolster, the abdomen is soft, and the thorax is curved and relaxed.

4. Rest your arms with slightly bent elbows around your head.

5. Feel the breathing movement in the area of the costal arches.

6. At first hold for 5–10 breaths; with practice gradually increase the time to several minutes.

7. To finish lift your pelvis, shift the bolster underneath your knees, then very gently lower your thorax, lumbar area, and pelvis onto the floor; rest your knees on the bolster; support your head if necessary; relax for a few breaths.

Exercise 2.6: Supported side-bending

Aims: relaxing the intercostal muscles; mobilizing the costovertebral joints.

1. Sit with straight legs with a bolster on your right side in line with your pelvis.

2. Bend your knees and lower them to the right side, keeping the feet left of your pelvis, and the left lower shinbone resting in the arch of your right foot.

3. Lower the right side of your ribcage onto the bolster, with the right hip remaining on the floor; while lying down lengthen the right side of your trunk slightly, even though it will be the shorter side when you are side-lying on the bolster (Figure 6.46). Your right arm is bending and supporting the head comfortably; if necessary, place a small pillow between the arm and the head.

4. Bring your left arm over your head so that it is relaxed (Figure 6.47).

5. Feel your left side lengthening with inhalation, softening with exhalation.

6. Stay there for 3–5 breaths to start, gradually increasing with practice.

7. To come back place your left hand on the floor in front and push yourself up from this hand; your left leg slides away slightly.

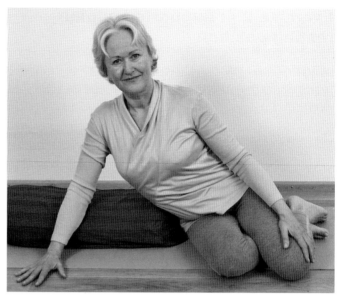
Figure 6.46

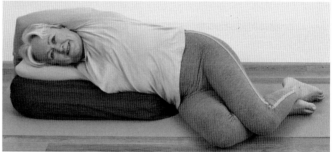
Figure 6.47

8. Sit straight; again, straighten your legs; take a slightly deeper breath and feel the difference between left and right.

9. Repeat points 1–7 with the bolster on your left side.

10. To finish sit in a symmetrical position for a few breaths and stay calm.

Stronger variation

For stronger side-bending, place the bolster across a mat and support your head with a folded towel or blanket; then follow points 1–10 (Figure 6.48).

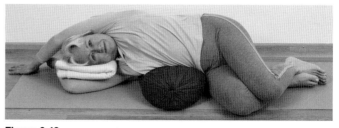
Figure 6.48

Exercise 2.7: Supported forward-bending

Aims: relaxing the intercostal muscles between the lower back ribs and relaxing the area between the shoulder blades.

1. Kneel on a soft support, thighs close together, buttocks on your heels.

2. Put a folded blanket on your thighs and in front of your knees on the floor.

3. Bend forwards and adjust the blanket so that your costal arches are resting on it.

4. Rest your forehead on the pillow so that your neck is relaxed.

5. Place your arms beside your head, elbows slightly bent (Figure 6.49).

6. Feel your middle back and the area between your shoulder blade widening with inhalation and softening with exhalation.

7. Stay there for 3–5 breaths initially; with practice gradually increase this time as far as reasonable.

8. To come back put your hands on the floor beside your knees and push yourself upright into a kneeling position.

9. Stay calm for a few breaths.

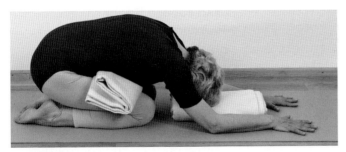

Figure 6.49

Hint

If you cannot kneel, perform the variation of coachman relaxation on a chair (see exercise 1.8). Place the folded blanket underneath your costal arches.

Exercise 2.8: Finetuning rotation

Aims: mobilizing and strengthening the thorax.

1. Sit on the floor cross-legged or kneel with your buttocks on the heels or on a sufficient support between your feet (Figure 6.50) or sit on a chair with your knees together (Figure 6.51).

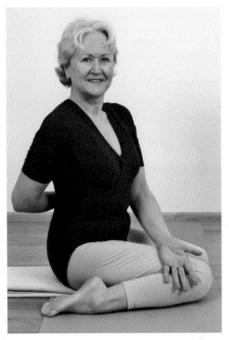

Figure 6.50

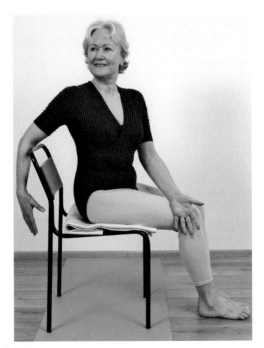

Figure 6.51

6 CHAPTER
The basic exercises
2. Basic exercises for the thoracic cage and ribs

2. Maintain a neutral lumbopelvic position throughout the exercise.

3. With an inhalation start lifting from your lower abdomen without changing the position on your sitting bones; lengthen your spine; gently lift your sternum and upper ribs, and lengthen between your neck and the back of your head, maintaining the position of the chin.

4. While exhaling turn to the right within your sensible range, maintain the lift.

5. Put the back of your left hand on your right thigh, the right arm around your back (Figure 6.50; in Figure 6.51 an alternative arm hold is shown).

6. While inhaling lift as described in point 3.

7. Exhaling, maintain this lift and turn a little further.

8. Turn your head softly and gently.

9. Perform points 6 and 7 3–5 times while keeping the rotation of your head soft and gentle.

10. Breathing naturally, stay 3–5 breaths in the maximum rotated, lifted position.

11. Maintaining the lift, reverse the rotation of your head and come back to the center while exhaling.

12. Repeat points 3–11 to turn to the left side.

13. After coming back to the center remain calm for a few breaths.

Refined work

1. Sit on a chair with your knees together (Figure 6.51) or on the floor cross-legged or kneeling with your buttocks on the heels or with a sufficient support between your feet (Figure 6.50).

2. Maintain a neutral lumbopelvic position throughout the exercise.

3. With an inhalation start lifting from your lower abdomen without changing the position on your sitting bones; lengthen your spine; gently lift your sternum and upper ribs; gently lengthen between your neck and the back of your head, maintaining the position of the chin. With an

exhalation put the back of your left hand on your right thigh, the right arm around your back and turn to the right until you just start feeling the limit of the rotation movement, maintaining the lift.

4. Inhaling again, observe the lifting described in point 3.

5. At the very end of the inhalation relax very slightly from the present limit of rotation.

6. Exhaling, maintain a neutral lumbopelvic position and the lifting, and turn further to the right until you just start feeling the new limit.

7. The head rotates only slightly so that the throat remains relaxed, with the eyes also relaxed.

8. Repeat points 4–7 3–5 times.

9. Breathing naturally, stay for 3–5 breaths in the maximum rotated, lifted position.

10. Maintaining the lifting, reverse the rotation of the head, and come back to the center while exhaling.

11. Repeat points 3–10 to turn to the left side.

12. After coming back to the center remain still for a few breaths.

Exercise 2.9: Four-point kneeling

Aims: mobilizing the upper and middle ribs, balance.

1. Kneel on a folded blanket to have a soft support for your knees and enough height so that the back is nearly horizontal; the knees are hip width apart, and the thighs are perpendicular; the lower legs are parallel, with the feet pointing backwards; put your hands on the floor, keeping your wrists underneath your shoulder joints.

2. Adjust the neutral lumbopelvic position.

3. Maintain this neutral position and control the costal arches, keeping them slightly inwards.

4. Lift your right arm horizontally; turn it so that the palm is facing the ceiling (Figure 6.52).

5. Hold for 3–5 breaths; lift your arm slightly higher as long as you can maintain the neutral lumbopelvic position and control the costal arches.

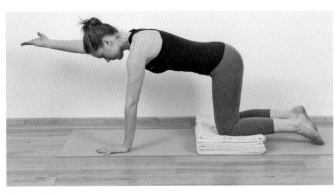

Figure 6.52

6. Bring the right hand down to the starting position.

7. Repeat points 2–6 for the left arm.

8. To finish bring your pelvis as close as possible towards your heels; rest your trunk on your thighs for a few breaths.

Refined work

Try different rotations of the lifted arm; feel the different areas of your ribcage you can reach.

3. Basic exercises for the thoracic spine

The thoracic spine has maintained the forward bending found in the embryological state. This kyphotic shape helps to protect the contents of the thorax, and so needs firmness. But it also needs to be flexible for good breathing movement. During inhalation the thorax moves so that the thoracic spine bends slightly backwards, and the distances between the individual vertebrae are increased. During exhalation the movement of the thorax is associated with a slight forward bending of the thoracic spine (see Chapter 5). Good mobility of the lower thoracic spine as well as the upper lumbar spine is important for the diaphragm.

The main movement of the thoracic spine is rotation. Depending on the direction of rotation, the movement is controlled by either the anterior or posterior part of the spinal segment if combined with sidebending. Therefore sudden side-bending and rotation movements should be avoided (Kingston 2001). If reactions like perspiring, trembling, or breathing changes occur, reduce the intensity of the exercises. Some of the exercises for the thoracic spine are similar to the rib exercises, with a slightly different focus. In both rib and thoracic exercises it is important to maintain a neutral lumbopelvic position to focus on the thoracic area.

Exercise 3.1: Mini-back-bend

Aim: mobilizing a specific area of the thoracic spine.

1. Lie on a rolled towel which is the diameter of your wrist supporting your spine up to the target segment. This segment bends backwards over the end of the roll.

2. If the roll is uncomfortable underneath your spine, make it thinner; if it is not effective, make it thicker; if necessary use a pillow underneath your head.

3. Hold the back of your head with your hands, the thumbs around its lower ridge; gently pull your head until you feel traction on the spinal segment that is lying over the end of the rolled towel (Figure 6.53).

4. Stay there for 3–5 breaths.

5. Depending on the result you can stay for a few more breaths.

6. Release your hands from your head.

7. Roll to the side and come up to sitting; sit in a neutral position for a few breaths and feel the breathing movement in the area you have been working on.

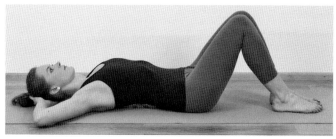

Figure 6.53

Exercise 3.2: Side-lying rotation

Aim: mobilizing the thoracic spine into rotation.

1. Lie on your right side, hips and knees comfortably bent at about 90°; the pelvis is perpendicular to the floor, and the left knee is exactly above the right knee; you may like to use a pad between your knees.

2. If needed, use a pillow underneath your head; the pillow must be broad enough so that the head stays on it during the rotation; if it is the right height for the back of the head, it may be too low for the side-lying; however, this is not a problem as the side-lying is only for a short period.

3. Shift your right arm and shoulder forwards in line with the shoulder girdle; this initiates the rotation (Figure 6.54).

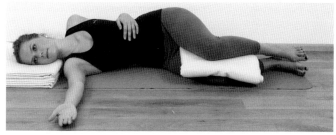

Figure 6.54

4. Place your left hand on the left costal arch.

5. Keeping your hips and knees in line as described in point 1, move your left arm and shoulder back towards the floor; combine this rotation with your exhalation. Stay calm during inhalation.

6. Maintaining your hips and knees as described in point 1, lower your left arm and shoulder again during exhalation a few times, until you can go no further in the rotation (Figure 6.55).

7. Gently rotate your head to the left, only as far as your neck and throat remain relaxed.

8. Feel the rotation of your head connecting to the rotation of your upper thoracic vertebrae.

9. Stay in this final position for 3–5 breaths; observe whether you can feel any further change while you exhale; feel if the position of your head is still right.

10. Come back to lying on your right side as described in point 1; stay there for 1–2 breaths.

11. Turn to the left side and repeat points 1–10 for this side.

12. To finish, turn onto your back and stay calm for a few breaths.

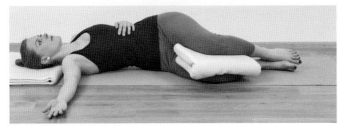

Figure 6.55

Exercise 3.3: Thoracic side-bending

Aims: mobilizing the thoracic spine into side-bending, strengthening the sides, balance.

1. Lie on your right side with a soft support for the hip; your left arm is resting on your left side, the right arm is outstretched forwards perpendicular to the body, and your head is resting on a pillow.

2. Lift your head into side-bending and slide your left hand on your left thigh towards your left foot as you exhale, remaining side-lying on your right hip (Figure 6.56). Hold for 1–2 breaths, then come back to the side-lying position while inhaling; with practice you can hold for up to 3 breaths.

3. Perform point 2 3–5 times, then rest for a few breaths on the right side; bend your knees if comfortable.

4. Turn on your left side; lie as described in point 1.

5. Repeat points 2 and 3 for the left side.

6. To finish lie on your back for a few breaths.

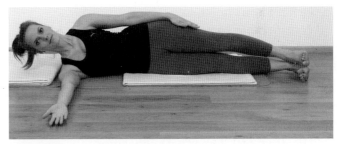

Figure 6.56

Stronger, supported side-bending

1. Lie on your right side, with your head resting on your outstretched right arm.

2. Keeping the right arm exactly in line with your right trunk side and staying side-lying on your right hip, lift your head; bend your right elbow to rest your head on the right hand, with your hand above the ear and the fingers pointing towards the back of the head (Figure 6.57). If this is too much side-bending for your cervical spine, place your left hand on the floor in front of your chest; slightly push yourself up from the left hand.

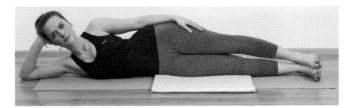

Figure 6.57

3. Stay there for 3–5 breaths, then straighten your right arm on the floor, and rest your head for a few breaths on it; bend your knees if comfortable.

4. Turn on your left side and repeat points 1–3 for the left side.

Exercise 3.4: The little boat

Aims: mobilizing and strengthening the thoracic area into forward-bending.

1. Lie on your back with your knees bent and your feet on the floor, feet and knees hip width apart, or alternatively rest your lower legs on a chair, your wrists or hands crossed behind your head, the fingertips as far as comfortable towards the opposite shoulder; this arm hold helps to keep the neck and throat relaxed and to focus the active movements on the thoracic spine (Figures 6.58 and 6.59).

2. Lift your right arm and shoulder as you exhale (Figure 6.60), lower with inhalation.

3. Lift your left arm and shoulder as you exhale, changing the hands over.

4. Perform points 2 and 3 3–5 times, changing the hands over.

5. Lift your right arm and shoulder as you exhale; hold the position for 2–3 breaths; lower with inhalation.

6. Repeat point 5 for the left side.

7. Repeat points 5 and 6, changing the hands.

8. Lift your head and both shoulders and shoulder blades away from the floor as you exhale (Figure 6.59):

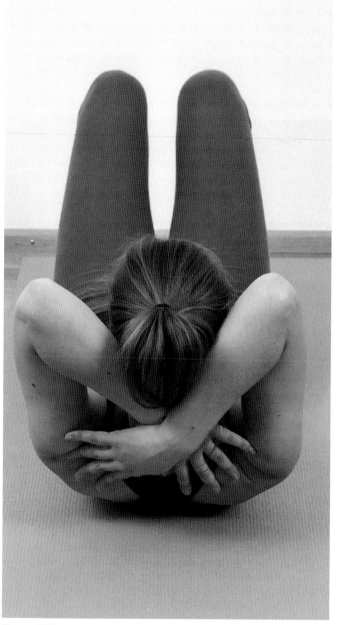

Figure 6.59

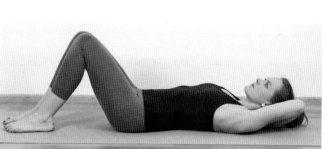

Figure 6.58

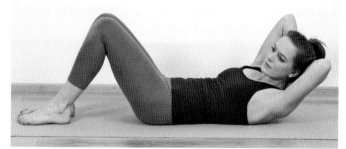

Figure 6.60

a. 3–5 times in a slow rhythmic movement coming back to the floor with inhalation

b. hold lifted for 3–5 breaths; lower your shoulders and head to the floor while inhaling

c. repeat a and b with the arms interchanged.

9. Release your hands; rest your arms at the sides of your body; lie on your back for a few breaths.

Exercise 3.5: Baby back-bends

Aims: mobilizing the thoracic spine into back-bending and strengthening the back of the thoracic area.

1. Lie on your stomach; use a folded blanket to give sufficient support for the hip bones and the knees; support your forehead so that the nose is free and the neck relaxed.

2. Your arms are lying at the sides of your body, palms facing the ceiling (Figure 6.61).

3. Slightly pulling your lower abdomen away from the floor, lift your arms and shoulders as you inhale, keeping the forehead on the support; lower the arms and shoulders as you exhale and relax your back and abdomen; if needed, stay calm for 1–2 breaths.

4. Perform point 3 3–5 times.

5. Slightly pulling your lower abdomen away from the floor, lift your arms and shoulders as you inhale, keeping your forehead on the support; hold the position for 3–5 breaths breathing naturally, and lower as you exhale; stay there for a few breaths and feel the softness between your shoulder blades.

6. As long as your neck and head are completely comfortable, you can perform points 3–5 lifting your head as well (Figure 6.62).

7. To finish stretch your right arm beside your head in line with your right trunk side; with the help of your left hand, turn on your right side; stay calm for a few breaths with your knees bent and your pelvis in the neutral position, then come up to sitting; if you prefer getting up from the left side, stretch your left arm beside the head first.

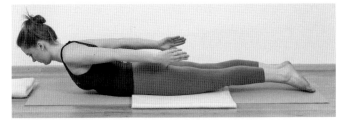

Figure 6.62

Refined work

The exercise can be performed with different rotations for the arms: palms facing the body, facing each other, facing the floor, and the ceiling. Start the way that feels most natural to you, then gradually try the other variations.

Variations for the arms

Variation a

Stretch your arms to the sides in line with your shoulder girdle and follow points 3–7 (Figure 6.63). Refine this variation by rotating your arms in different ways, such as palms to the floor and palms facing the ceiling.

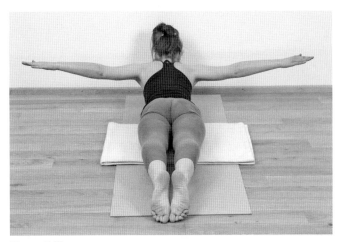

Figure 6.63

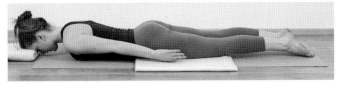

Figure 6.61

Variation b

Stretch your arms over your head and follow points 3–7 (Figure 6.64). Refine by rotating your arms in different ways: palms facing each other, palms towards the floor or towards the ceiling. By changing the rotation of your arms you can feel the effect on your shoulder blades, the area between the shoulder blades, and the thoracic spine.

As a subtle variation that is less demanding but develops awareness: lift only the right arm; feel the least action you need to do to have an effect on the thoracic area; try different rotations of the arm; repeat with your left arm.

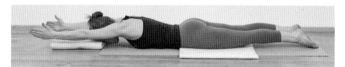

Figure 6.64

Exercise 3.6: Sitting twist

Aims: mobilizing the thoracic spine into rotation, balance of mobilizing and strengthening the thoracic spine.

1. Sit cross-legged on the floor or on a pillow or sit on a chair with the knees and feet together.

2. Adjust the pelvis to the neutral position so that your spine is in a natural, upright position; rest your hands on your thighs.

3. With inhalation straighten up further, from your pelvic floor towards your chest, lengthening from the neck to the back of your head, and maintaining the position of the chin, with shoulders relaxed.

4. Remaining firm on your sitting bones and maintaining the lift as described in point 3, turn to the right while exhaling, keeping the left hand on the right thigh (Figure 6.65), the right fingertips on the floor or on the chair or a brick; alternatively you can put your right arm around your back with the back of your hand on the body.

5. Perform the lifting as described in point 3 as you inhale and gently rotate further with each exhalation 3–5 times; maintain the rotation you have reached whenever you inhale again.

6. Turn your head to the right as far as the neck and throat are comfortable; keep your eyes soft;

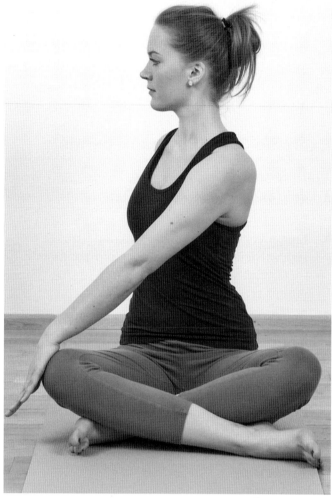

Figure 6.65

stay there for 1–2 breaths; feel the rotation of your head connecting to the rotation of your upper thoracic vertebrae.

7. Maintain the lifted position while you come back to the center.

8. Rotate to the left, as described in points 3–7.

9. To finish sit straight for a few breaths.

Refined work

Perform the sitting twist as described above; refine by visualizing the rotation for one vertebra after another, starting above the pelvis to below the neck; during one exhalation about 2–4 vertebrae can be covered. Feel the rotation of your head connecting to the area between your shoulder blades.

Exercise 3.7: Leaning over the back of the chair

Aim: mobilizing the thoracic spine into back-bending.

1. Use a chair which supports the lower half of your back.

2. Put a soft pad over the back of the chair.

3. Sit on the chair; slide forwards or backwards or support the buttocks with a pillow until the segment of your thoracic spine you want to reach is at the upper end of the back of the chair (Figure 6.66).

4. Maintain the neutral lumbopelvic position throughout the exercise and hold your head with your interlocked fingers, the thumbs underneath the lower ridge of the back of the head; adjust your head so that the throat remains relaxed.

5. Using the head and the arms as levers gently pull to get to the thoracic segment you want to reach; keeping this segment on the upper end of the back of the chair gently add the following movements, holding each for 2–3 breaths:

   a. leaning back slightly further

   b. side-bending right and left

   c. rotating right and left

   d. gently combining the different movements.

6. Depending on the results, you can repeat points 4 and 5 once or twice, changing the interlocking of your fingers.

7. If you want to work like this on a lower segment of your thoracic spine sit closer to the back of the chair or use a higher support for your buttocks.

8. If you want to reach a higher segment of your thoracic spine, sit further away from the back of the chair.

9. To finish remain seated for a few breaths and feel the breathing movement in the area you worked on.

Hint

With increasing practice you can refine and vary the movements as described in points 4 and 5 to make the exercise more effective with less force.

Exercise 3.8: Strong back

Aim: strengthening the thoracic area.

1. Sit on a chair, slightly away from its back; alternatively you can use a wall if you sit on a stool.

2. Move your bent elbows backwards, only a few centimeters behind the plane of your back; maintain a neutral lumbopelvic position and lift your thorax (Figure 6.67).

3. Readjust the distance from the back of the chair or the wall so that the elbows are just touching the back of the chair or wall.

4. Maintaining a neutral lumbopelvic position and the lifted thorax push the back of the chair or the wall with your elbows with one-third of your full strength; hold for 2–3 breaths.

5. Relax your arms for 2–3 breaths; place your hands on your thighs.

6. Move 2–3 cm forwards on the chair, or bend forwards slightly from the hips.

7. Moving your bent elbows backwards again, they will be slightly higher when they reach the back rest (Figure 6.68).

8. Repeat points 4 and 5.

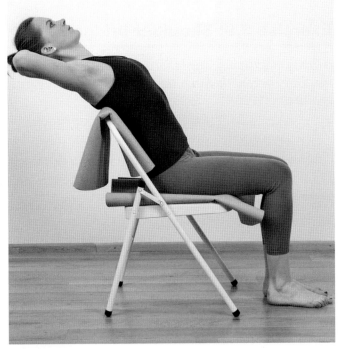

Figure 6.66

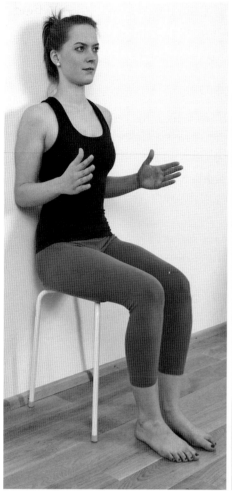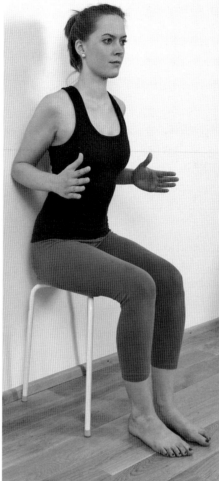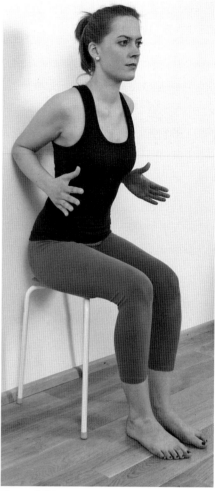

Figure 6.67   Figure 6.68   Figure 6.69

9. If you can bring your elbows slightly more backwards and higher, do so; move 2–3 cm forwards or bend further forwards from your hips (Figure 6.69) and repeat points 4 and 5; otherwise repeat points 4 and 5 in your previous arm position (Figure 6.68).

10. Then rest your hands on your thighs, relax your arms, and feel your breathing movement between your shoulder blades for a few breaths.

Refined work

Practice pushing your bent elbows to the back of the chair; play with different distances from the back of the chair, different directions, and distances of your elbows and different amounts of pressure to find the best effect.

Exercise 3.9: Shoulder bridge

Aims: mobilizing the thoracic spine into back-bending, strengthening the thoracic area against gravity.

1. Lie on your back, knees and feet hip width apart, knees bent, feet one foot length away from the buttocks, soles of the feet on the floor; elbows bent, as close as possible to the sides of your trunk, fingers pointing towards the ceiling.

2. Keeping your throat relaxed, lift your pelvis as long as you can maintain the neutral lumbopelvic position (Figure 6.70); to help in keeping the throat relaxed, move the chin a tiny bit away from the sternum.

3. To lift further press your elbows into the floor, again keeping a soft throat; move the hands apart

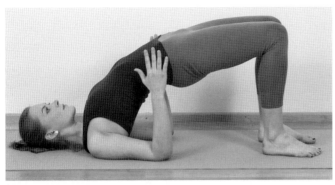

Figure 6.70

and the elbows closer together, corresponding to an external rotation of the arms; this makes the effect even stronger.

4. Hold for 3–5 breaths.

5. To come down lower yourself vertebra by vertebra, starting with the first thoracic vertebra, and finishing with the pelvis.

6. Repeat points 2–5 once or twice.

Refined work

To refine the exercise reduce the pushing force from the elbows; consciously lift the vertebrae instead, starting with the lowest cervical vertebra, then moving onto the thoracic vertebrae, one after another. With increasing practice you can continue to refine for greater effect.

Resting pose

Aim: relaxing the thoracic area.

Support your pelvis and middle back on a bolster, so that the shoulders and back of your head are resting on the floor (Figure 6.71). Choose the height of the bolster so that your abdomen and back are relaxed.

If the bolster is too high use a folded blanket instead; you can adjust the height of the blanket exactly to your need. Adjust yourself so that your throat is soft and you feel relaxed in the back and in the abdomen.

With increasing practice you can gradually increase the height of the bolster to feel relaxed in the pose. Stay for 5–10 breaths in the beginning, gradually increasing to several minutes with practice. You can choose either of the arm positions besides the trunk, in line with the shoulder girdle, or loosely around the head or any combination.

To finish lift your pelvis slightly to remove the bolster or blanket, lower your spine like a pearl necklace one vertebra after another. Then lie on your back for a few breaths.

Exercise 3.10: Four-point kneeling

Aims: mobilizing the thoracic spine, strengthening the thoracic area, balance.

1. Kneel on a folded blanket to have a soft support for your knees and enough height so that your back is nearly horizontal; the knees are hip width apart, and the thighs are perpendicular; the lower legs are parallel, with the feet pointing backwards; put your hands on the floor, keeping your wrists underneath your shoulder joints (Figure 6.72).

2. Adjust the neutral lumbopelvic position.

3. Keeping your pelvis neutral, lift your right arm horizontally in line with the right side of your trunk as you inhale (Figure 6.73).

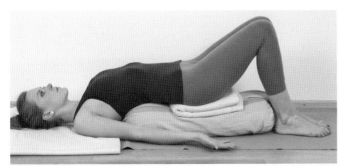

Figure 6.71

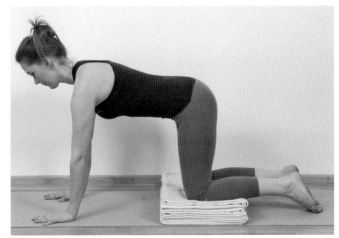

Figure 6.72

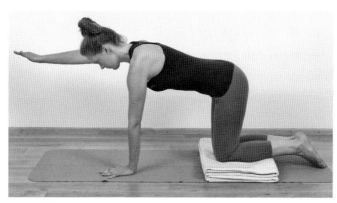

Figure 6.73

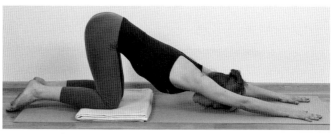

Figure 6.74

4. With the palm facing the floor first, then perpendicular facing the left side, then facing the ceiling, hold each position for about one breath.

5. Bring the right hand back to the starting position as you exhale; stay there for 1–2 breaths.

6. Repeat points 3–5 for the left arm.

7. Perform points 3–6 2–3 times.

8. To finish lower your pelvis towards your heels as far as comfortable; bend your trunk and head down; keep your arms in a relaxed position, and stay there for a few breaths (see exercise 1.9, Figure 6.16).

Refined work

Follow points 1–8. In addition lift the opposite leg to challenge the balance more. Lift your arm as high as you can while maintaining a neutral lumbopelvic position (see exercise 1.14, Figure 6.31).

Exercise 3.11: Cat stretch

Aim: mobilizing the thoracic spine.

1. Start in the four-point kneeling position, with your knees on a soft support.

2. Maintaining the thighs perpendicular to the floor and a neutral lumbopelvic position, walk your hands forwards until your trunk and arms are in one line (Figure 6.74).

3. If possible rest your forehead on the floor; otherwise use a pillow.

4. Stay there for 3–5 breaths.

5. Then walk your arms a little closer towards your knees and rest your elbows on the floor for a few breaths, keeping your hands in line with the elbows.

6. Again straighten your arms as described in point 2.

7. Maintaining the position of the pelvis bend your right elbow towards the floor as you exhale and turn your head slightly to the left as far as is comfortable for the neck and throat (Figure 6.75).

8. Stay there for 2–3 breaths; feel the breathing movement in your thorax.

9. Stretch your right arm, bring your head back to the center, and stay there for 1–2 breaths.

10. Repeat points 7–9 for the left side.

11. Perform points 7–10 2–3 times.

12. To finish lower your pelvis as close as you can to your heels, bend your trunk and head down, keeping your arms in a relaxed position; stay calm for a few breaths (see exercise 1.9, Figure 6.16).

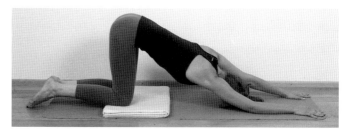

Figure 6.75

4. Basic exercises for the shoulder girdle and the cervicothoracic junction

The shoulder girdle consists of the two clavicles and the scapulae. The glenohumeral joints, the ball and socket joints connecting the scapula and the humerus, are the most mobile and least stable joints in the body. Before prescribing a specific exercise program for the shoulder girdle a thorough diagnosis should be focused on finding out whether the restriction is in the scapulothoracic area or whether it is compensation for weakness or hypermobility in the glenohumeral joint. In such cases mobilizing the glenohumeral joint further would cause discomfort, whereas it is often helpful to improve the mobility of the scapulae. Stable shoulder blades help to protect in weight-bearing. The clavicles are moved in most shoulder exercises as well.

The shoulder girdle is connected to many other structures, from the skull to the pelvis. It is worth considering these areas as well, particularly if there is no improvement from working on the shoulder girdle itself. A frequent cause of shoulder problems is restriction in the upper ribs. Then it is sensible to include rib-mobilizing exercises. As the anatomical structures and functions of the cervicothoracic junction are closely related to the shoulder girdle, we will give a summary of these two areas here.

The shoulder girdle has a wide range of movement possibilities. We shall consider movements with the main emphasis on the glenohumeral joints, and on the scapulae. Flexion (forward and upward movement of the arms) and abduction (movement of the arms to the side and upwards) are summarized as elevation of the shoulder by some authors (Kingston 2001). But rotation of the arms is different. If you start, for example, with the arms downwards and the palms facing the thighs, after raising the arms by moving them forwards and upwards, the palms are facing each other (see Codman's paradox, Magee 1997). After raising the arms by moving them to the sides and upwards, the backs of the hands are facing each other. The last phase of elevation needs extra movement of the cervicothoracic area and the upper thoracic spine. If both arms are elevated there is some back-bending, whereas when you elevate one arm there is side-bending in this area.

Exercise 4.1: Pendulum exercises standing

Aims: *mobilizing the shoulder joints, particularly encouraging fluid transport.*

1. Stand with your feet one step apart, one foot forward, one foot backwards, the front leg slightly bent, in a natural position.

2. To adjust your pelvis as if you are going to walk, slightly lift your back heel and then bring it back to the floor.

3. Swing your arms in opposition in a natural rhythm like a pendulum up to 1 minute; be aware of the weight of your arms (Figure 6.76).

4. Change your feet and again swing your arms as described in point 3.

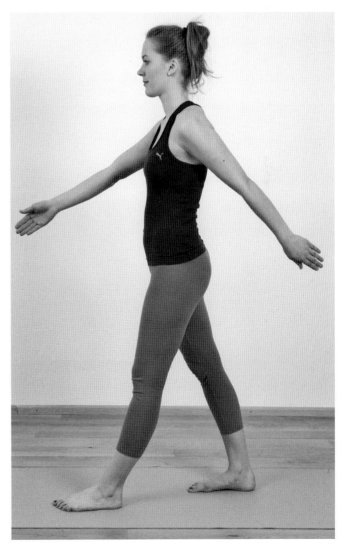

Figure 6.76

Hint

Practice the pendulum movements while walking.

Refined work

1. Stand sideways to a table or chair so that you can rest your right hand on it, with your feet apart up to one leg length, and the right foot in front.

2. Bend forward and rest your right hand or elbow on the chair or table so that your posture is comfortable (Figure 6.77).

3. Swing your left arm so that it can move in lines in different directions and in circles for 1–2 minutes; try different rotations of your arm, such as palm forward, towards the body, and backwards.

4. Then come back, and turn around.

5. Now the table or chair is on your left side.

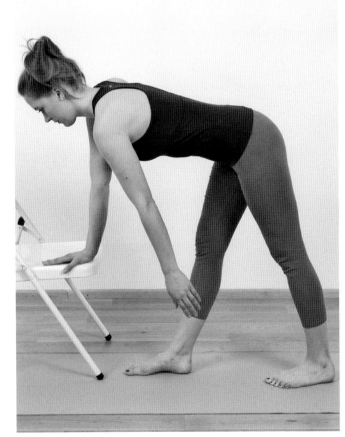

Figure 6.77

6. Move your feet apart, up to one leg length, with the left foot in front.

7. Repeat points 2 and 3 for the right arm.

Exercise 4.2: Scapular movements

Aims: mobilizing the shoulder blades, relaxing the periscapular area, coordination.

1. Sit cross-legged on the floor or sit on a chair with your knees and feet parallel; adjust the neutral lumbopelvic position.

2. Maintaining the neutral position and the head well balanced, move your shoulder blades in different directions, each for 3–5 breaths:

   a. forwards (apart from each other) and backwards (closer together)

   b. up and down

   c. circular (clockwise and counterclockwise).

   After each movement stay for a few breaths; feel the breathing movement between your shoulder blades and the relaxation of your shoulders.

Hints

• Moving the shoulders opposite and equally trains your coordination.

• You will be more aware of the movement if a partner puts his hands on your shoulder blades and follows your movements.

• Also performing the scapular movements leaning on a wall helps to refine awareness.

Exercise 4.3: Spider monkey 1

Aim: gentle mobilization of the shoulder girdle.

1. Sit on the floor with your knees together, the feet beside your hips, or sit on a chair with your knees and feet hip width apart and parallel; adjust the pelvis to the neutral position.

2. Relax your neck, throat, and shoulders.

3. Stretch your right arm and turn it inwards; bend it and move it around your back to hold your left upper arm (Figure 6.78); if you cannot reach your left upper arm use a belt around your arm and hold the belt with the right hand; your left

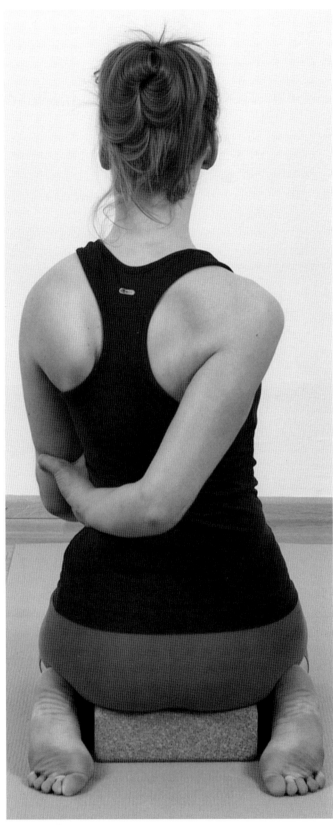

Figure 6.78

hand is on your left thigh, or if possible on the right one.

4. Continue holding your left arm with the right hand and move the left arm forwards as far as the right shoulder can take the backwards movement.

5. Turn your head to the left very gently.

6. Hold for 3–5 breaths.

7. Then release; rest your hands on your thighs for 1–2 breaths, with the palms up or down as you like.

8. Repeat points 2–7 for the left arm.

Exercise 4.4: Spider monkey 2

Aims: mobilizing the shoulder girdle and the cervicothoracic junction.

1. Sit on the floor or on a chair as described in exercise 4.3, point 1.

2. Relax your neck, throat, and shoulders.

3. Stretch your right arm and turn it inwards; bend it and move it around your back to hold your left upper arm; if you cannot reach your left upper arm use a belt around it and hold the belt with the right hand; the left hand is on your right thigh (Figure 6.79).

4. Continue holding your left arm with the right hand and move the left arm forwards as far as the right shoulder can take the backwards movement.

5. Feel the length of your spine while you inhale; turn your thorax to the right with exhalation.

6. Keeping your right shoulder back as much as possible and your sternum lifted, turn your head to the left, opposite to the rotation of the thorax, as far as is comfortable for your neck and throat.

7. Hold for 3–5 breaths.

8. Maintaining the length of your spine and the sternum lifted, come back to the center, release your arms, and stay there for 1–2 breaths.

9. Repeat points 2–8 for the left arm.

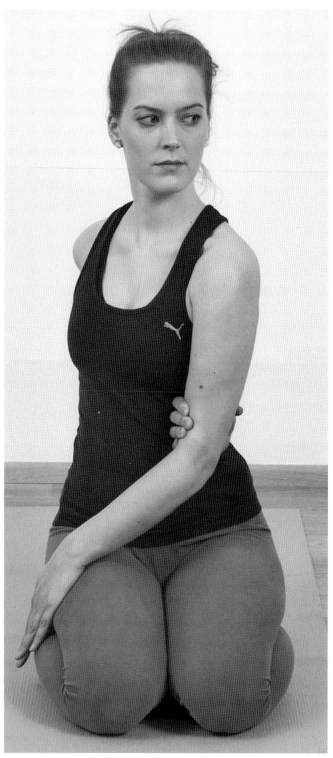

Figure 6.79

Exercise 4.5: Turning the head

Aim: mobilizing the cervicothoracic junction.

1. Sit cross-legged on the floor on a firm pillow or sit on a chair, with knees and feet together.

2. Adjust the pelvis to the neutral position so that your spine is in a natural, upright position.

3. Lift further with the inhalation from your pelvic floor towards your chest, gently lengthening from the neck to the back of your head, maintaining the position of the chin; shoulders are relaxed.

4. Remaining firm on your sitting bones, maintaining the lift as described in point 3, and with the back of the left hand on the right thigh and the right hand behind your pelvis, turn to the right while exhaling (Figure 6.80).

5. Maintaining the lift described in point 3 while inhaling, gently turn further with exhalation, 2–3 times; move your right shoulder back and let it sink towards the floor.

6. Gently turn your head to the right.

7. Keeping the right shoulder back and towards the floor, turn your head to the left as far as the neck and throat are comfortable, maintaining the vertex of the head in the center; keep your eyes soft, and stay there for 2–3 breaths.

8. Maintain the lifted position while you come back to the center.

9. Rotate to the left as described in points 3–8.

Hint

Keeping the superficial throat muscles soft while turning the head strengthens the deep stabilizing muscles of the cervical spine.

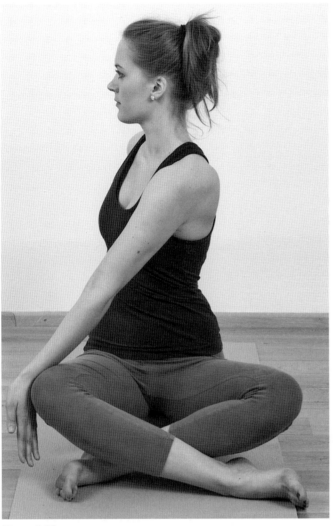

Figure 6.80

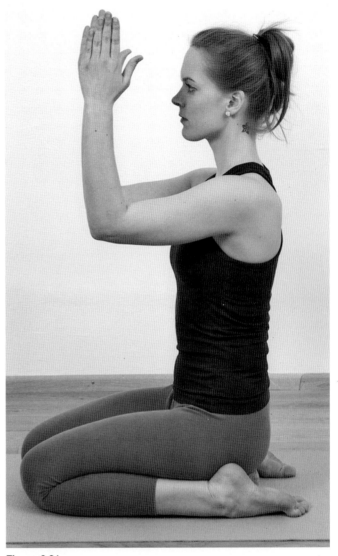

Figure 6.81

Exercise 4.6: Arms around each other

Aims: mobilizing the shoulder blades, stretching the area between the shoulder blades, coordination.

1. Sit on the floor on a firm pillow, knees together, feet beside your hips; or sit on a chair, with your knees and feet hip width apart and parallel; adjust your pelvis in a neutral position and keep your head straight as if balancing a book on the crown of your head.

2. Maintaining the stability of the pelvis, raise your arms, with your elbows at the height of your sternum (Figure 6.81).

3. Bring your right elbow in the plane of the sternum, move your left elbow underneath the right one, and wind the left lower arm and hand around the right one (Figure 6.82).

4. If this is not possible hold a belt between both hands (Figure 6.83).

5. To increase the stretch, slightly raise your elbows several centimeters, maintaining the length of your spine and the position of your head.

6. Breathe naturally even if the upper chest is compressed.

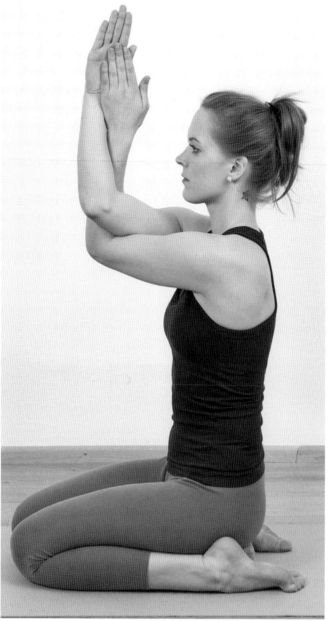

Figure 6.82

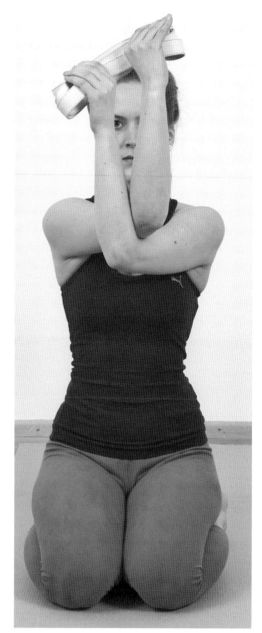

Figure 6.83

7. Feel the stretch between your shoulder blades as you inhale; feel the relaxation in this area as you exhale.

8. Maintain the posture for 3–5 breaths.

9. Release the arms with an exhalation, and feel the widening in your upper chest with inhalation.

10. Repeat points 2–9 with the arms interchanged.

Exercise 4.7: Elevating arms in three steps

Aims: mobilizing the shoulder girdle and the cervico-thoracic junction.

1. Sit on the floor on a firm pillow, knees together, feet beside your hips; or sit on a chair, with your knees and feet hip width apart and parallel; adjust your pelvis in a neutral position and keep your head straight as if balancing a book on the crown of your head.

2. Maintain the neutral pelvic position throughout the exercise.

3. Raise your arms to the side as long as the shoulders are not lifting (Figure 6.84).

4. To elevate the arms further while you inhale, also let your shoulder blades move upwards (Figure 6.85).

5. Turn your arms so that the palms are facing each other to lift the arms further with another inhalation. When you have reached the limit of this elevation, keeping the pelvis neutral, lift your upper sternum; this gives some back-bending in the cervicothoracic junction and the upper thoracic spine, necessary for the full elevation of the arms (Figure 6.86).

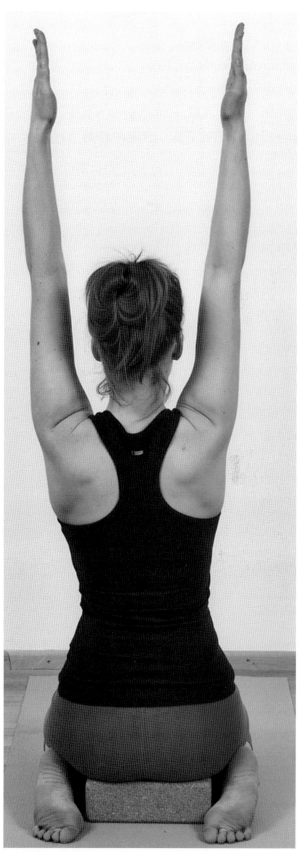

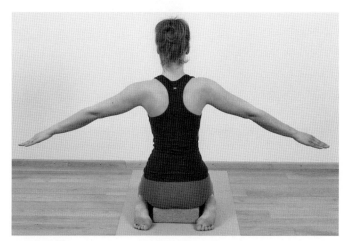

Figure 6.84

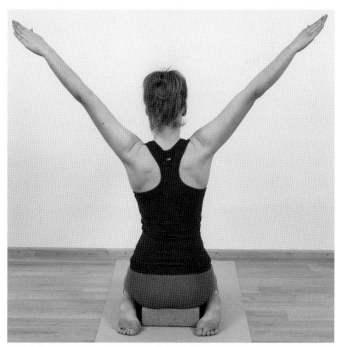

Figure 6.85

Figure 6.86

6. Stretch your arms even further upwards until you reach your final limit.

7. Hold for 2–3 breaths, then release your arms while you exhale; rest your hands on your thighs and relax your shoulders.

8. Perform points 2–7 2–3 times.

Exercise 4.8: Elevating the arms

Aims: mobilizing the shoulder girdle and the cervicothoracic junction.

1. Sit cross-legged on a firm pillow on the floor or sit on a chair, with knees and feet hip width apart and parallel.

2. Interlock your fingers, stretch your elbows, and bend your wrists, so that the palms are facing you.

3. Maintaining the neutral lumbopelvic position and your costal arches in the natural position, raise your arms over your head as you inhale.

4. When you reach the limit, maintain the neutral lumbopelvic position and lift your sternum to get the full elevation of the arms.

5. Keep your elbows straight and the wrists fully flexed (Figure 6.87).

6. Hold for 3–5 breaths.

7. Bring your arms down horizontally, internally rotate your arms so that the palms are away from you, with the thumbs stretched and the tips of the thumbs slightly touching (Figure 6.88).

8. Maintaining the neutral lumbopelvic position and your costal arches in the natural position, raise your arms above your head as you inhale, the palms facing the ceiling; lift your sternum for full elevation of your arms (Figure 6.89).

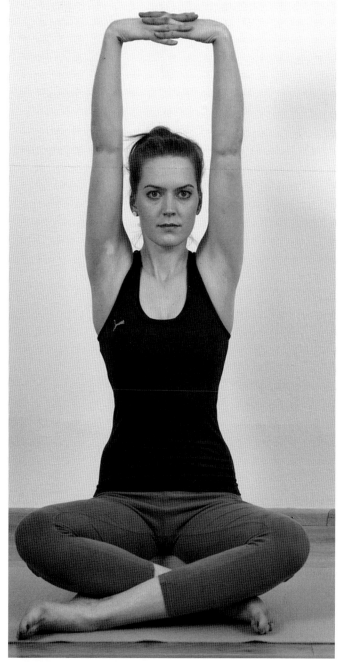

Figure 6.87

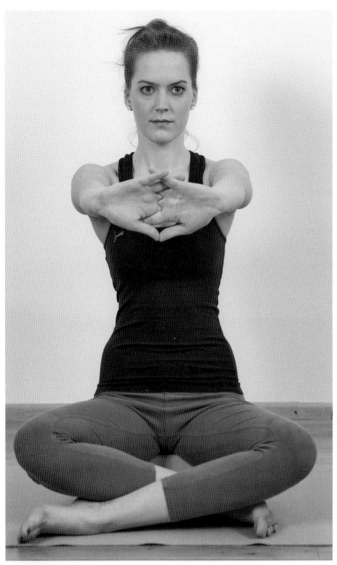

Figure 6.88

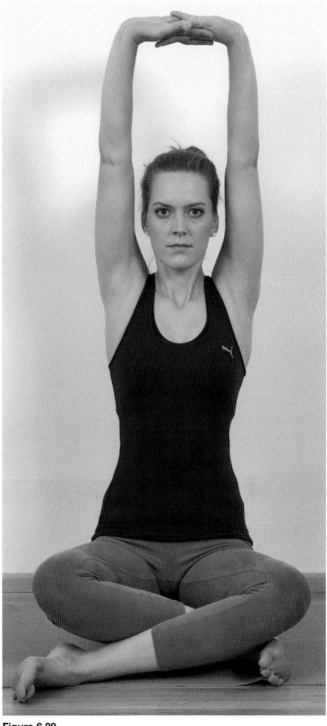

9. Hold for 3–5 breaths.
10. Release the hand hold; move your arms to the sides and down.
11. Stay there for a few breaths; relax your shoulders.
12. Interlock your fingers the other way around and repeat points 2–11.

Figure 6.89

Exercise 4.9: Strong shoulders

Aim: strengthening all structures of the shoulder girdle.

For all parts of this series of exercises it is essential to maintain the neutral lumbopelvic position and keep the costal arches in a natural position to get the best effect for the shoulder girdle.

For a general strengthening the whole series of exercises is recommended. If you want to focus on a special area, you can select the relevant parts.

Part 1

1. Sit on the floor on a firm pillow, knees together, feet beside your hips, or sit on a chair, with your knees and feet hip width apart and parallel; adjust your pelvis in a neutral position and keep your head straight as if balancing a book on the crown of your head.

2. Keeping your shoulders slightly down, and your head in a position so that the neck and throat stay relaxed, fold your hands at the level of your sternum and feel the contact of your palms, thumbs, and fingers; keep your fingers and thumbs straight (Figure 6.90).

3. Press your palms together with one-third of your full strength for 2–3 breaths, keeping your shoulders down; keeping the contact of your palms, release the pressure.

4. Perform point 3 3–5 times.

5. Release the hands; rest them on the thighs for a few breaths.

Part 2

1. Sit on the floor or on a chair as described in part 1 point 1.

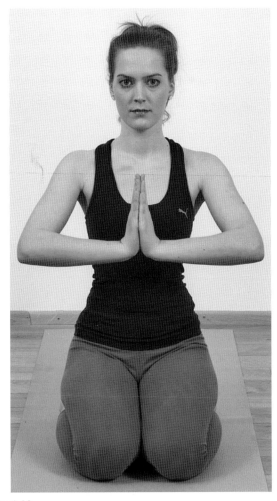

Figure 6.90

2. Put a belt around your arms, just above the elbows, so that the elbows are shoulder width apart.

3. Raise your elbows to the height of your shoulders, fingers pointing towards the ceiling (Figure 6.91).

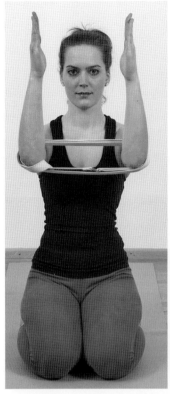
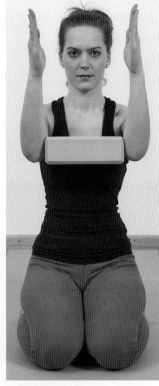

Figure 6.91   Figure 6.92

2. Hold a brick or book between your elbows.

3. Raise your elbows to the height of your shoulders, fingers pointing towards the ceiling (Figure 6.92).

4. Press your elbows against the brick or book with one-third of your full strength for 2–3 breaths; release the pressure, still holding the brick or book.

5. Perform point 4 3–5 times, each time at a different height for the elbows, above and below 90°.

6. Carefully lower your elbows to release the brick.

Part 4

1. Stand or sit close to a wall; move your bent elbows backwards, as close together as possible, keeping the lower arms parallel.

2. Maintaining the neutral lumbopelvic position, your sternum slightly lifted and your shoulders down, press the elbows against the wall with one-third of your full strength for 2–3 breaths for each of the following variations (this is a complex movement as the elbows are moving backwards and together):

    a. the elbows just slightly further back than your back (Figure 6.93)

    b. adjusting the distance from the wall, bring your elbows slightly further back and higher (Figure 6.94)

    c. moving still further away from the wall, bring your elbows further back and higher (Figure 6.95).

4. Press your elbows against the belt with one-third of your full strength for 2–3 breaths; release the pressure; maintain the posture.

5. Perform point 4 3–5 times, each time at a different height for the elbows, above and below shoulder level.

6. Release your arms.

Part 3

1. Sit on the floor or on a chair, as described in part 1 point 1.

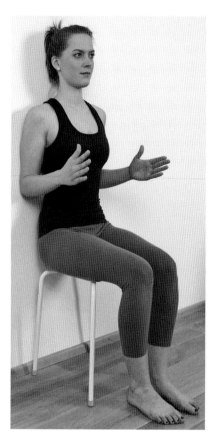

Figure 6.93

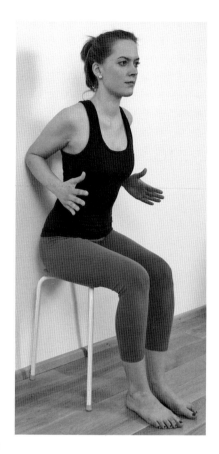

Figure 6.95

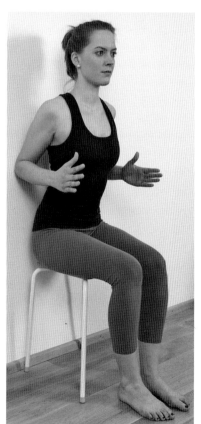

Figure 6.94

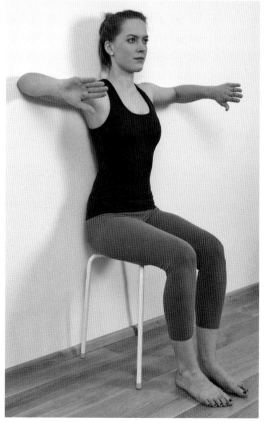

Figure 6.96

3. For the last attempt be close to the wall; lift your elbows sideways to shoulder height and press them to the wall with one-third of your full strength for 2–3 breaths (Figure 6.96).

4. Perform point 3 2–3 times; for the repetitions change the rotation of your arms so that the hands are higher and closer to the wall.

Hint

A more sensitive approach to this exercise is possible with a partner helping to resist the movement of the elbows rather than a wall.

Exercise 4.10: Four-point kneeling

Aims: mobilizing the shoulder joints, strengthening the rotator cuff and the muscles moving the shoulder blades, balance, coordination, synchronization.

1. Kneel on a folded blanket to have a soft support for your knees and enough height so that the back is nearly horizontal; the knees are hip width apart, and the thighs are perpendicular; the lower legs are parallel; place your hands on the floor, with the wrists underneath the shoulder joints (Figure 6.97).

2. Adjust the neutral lumbopelvic position.

3. With an inhalation raise your right arm forwards with the palm facing the floor as far as you can maintain the neutral lumbopelvic position, keeping the costal arches in a natural position, and both shoulders at the same height; also hold your head in line with your spine (Figure 6.98).

4. Hold for 2–3 breaths; refine this movement by raising the arm slightly higher; exhaling, bring the right hand back to the floor.

5. Repeat points 2–4 with your left arm.

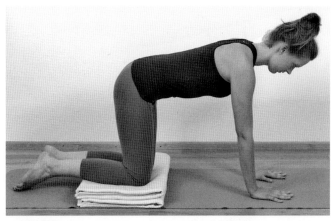

Figure 6.97

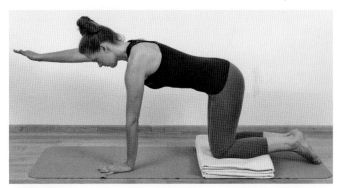

Figure 6.98

6. Repeat points 2–5 twice with the following variations:

   a. palm of the raised arm perpendicular, thumb towards the ceiling (Figure 6.99).

   b. palm of the raised arm facing the ceiling (Figure 6.100).

7. To finish bring your buttocks as close as possible towards your heels, bend forwards and rest your arms on the floor so that the shoulders are relaxed; stay calm for a few breaths.

Refined work

Perform points 1–6; in addition to raising the arm, raise the opposite leg horizontally (Figure 6.101). Try different speeds for combining and synchronizing the arm and leg movements. Finish as described in point 7.

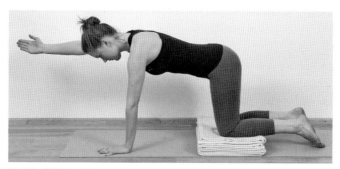

Figure 6.99

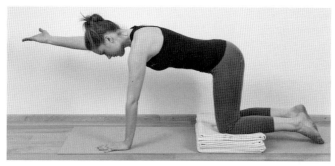

Figure 6.100

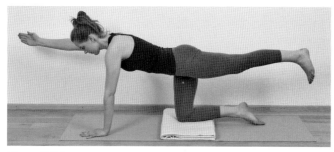

Figure 6.101

Exercise 4.11: All-embracing shoulder work

Aims: mobilizing the cervicothoracic area and relaxing the muscles around this area, combining different movements of the shoulder joints and the shoulder blades, coordination, synchronization.

1. Sit on the floor on a firm pillow, knees together and feet besides your hips; or sit on a chair, knees and feet hip width apart and parallel; adjust your pelvis to the neutral position.

2. Raise your right arm in front of you; externally rotate it, bend your elbow and raise it to rest the right hand over the cervicothoracic junction or between the shoulder blades.

3. With your left hand move the right elbow further up; the right hand will slide further down towards the thoracic spine.

4. Stretch your left arm, internally rotate it, bend the elbow; bring the back of the left hand along your back as high as possible.

5. Maintaining the neutral position of your pelvis, catch your hands and hold for 3–5 breaths (Figure 6.102).

6. If the hands cannot catch or the catching causes shoulder pain, hold a belt between your hands; it is useful to put this belt over your right shoulder before starting point 2 (Figure 6.103).

7. Then release the arms and stay there for 1–2 breaths, relaxing your shoulders.

8. Repeat points 2–7 starting with your left arm.

9. Perform points 1–8 once or twice.

Refined work

Perform points 1–8. Refine further and further:

- Lifting the upper arm slightly higher gives some side-bending action for the cervicothoracic junction and the upper thoracic spine; feel this with the hand that is touching this area.

- Moving the upper arm and the other shoulder slightly further backwards gives some back-bending for the cervicothoracic junction and upper thoracic spine; feel this with the hand that is touching this area.

- Maintaining the position perform subtle slow movements with your shoulder blades.

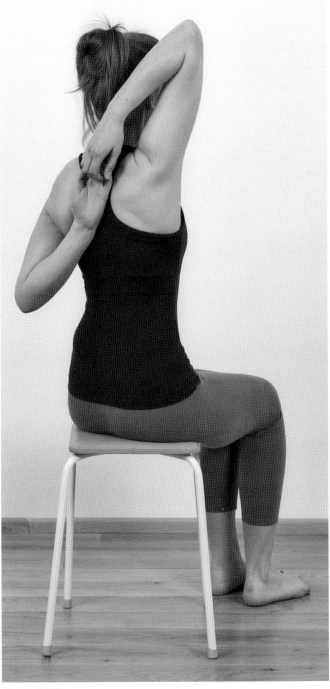

Figure 6.102

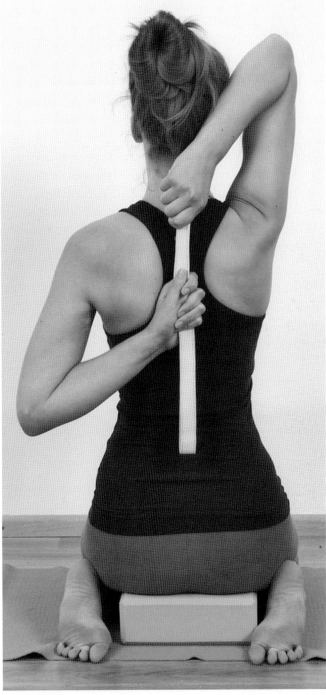

Figure 6.103

Exercise 4.12: Thoracic outlet

Aims: *gently mobilizing the cervicothoracic junction and the area to the upper sternum.*

1. Place the fingertips of one hand over the first thoracic vertebra, and the fingertips of the other hand left and right of the upper sternum, underneath your clavicle (Figure 6.104).

2. Feel the movement underneath your fingertips with inhalation and exhalation. With inhalation there is a subtle segmental back-bending in the upper thoracic spine; the upper ribs and the sternum are rising.

Hint

This exercise goes well with exercise 3.1, mini-back-bend, with the rolled towel ending at the first thoracic vertebra.

If you practice the shoulder stand you may find this exercise helpful preparation.

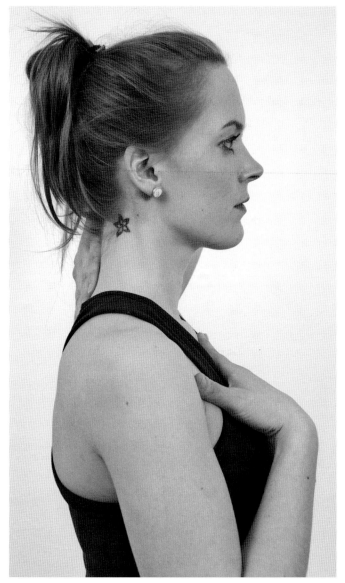

Figure 6.104

5. Basic exercises for the cervical spine, head, and temporomandibular joint

We have summarized these three areas together as there is a close connection between them. The head, neck, and jaw are called the stomatognathic system. All the muscles connecting these areas as well as the shoulder girdle are in constant, dynamic cooperation. "The efficiency of this balancing system contributes to effective function of the mouth, throat, cervical spine and head, as well as the thorax and upper limb" (Stone 1999, p. 227). The hyoid bone plays a central role in this system; it connects the shoulder girdle, mandible, and cranium.

Where there are problems with the temporomandibular joint a dental investigation should be carried out first. In addition gentle local mobilization often releases tension. In many cases the posture and movement patterns of other areas of the body are involved and have to be corrected. The mandible can move up and down, forwards and backwards, and to both sides. All these movements are combined in chewing. When you open your mouth the mandible moves forwards; it moves backwards when the mouth is closed.

These complex connections require particular mindfulness for the position and movements of the head. The head should be kept in the midline as far as possible, and the movements should be performed in a gentle, mindful way. Particularly vulnerable areas of the upper cervical spine are the ligaments and the vertebral artery. If there is any dizziness or there are neurological signs and symptoms, stop the exercise immediately. If the symptoms continue then medical investigation should be sought as quickly as possible. To protect this vulnerable area during exercising we recommend awareness during any exercise, precise positioning of the head, particularly in back-bending, rotations, and inversions, and strengthening the cervical muscles (Roth 2009). Refining the head movements, particularly rotation, so that the superficial throat muscles stay relaxed, strengthens the deep stabilizing muscles and protects the cervical spine.

Exercise 5.1: Atlas and axis

Aim: mobilizing the upper cervical spine.

1. Lie on your back with your abdomen and lumbar area relaxed, your shoulders relaxed and your head resting comfortably; use a pillow for your head if necessary (Figure 6.105).

2. Very gently roll your head to the right as you exhale; with the inhalation bring it back to the center, gently lengthening the neck (Figure 6.106).

3. Very gently roll your head to the left as you exhale; with the inhalation bring it back to the center, gently lengthening the neck.

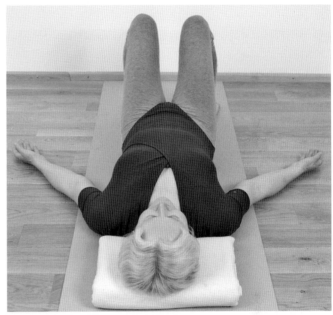

Figure 6.105

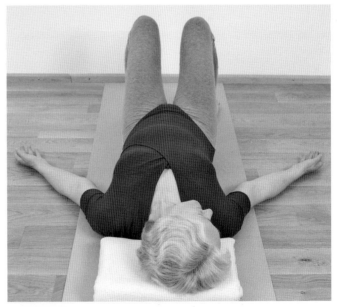

Figure 6.106

4. Perform points 2 and 3 3–5 times, then rest for a few breaths.

Refined work

1. Lie on your back with your abdomen and lumbar area relaxed, your shoulders relaxed and your head resting comfortably; use a pillow if necessary.

2. With an exhalation raise your head as far as comfortably possible (Figure 6.107).

3. Hold the position with the inhalation.

4. With the next exhalation gently turn your head to the right, then to the left, then to the center, keeping your vertex in the center (Figure 6.108).

5. With the next inhalation bring your head down, gently lengthen your cervical spine, and relax for 1–2 breaths.

6. Perform points 2–5 3–5 times.

7. Relax with your head in the center for a few breaths.

Exercise 5.2: Long neck

Aim: keeping the cervical spine long against gravity.

1. Sit straight on the floor or on a chair; put a book or a small bag filled with flour or rice or another suitable item on the crown of your head (Figure 6.109).

2. Feel the lifting and lengthening when you inhale, as if you are lifting the item on your head higher; maintain this lifting during exhalation.

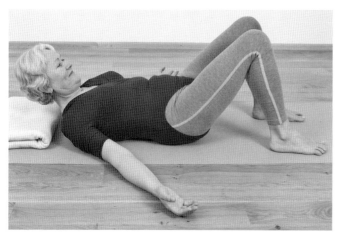

Figure 6.107

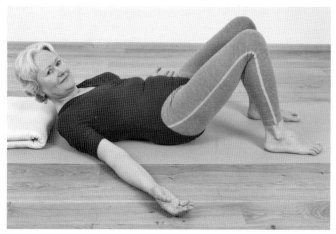

Figure 6.108

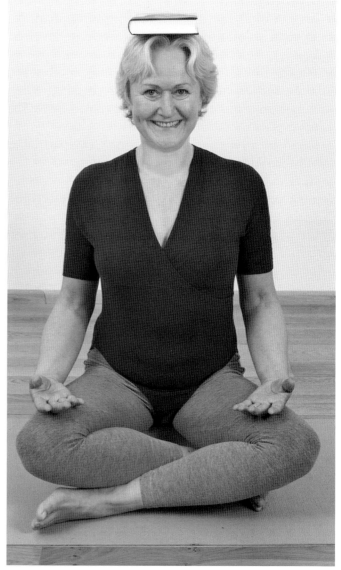

Figure 6.109

3. Maintaining the pelvis neutral and the shoulders relaxed, constantly finetune the position of your head so that the weight on the crown of your head remains stable.

4. Maintain this lifting for 3–5 breaths or longer if it feels right.

Exercise 5.3: Mobile head on the spine

Aims: mobilizing the atlanto-occipital joint, creating space between the first cervical vertebra and the base of the skull.

1. Sit in an upright position on the floor or on a chair.

2. Balance your head on the cervical spine.

3. Gently move your head forwards and backwards in a slow, rhythmic movement, 3–5 times. Keep the chin at the same height; look at a fixed point at eye level (Figures 6.110 and 6.111).

4. Keeping your shoulders relaxed, slightly bend your head forwards and perform a subtle side-bending movement with your head, as if pulling one ear slightly away from the side of the neck. Practice on both sides, 3–5 times (Figure 6.112).

5. Place one index finger in front of your hyoid bone, exactly between your chin and throat (Figure 6.113).

6. Gently bend your head forwards and backwards, using the index finger as a pivot; find the rhythm and the quality of movement so that it feels smooth.

7. Perform point 6 3–5 times.

8. Hold your head with both hands, with the thumbs supporting the mandible, the index and middle fingers on the lower ridge at the back of your head (Figure 6.114). Gently lean the lower ridge at the back of your head on the index and middle fingers as you inhale, maintaining the position of the chin. Feel the subtle lengthening of the upper neck; feel as if the base of the skull is supported by a small, soft pillow; release with exhalation.

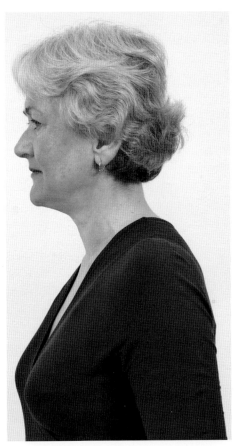

Figure 6.110

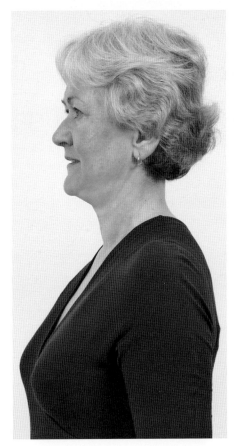

Figure 6.111

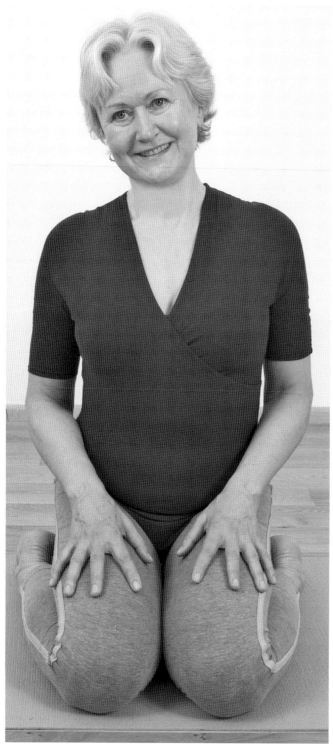

Figure 6.112

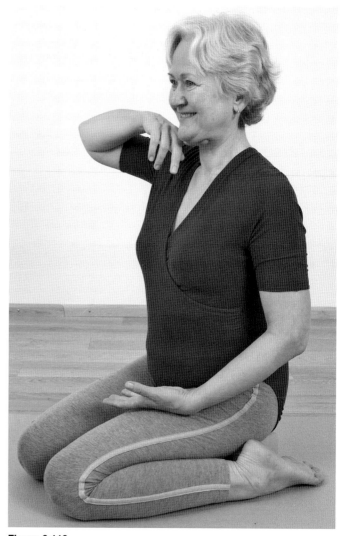

Figure 6.113

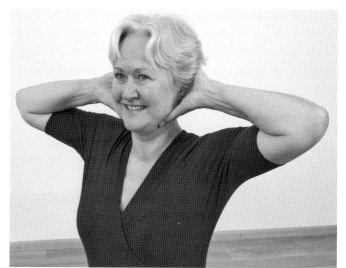

Figure 6.114

9. Repeat point 8 3–5 times.

10. Also observe the effect of this movement on your upper chest; the sternum and upper ribs are slightly raising.

11. Release your hands.

12. Sit quietly for a few breaths and feel like the base of the skull is supported by a small, soft pillow.

Exercise 5.4: Turn and bend

Aim: mobilizing the atlanto-occipital joint.

1. Stand or sit straight.

2. Feel the lengthening of the cervical spine when you inhale.

3. Lifting from the lower abdomen, raise your straight arms to the side, parallel to the floor.

4. While you exhale turn your head to the right, keeping the lengthening in your cervical spine.

5. Keep your shoulders down, and extend your arms and shoulder blades further. With another exhalation, gently tilt your head forwards and backwards as far as comfortable, keeping your cervical spine long and stable (Figures 6.115 and 6.116). With the inhalation, control this stability and keep your head upright.

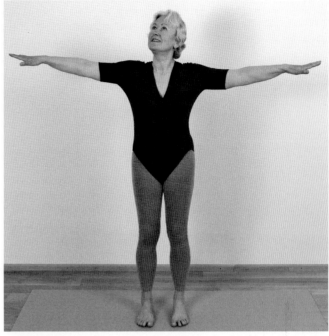

Figure 6.116

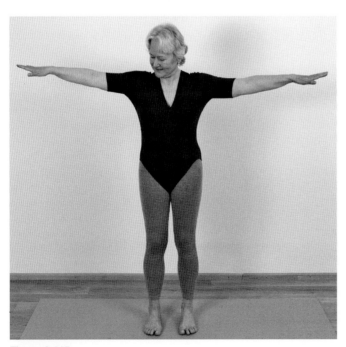

Figure 6.115

6. Perform point 5 3–5 times.

7. While you exhale turn your head to the left, keeping the lengthening in your cervical spine.

8. Repeat points 5 and 6 for this rotation of your head.

9. Bring your head back to the center, relax your arms, and stay calm for a few breaths.

Exercise 5.5: Gentle side-bending

Aim: mobilizing the cervical spine.

1. Sit on the floor or on a chair in an upright position (Figure 6.117).

2. Feel the space between your upper cervical spine and the base of your skull as if a small pillow is supporting your skull.

3. Keep your shoulders and arms relaxed. Very slightly bend your head forwards. With an exhalation gently bend your head to the right, your right ear towards the right shoulder, so that you feel a gentle stretch from your left ear to your left shoulder. Feel this stretch particularly during exhalation (Figure 6.118).

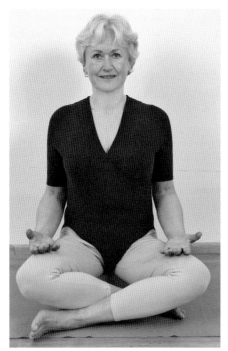

Figure 6.117

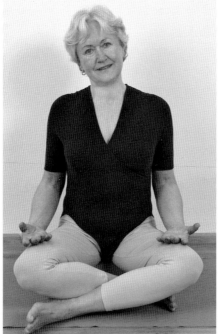

Figure 6.118

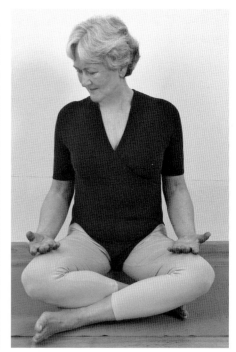

Figure 6.119

4. Hold point 3 for 2–3 breaths.

5. Bring your head back to the center and repeat point 3 and 4 to the left side.

6. Perform both sides 2–3 times.

7. Stay with your head in the center for 1–2 breaths.

8. Keeping your shoulders relaxed, again bend your head to the right as you exhale, with your right ear towards your right shoulder.

9. When you feel the soft, gentle stretch from your left ear to your left shoulder, turn your head towards your right armpit, feeling the soft, gentle stretch slightly more backwards now (Figure 6.119).

10. Hold for 2–3 breaths.

11. To bring your head back to the center keep it bent and move it to the center first, then raise it upright.

12. Repeat points 8–11 on the left side.

13. Perform both sides 2–3 times.

14. To finish stay calm with your head in the center for a few breaths.

Exercise 5.6: Strong neck

Aim: general strengthening of the cervical spine.

1. Sit on the floor or on a chair in an upright position.

2. Put one hand on your forehead to resist the forward bending of your head (Figure 6.120).

3. Apply no more than 10–30% of your full strength, so that you can continue normal breathing; hold the resisted position for 2–3 breaths; release your hand, and relax your arms for 2–3 breaths, lengthening your cervical spine.

4. Perform points 2 and 3 2–3 times; use the other hand for a repetition.

5. Put both hands with the fingers interlocked on the back of your head to resist the back-bending of your head (Figure 6.121).

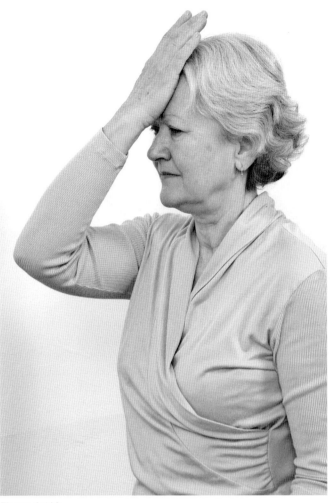

Figure 6.120

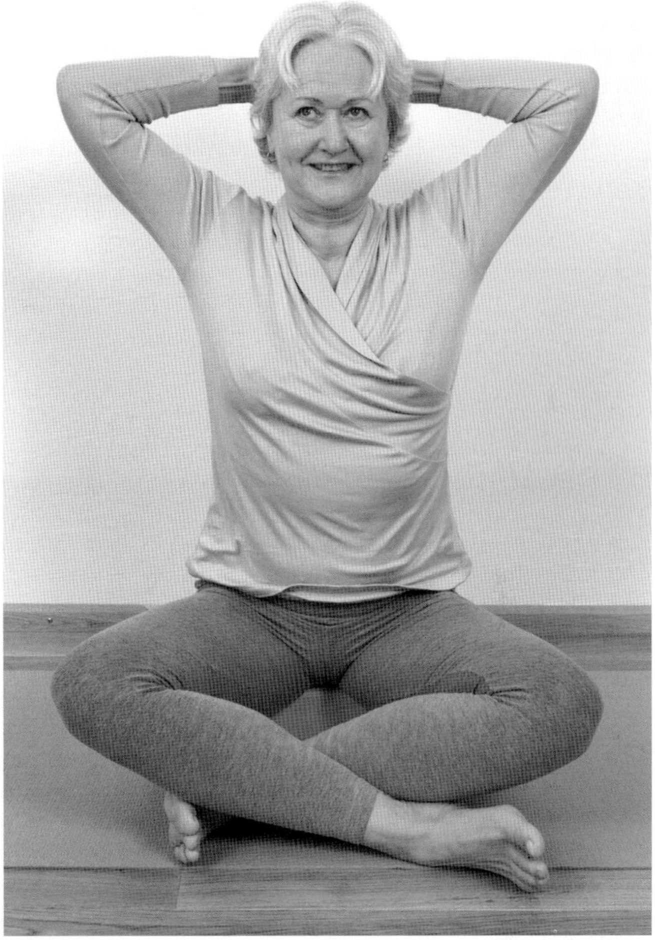

Figure 6.121

6. Apply no more than 10–30% of your full strength, so that you can continue normal breathing; hold the resisted position for 2–3 breaths; release your hands, and relax your arms for 2–3 breaths, lengthening your cervical spine.

7. Perform points 5 and 6 2–3 times.

8. Bring your left hand over your head, and hold it above your right ear (Figure 6.122).

9. Resist the side-bending of your head to the right with no more than 10–30% of your full strength, so that you can continue normal breathing; hold the resisted position for 2–3 breaths; release your hand, and relax your arms for 2–3 breaths, lengthening your cervical spine.

10. Perform points 8 and 9 2–3 times.

11. Repeat points 8–10 for the other side.

12. Put your right hand on your forehead and your left hand on the back of your head; in this way the rotation of your head to the right is resisted by the palms (Figure 6.123).

13. Hold for 2–3 breaths, then release your hands.

14. Perform points 12 and 13 2–3 times.

15. Change your hands and perform points 12–14 in the other direction.

16. To finish remain seated and be calm for a few breaths.

6 CHAPTER
The basic exercises
5. Basic exercises for the cervical spine, head, and temporomandibular joint

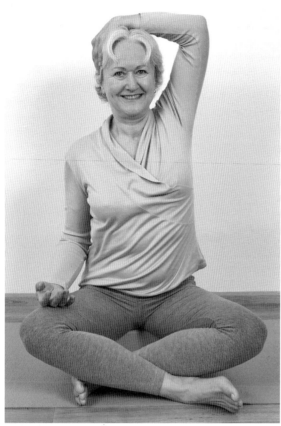

Figure 6.122

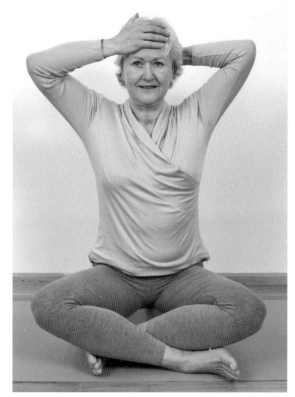

Figure 6.123

Exercise 5.7: Relaxed jaw

Aim: mobilizing the temporomandibular joint. Breathe naturally through your nose throughout this exercise.

1. Sit on the floor or on a chair in an upright position.
2. Relax your tongue on your mandible.
3. Slightly open your mouth.
4. Keeping your shoulders relaxed and your head upright, gently move your chin forwards and backwards 3–5 times.
5. Close your mouth.
6. Perform the following so that it feels smooth and round: chin slightly forwards, open your mouth, chin down; chin backwards; close your mouth, chin up; continue normal breathing.
7. Perform point 6 3–5 times.
8. To finish close your mouth, relax your tongue, stay calm for a few breaths and feel the relaxation in your jaw.

Variation

To increase awareness of the movement of the jaw, place your fingerpads flat in front of your ears, so that you feel the movements of the condylar processes of your lower jaw. Refine the exercise described in points 2–7 so that the movement becomes smooth and both processes move at the same time. For more extensive awareness you can put your index fingers gently into the outer auditory canal.

Refined work

1. Sit on the floor or on a chair in an upright position.
2. Relax your tongue on your mandible.
3. Keeping your mouth closed, slightly lift your upper teeth away from your lower teeth; as you exhale feel the space between your tongue and palate increasing and feel the relaxation of your jaw, tongue, and ears.
4. Hold for 3–5 breaths.
5. To finish stay calm for a few breaths.

Hint

This mindful finetuning can be integrated into many positions and exercises.

Exercise 5.8: Moving the tongue

Aims: general mobilization and relaxation of the jaw and tongue.

Variation a

1. Sit in an upright position.

2. Keeping your mouth closed or only slightly open perform circular and figure-of-eight movements with your tongue, about one movement per breath; perform the movements in both directions.

3. Continue for 5–10 breaths.

4. Relax your tongue in its natural position on the mandible, and continue normal breathing.

5. Touch your teeth with the tip of your tongue several times, moving your tongue along the upper and lower teeth, for 3–5 breaths.

Variation b

1. Sit in an upright position.

2. With an exhalation stretch your tongue as far out and down as possible; hold for 3 breaths; continue normal breathing through your nose.

3. Relax the tongue in its natural position on the mandible.

4. Perform 2–3 times.

Variation c

1. Sit in an upright position.

2. At the end of an exhalation stretch your rolled tongue between your lips (Figure 6.124).

3. Gently inhale through the rolled tongue; the flow is so gentle that your tongue does not become dry.

4. At the end of inhalation relax your tongue to its natural position on the mandible.

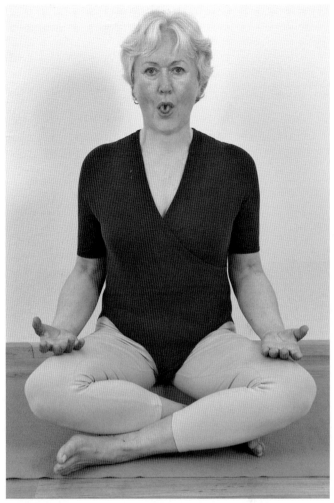

Figure 6.124

5. If you feel more comfortable take 1–2 normal breaths before you repeat the technique.

6. Perform points 2–5 5–6 times.

7. To finish stay calm for a few breaths and feel the relaxation in your jaw, tongue, ears, and upper neck.

Hint

If you cannot roll your tongue perform points 2–7 with your tongue flat between your lips.

Recommendation

Laughing is a very good exercise for the whole face. Combine it with performing the tongue exercises in front of a mirror or in a group.

Exercise 5.9: Sensitive nose

1. Sit in a comfortable position on a chair or on the floor.

2. If you need to, use a back rest.

3. Bring your elbows slightly forwards, your thumbs on your mandible, your ring fingertips gently in the deepening on the sides of the nose below the nasal bone (Figure 6.125).

4. Find the softest contact of your ring fingertips with the sides of your nose to make the nasal passages slightly narrower so that the flow of your breath becomes subtle.

5. Hold for 5–10 breaths.

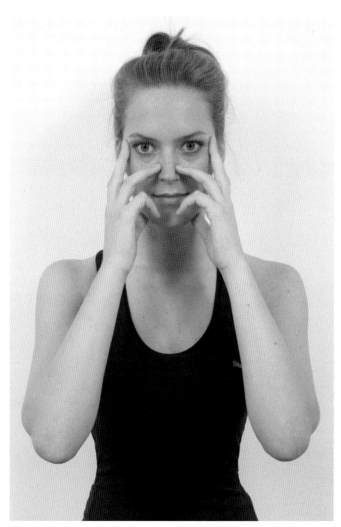

Figure 6.125

6. At the end of an inhalation remove the fingertips from the nose, and rest your hands on your thighs for a few breaths; feel the inhalation and exhalation inside your nose.

Exercise 5.10: Moving the eyes
(Figure 6.126)

1. Sit so that you can hold your head upright.

2. As you exhale turn your eyes as far as possible to the right; release as you inhale.

3. As you exhale again, turn your eyes as far as possible to the left; release as you inhale.

4. Perform points 2 and 3 3–5 times.

5. As you exhale look down; release your eyes as you inhale.

6. As you exhale look up; release as you inhale.

7. Perform points 5 and 6 3–5 times.

8. Move your eyes in all diagonal directions as described for the other movements.

9. Finish moving your eyes 3–5 times in figure of eight, in both directions.

10. Remain seated for a few breaths and relax your eyes.

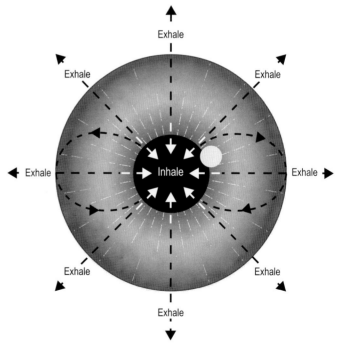

Figure 6.126 Eye movements.

Exercise 5.11: Palming

Aim: relaxation of the eyes.

1. Prepare a folded blanket for your elbows.
2. Sit on a chair in front of a table.
3. Adjust the folded blanket so that you can rest your elbows on it. The palms are at the level of the eyes.
4. Slightly bend forward from your hips, keeping the trunk straight.
5. Close your eyes, put your right hand on your right eye, your left hand on your left eye; the heels of your hands are on the cheekbones below the eyes, while the fingers are crossing on the forehead (Figure 6.127).
6. Look into the darkness.
7. Hold for 1–3 minutes; with practice you can hold this position for up to 10 minutes.

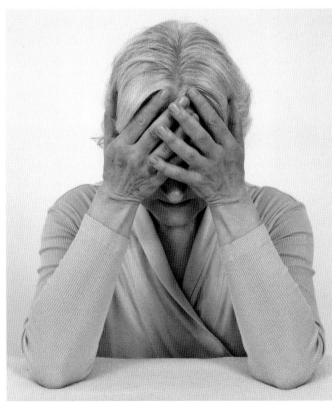

Figure 6.127

8. Keep your eyes closed when you come back to the upright sitting position and rest your lower arms and hands on the table.
9. Stay there for a few breaths.
10. Still feel the calmness in your eyes when you open them.

Exercise 5.12: Attentive ears

The exercises for the temporomandibular joint are relevant to the ears, but there is no actual ear exercise. Therefore we suggest a manual treatment technique that you can do yourself.

1. Sit comfortably straight.
2. Gently move your arms forwards from your shoulder joints till the elbows are at the level of the shoulders.
3. Put the index, middle, and ring fingers or the palms flat on the outer ear; apply as much gentle pressure as is comfortable.
4. Move your outer ear with the fingers or palms gently in a circular movement, 5–10 times clockwise, 5–10 times counterclockwise.
5. Rest your arms and hands for a few breaths.
6. Raise your arms to the sides, elbows to shoulder level.
7. Put your index fingers into the outer auditory canal; gently massage the wall of the canal with your index fingers for 3–5 circles each way.
8. Gently put your palms on your outer ear to close your ears; remove the hands quickly. Perform this only once
9. Relax your arms for a few breaths.
10. Gently move your arms forwards from your shoulder joints until the elbows are at shoulder level.
11. Cover your ears with your palms; listen to the inner sound for a few breaths.
12. Relax your arms, remain seated for a few breaths; you can feel as if fingers in your outer auditory canals are pulling you slightly upwards.

6. Basic exercises for elbows, wrists, and hands

The elbow and wrist are closely connected in terms of both joint mechanics and soft-tissue structures. The elbow joint is an ingenious construction which works as a hinge yet also gives rotational mobility. It consists of three joints. The articulations between the humerus and ulna and the humerus and radius make flexion and extension possible. The articulation between the radius and ulna makes supination and pronation possible; it is a rotation of the radius within the annular ligament. The shape of the bones meeting at the elbow joint gives the elbow stability. The valgus is a frequent deviation at the elbow joint. In general it is stronger in females than in males. To stabilize it we recommend relaxing slightly from full extension or using a belt around the elbows in weight-bearing exercises. Both help to strengthen the flexor and extensor muscles working on the elbow joint in a balanced way.

"The wrist is an extremely delicate structure that requires mobility and yet stability" (Hartman 2001, p. 219). The carpal bones with all their articulations allow a wide variety of hand movements and skills. How many useful and beautiful things have been made by human hands, how much can be expressed by the hands, and how important the hands are for communication and touching. Exercises for the hands have been developed into a refined art in Indian dancing.

The aim of the exercises in this chapter is to maintain or improve the functions of the hands, give them sufficient mobility, but also to learn to use the muscles of the arms, hands, and fingers in a balanced way. This is particularly important as muscles do not stabilize the wrist: none of the 10 tendons around the wrist is attached to any of the carpal bones. If a patient has fallen on the extended wrist and has ongoing pain the wrist should be investigated for a possible fracture of the carpal bones.

The elbow, shoulder girdle, and cervical spine should also be considered in problems with the hands or wrists; problems with the elbow can also be caused by the shoulder girdle or the cervical spine.

Exercise 6.1: Shake hands

Aims: mobilizing and relaxing the wrist and hand.

1. Sit in an upright position on the floor or on a chair.

2. Bend your right elbow so that your right hand is in front of your abdomen.

3. Hold the right wrist with your left hand underneath (Figure 6.128) and shake the hand for 3–5 breaths in a natural rhythm; the right hand is completely passive.

4. Hold the little finger side of the right hand with your left hand (Figure 6.129) and shake the right

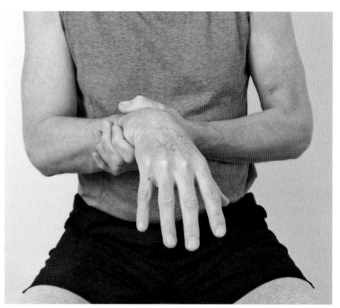

Figure 6.128

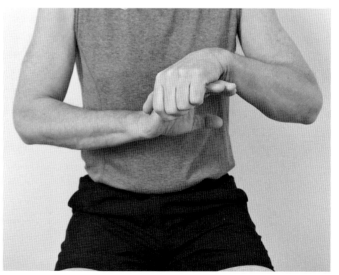

Figure 6.129

hand for 3–5 breaths in a natural rhythm; your right hand remains completely passive.

5. Repeat points 2–4 for the left hand.

Refined work

- Hold different parts of the wrist to reach different parts of the wrist joint.
- Hold different parts of the little finger side of the hand to reach different parts of the hand (Figures 6.129 and 6.130).

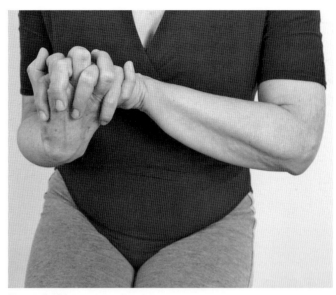

Figure 6.131

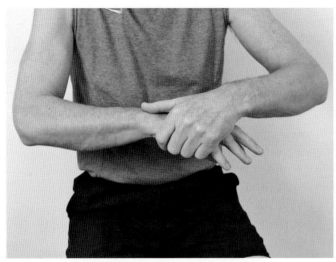

Figure 6.130

Exercise 6.2: Wrist circumduction

Aim: mobilizing the wrist joint.

1. Sit in an upright position on the floor or on a chair.

2. Rest your right upper arm and elbow on your right-side ribs, with the right hand in front and away from the abdomen.

3. Interlock your left and right fingers (Figure 6.131).

4. Keep your right elbow on your right-side ribs and, keeping the height of the right lower arm, make circular movements with your right hand for 3–5 breaths (Figure 6.132); make the movements round and smooth.

5. Repeat points 2–4 for the left wrist.

6. Finish sitting for a few breaths, resting the back of your hands on your thighs.

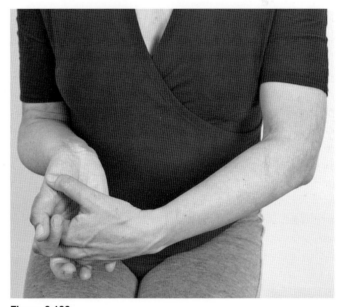

Figure 6.132

Exercise 6.3: Carpal tunnel stretch

Aim: stretching the carpal tunnel.

1. Sit in an upright position on the floor or on a chair.

2. Rest your right elbow on your right-side ribs, with the hand in front of your abdomen and the palm facing forwards.

3. Hold your right hand with the left hand, the thumb on the back of the hand, to stretch the

113

wrist to the limit (Figure 6.133); if there is discomfort, or tingling or numbness, ease off until this sensation goes away.

4. Hold for 3–5 breaths, then release gently.

5. For a more powerful extension of the wrist and stretch of the carpal tunnel put your left thumb on the back of your right wrist and repeat points 3 and 4 (Figure 6.134).

6. Relax your hands for 2–3 breaths.

7. Repeat points 2–6 for your left wrist.

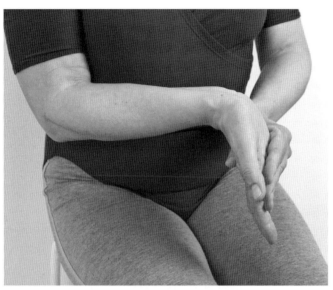

Figure 6.133

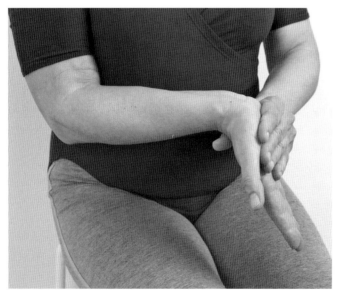

Figure 6.134

Exercise 6.4: Strong and flexible wrists

Aims: mobilizing and strengthening the wrists, stretching the carpal tunnel.

1. Sit on a chair in an upright position, resting your lower arms on a table (Figure 6.135); or sit on the floor in an upright position, knees bent, feet on the floor, resting your elbows on your knees (Figure 6.136).

2. Fold your hands; palms, left and right thumb, left and right fingers are straight and in contact with each other; lower your wrists as far as possible, ease off slightly from the limit of stretch.

3. Maintain the contact of the palms, fingers, and thumbs; hold the elbows and wrists at the same level, with the shoulders relaxed; use the right wrist as a pivot and with an exhalation move both hands together slightly to the right until you reach the limit of movement in the right wrist. Inhaling, release the hands to the center. Using the left wrist as a pivot, with an exhalation move both hands together slightly to the left until the movement barrier in the left wrist is reached. Inhaling, release the hands to the center.

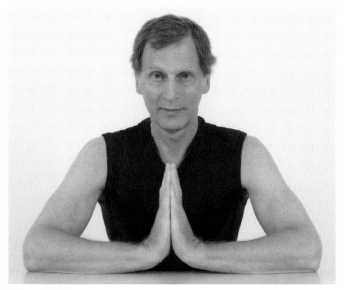

Figure 6.135

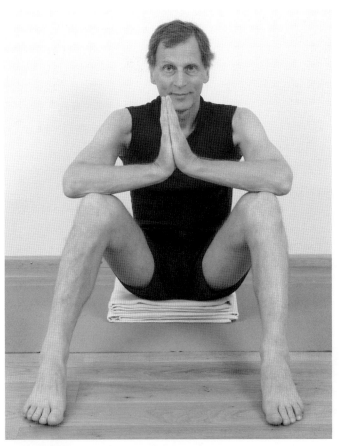

Figure 6.136

Exercise 6.5: Integrated wrist mobilization

Aim: *mobilizing the wrists into full flexion and extension.*

1. Sit in an upright position on the floor or on a chair.

2. Interlock your fingers; first hold your arms horizontally, with the palms facing you, the wrists fully flexed, and the tips of the thumbs touching (Figure 6.137).

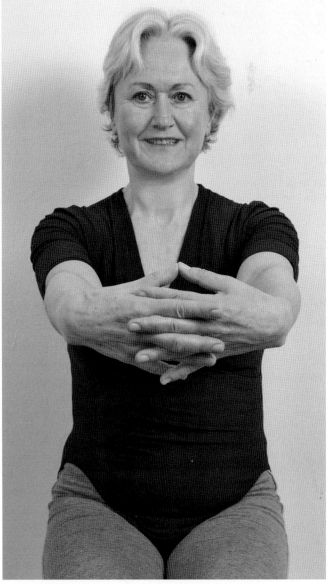

4. Perform point 3 3–5 times.

5. Maintaining the elbows and wrists at the same level, with shoulders relaxed, move both hands to the right until you reach the limit of movement, applying appropriate pressure with the left hand. Maintain this position; press your right hand against your left hand with one-third of your full strength; hold this for 3 breaths. When you release the pressure with your right hand you will probably be able to move both hands slightly more to the right to the new limit. Again, for 3 breaths press your right hand towards your left hand. After releasing feel the new limit. Depending on the result you may want to repeat once again.

6. Relax your hands for a few breaths.

7. Then repeat points 5 and 6 on the left side.

Figure 6.137

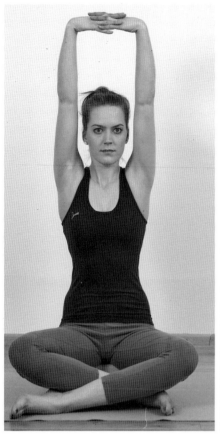

Figure 6.138

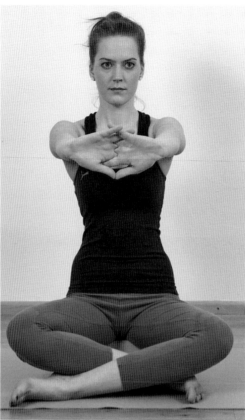

Figure 6.139

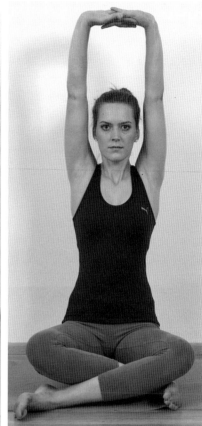

Figure 6.140

3. Keeping your pelvis neutral, elevate your arms (Figure 6.138).

4. After reaching the limit, slightly move your upper thoracic spine inwards to lift your sternum; this makes you raise your arms even further, to the maximum. Hold for 3–5 breaths.

5. Bring your arms back to the horizontal position; internally rotate the arms to turn your hands around so that the palms are facing away from you; stretch your thumbs away from your index fingers, with the tips of the thumbs touching, so that the palms and carpal tunnels are stretched (Figure 6.139).

6. Keeping your pelvis neutral, raise your arms again so that the palms are facing towards the ceiling; fully stretch the elbows. After reaching the limit, slightly move your upper

thoracic spine inwards to lift your sternum; this makes you raise your arms even further, to the maximum (Figure 6.140).

7. Hold for 3–5 breaths.

8. Release the hands, lower the arms to the sides and then down.

9. Stay calm for a few breaths, relaxing your arms and wrists.

10. Interlock the fingers the other way around and repeat points 2–9.

Hint

When you interlock your fingers, observe which way you interlock them. You probably automatically use the same side every time. Practice both ways, particularly the less usual one.

Exercise 6.6: All-round elbow movement

Aims: mobilizing the elbow joint, coordination.
There are three sequences of movements. The range is from the fully bent elbow to the fully stretched elbow. During movement within one range the position changes between supination and pronation several times. Also the hand holds can be varied: from the fist positions we have selected the flexed and extended wrist, from the positions with straight fingers we have selected a slightly extended wrist. Each example is shown in supination and pronation. You can practice both hand holds with a variety of angles for the wrists, depending on your restrictions. We have also shown different angles of the elbows; each is only one part of the whole movement.

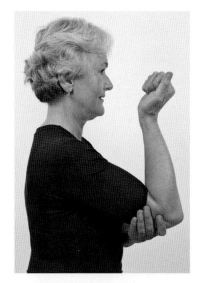

Figure 6.141

1. Sit in an upright position on the floor or on a chair.

2. Bend your right elbow and hold your arm close to the elbow with your left hand.

3. Make a loose fist, and slightly extend the wrist (this exercise can be practiced with different angles of wrist extension).

4. Alternate between supinating (turn the lower arm so that the thumb is pointing outwards; Figure 6.141) and pronating (turn the lower arm so that the thumb is pointing inwards: Figure 6.142), gradually increasing the angle of the elbow; repeat this supination and pronation several times until the elbow is fully stretched.

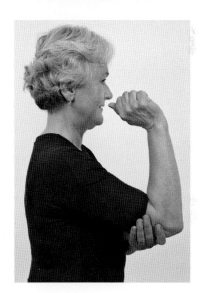

Figure 6.142

5. Reverse the movement, continuing supination and pronation until the elbow is fully bent again.

6. Repeat points 4 and 5 with your wrist flexed (Figures 6.143 and 6.144).

7. Stretch your fingers and thumbs and repeat points 4 and 5 (Figures 6.145 and 6.146). This can also be practiced with different degrees of flexion and extension of the wrist.

8. Repeat points 2–7 for your left wrist.

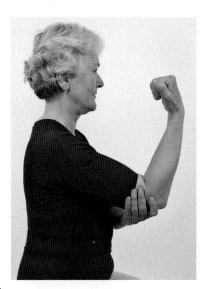

Figure 6.143

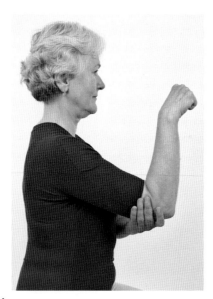

Figure 6.144

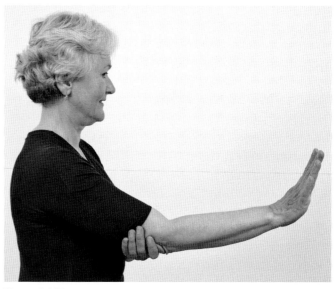

Figure 6.146

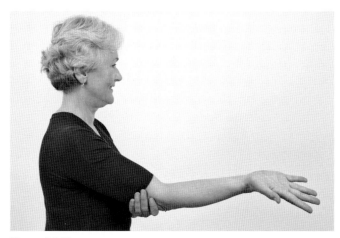

Figure 6.145

Variations

- Perform movements 2–8 with both hands at the same time.
- Try different speeds for the movements.

Exercise 6.7: Four-point kneeling variations

Aims: strengthening the hands, wrists, and elbows, coordination, mobilizing the interphalangeal joints.

1. Go into the four-point kneeling position (see exercise 1.14).
2. Hyperextend and slightly bend your elbows and find the best balance for your arms.
3. Hold this balance for 3–5 breaths.
4. Keeping your elbows unchanged and the palms on the floor, hyperextend your fingers and thumbs (Figure 6.147).
5. Hold for 1–2 breaths; feel the effect on the wrists and arms.

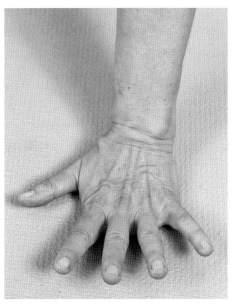
Figure 6.147

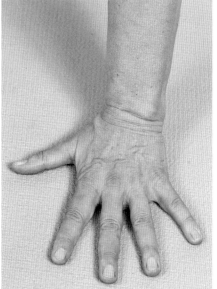
Figure 6.148

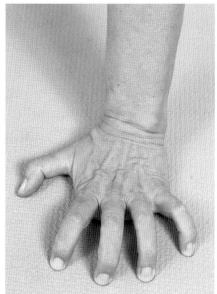
Figure 6.149

6. Then relax your fingers and thumbs on the floor for 1–2 breaths.

7. Repeat points 4–6 3–5 times.

8. Keeping the elbows unchanged and the palms on the floor, press the straight fingers and thumbs into the floor (Figure 6.148).

9. Hold for 1–2 breaths; feel the effect on the wrists and arms.

10. Then relax your fingers and thumbs on the floor for 1–2 breaths.

11. Repeat points 8–10 3–5 times.

12. Keeping the elbows unchanged and the palms on the floor, slightly bend all joints of your fingers, press the pads of the fingers into the floor, to get a slight isometric contraction of the palms, fingers, and thumbs (Figure 6.149); hold for 3–5 breaths; repeat once or twice.

Hint

If your elbows are weak, put a belt around them and push your elbows against the belt.

Refined work

Practice the movements for the fingers and thumbs for each finger individually or for two adjacent fingers at the same time; try different speeds, also try very fast.

7. Basic exercises for the pelvis

The pelvis consists of two innominate bones, each containing three fused bones: the ilium, ischium, and pubis. Together with a complex system of soft tissues the pelvis protects the pelvic and abdominal organs; in women the pelvis also helps to carry a baby and give birth. The pelvis has to absorb complex, asymmetric forces from below and weight-bearing from above. The joints of the pelvis are the symphysis pubis and the sacroiliac or iliosacral joints, depending on which bone we consider to be stable and which is moving.

Probably no other area of the body has been debated as much as the sacrum and its joints with the ilia. There are countless varieties of shapes of the sacrum and joint planes and movement (Kapandji 2008). Mobility reduces with age, probably due to increased calcification of the ligaments. There is generally less mobility in men than in women. In women hormonal changes also influence ligamentous stability. Both the innominate bones and the sacrum can be moved passively and actively. For active movements there are muscles attached at the innominates and the sacrum. The sacrum can also function in a wide range of directions. The anteroposterior angle of the sacrum is connected to the spinal curves. Vertebral columns with more pronounced curves are frequently more mobile than less curved columns on a sacrum which is nearly vertical, but both can function well.

We have given some mobilizing exercises for the pelvic joints and a stabilizing exercise for the hips, which also stabilizes the iliosacral joints. Due to the delicate structural and functional nature of this area it is recommended that exercises are performed carefully. For stabilizing, adjust the pelvis into a neutral position balanced between tilting forwards and backwards, and particularly avoid side-shifting and torsion of the pelvis during the more complex exercises. This also protects the iliosacral joints, if they are hypermobile. Exercises 7.2, 7.3, and 7.6 were inspired by the book *Back Care Basics* (Pullig Schatz 1992).

We have not given any specific pelvic floor exercises, as the pelvic floor is included in virtually all classical yoga āsanas and in many basic exercises. As with the abdominal muscles and all other muscle groups, it is essential to strengthen, stretch, and relax the muscles of the pelvic floor. This is achieved through a well-balanced yoga practice.

Exercise 7.1: Mobilization of the iliosacral joints

Aims: mobilizing the iliosacral joints, moving the ilium posteriorly.

1. Lie on your back; use a suitable pillow underneath your head, if you need it.

2. Keeping your left leg straight, bend your right knee towards the right side of the chest so that the hip comes off the floor (Figure 6.150); hold the back of your thigh with both hands.

3. Hold for 2–3 breaths, then release slightly, keeping the position of your hands, and stay there for 1–2 breaths.

4. Rest your right arm on the floor; keeping your left shoulder relaxed, with your left hand hold around the back of your right thigh close to the knee or around the top of your shin; bring your right knee closer to the chest, slightly adducting towards the left side of your chest; the right hip comes further away from the floor (Figure 6.151).

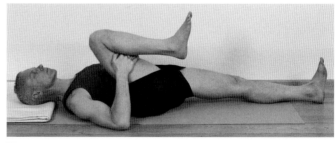

Figure 6.150

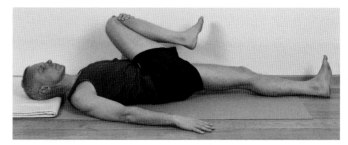

Figure 6.151

5. Hold for 2–3 breaths, then release slightly, keeping the position of your right hand, and stay there for 1–2 breaths.

6. Bring your right knee closer to your chest, adducting more towards your left shoulder; the right hip comes further away from the floor.

7. Hold for 2–3 breaths, then release your hands and come back into a symmetric position, either with your legs bent or straight, whichever feels more comfortable; feel whether there is any difference in how the left and right hip are on the floor.

8. Repeat points 2–7 for the left leg.

Refined work for points 2 to 6

To increase the effect on your pelvis, move the shin-bone area slightly towards your head.

Exercise 7.2: General mobilization of the iliosacral joints

Aim: general mobilization of the iliosacral joints.

1. Lie on your back; use a suitable pillow underneath your head, if you need it.

2. Bend both legs, keeping the soles of the feet on the floor, about one foot length away from the buttocks, so that it feels right for the knees.

3. Put your left foot onto the central line, and cross your right leg over your left thigh (Figure 6.152).

4. Keeping your head and shoulders still on the floor, move your legs to the left and to the right, so that there is movement over the iliosacral

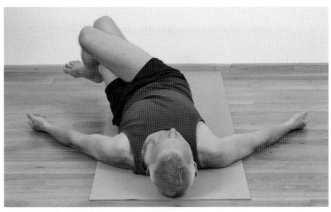

Figure 6.153

joints; do 1–2 movements during one inhalation and exhalation, for 3–5 breaths (Figure 6.153).

5. Release your legs to the position described in point 2.

6. Put your right foot onto the central line, and cross your left leg over the right one; repeat points 4 and 5.

7. To finish stay calm for a few breaths with the legs straight or bent.

Exercise 7.3: More complex mobilization of the iliosacral joints

Aim: general mobilization of the iliosacral joints.

1. Lie on your back, with your knees bent and feet on the floor.

2. Bring the soles of your feet together and let your knees fall apart (Figure 6.154).

3. Move the heels as close as possible towards the pelvis, as appropriate for your hips and knees; keep your shoulders and head relaxed.

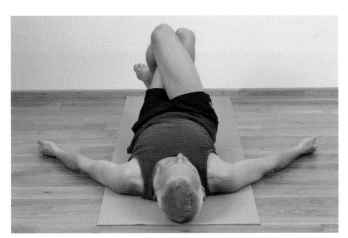

Figure 6.152

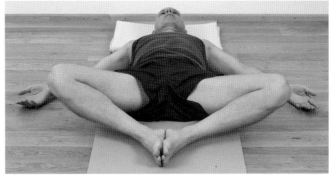

Figure 6.154

4. Circle your whole pelvis horizontally as if you are moving on a circle around your sacrum.

5. Perform 2–3 circles clockwise, and 2–3 counterclockwise.

6. Perform points 4 and 5 3–5 times.

7. To finish bring your knees together, with your feet hip width apart, and remain calm for a few breaths.

Hint

After practicing this exercise for a few months you may be able to correct wrong position and movement patterns.

Exercise 7.4: Lying on your sacrum

Aims: mobilizing the iliosacral joints, anterior movement of the ilia, balance.

1. Prepare a firmly rolled towel which is the diameter of your wrist; alternatively, for a stronger effect, use a brick.

2. Lie on your back with your knees bent and the soles of the feet on the floor.

3. Lift your pelvis and put the rolled towel or brick underneath your sacrum exactly in line with the spine.

4. Lower your sacrum onto the roll or brick so that your abdomen and lumbar area are soft.

5. Keeping your left leg bent, and your sacrum still on the towel or brick, slide your right heel away to straighten your right leg so long as you are comfortable in the back of your pelvis and lumbar area (Figure 6.155). If this is not possible with the roll or brick, reduce the height.

6. Hold for 3–5 breaths.

7. Bend your right knee to the starting position so that the soles of both feet are on the floor; relax your abdomen.

8. Repeat points 5–7 for the left leg.

9. Perform points 5–8 2–3 times.

10. To finish lift your pelvis, remove the towel or brick, and gently lower your back; stay calm for a few breaths.

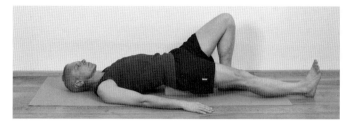

Figure 6.155

Exercise 7.5: Psoas stretch

Aims: stabilizing the pelvis, stretching the psoas and the groins.

1. Prepare a firmly rolled towel which is the diameter of your wrist; alternatively, for a stronger effect, use a brick.

2. Lie on your back with your knees bent and the soles of the feet on the floor.

3. Lift your pelvis and put the rolled towel or brick underneath your sacrum exactly in line with your spine.

4. Lower your sacrum onto the towel or brick so that your abdomen and lumbar area are soft.

5. Bend your right knee towards your chest; holding the top of the shin with both hands and keeping your sacrum still on the towel, straighten your left leg (Figure 6.156). Bring your right knee closer towards your chest. As soon as your left knee starts bending, push your left heel further away so long as you are comfortable in the back of your pelvis and lumbar area; adjust the distance of your right knee from your chest so that you can straighten your left leg.

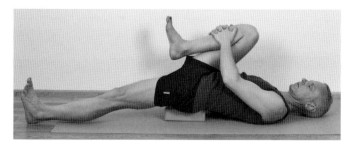

Figure 6.156

6. Hold for 3–5 breaths.

7. Put your right foot on the floor, with the right knee bent.

8. Bend your left knee towards your chest; holding the top of the shin with both hands, keep your sacrum still on the roll or brick, and straighten your right leg. Bring your left knee closer towards your chest. As soon as your right knee starts bending, push your right heel further away so long as you are comfortable in the back of your pelvis and lumbar area; adjust the distance of your left knee from your chest so that you can straighten your right leg.

9. Hold for 3–5 breaths, then release the position.

10. Lie with your sacrum on the rolled towel, your knees bent, and the soles of your feet on the floor.

11. Keeping your sacrum still on the towel or brick, slide both heels away to straighten both legs; slightly tilt your pelvis backwards. If there is any discomfort in the back of the pelvis or the lumbar area, bend your knees, and rest the soles of your feet on the floor.

12. Hold for 3–5 breaths.

13. Bring your feet back to the starting position with the soles on the floor; slightly lift the pelvis, remove the towel or brick, and lower the back of your pelvis on the floor; if you can keep your abdomen and lumbar area soft, straighten and relax your legs; stay calm for a few breaths.

Exercise 7.6: Correcting pelvic torsion

Aim: derotating the pelvis.

To test which side of the pelvis is more posterior or backwards, to which side it is rotated:

1. Lie on your back.

2. Bend both knees, keeping the soles of your feet on the floor, and knees and feet together.

3. Rock both knees in a slow rhythm to the left and to the right.

4. If you feel more weight in your right hip when rocking to the right than in your left hip when rocking to the left, your right side

is more posterior; otherwise your left side is more posterior.

We are describing here the exercise for a posterior right side; if your left side is more posterior, swop left and right in the description:

1. Lie comfortably on the floor, using a pillow for your head if you need it.

2. Bend your right leg, with the knee towards your chest; hold the back of the thigh or the top of the shin with both hands; if there is any irritation in the knee hold the back of your thigh.

3. Keeping the shoulders relaxed on the floor, pull your right leg closer towards your chest.

4. Raise your left leg, externally rotate and abduct it about the width of your foot to the left and slowly lower it to the floor; the weight of the left leg turns your pelvis to the left – opposite to the diagnosed rotation of your pelvis (Figure 6.157).

5. Bring your left leg back to the starting position in line with the left side of your body.

6. Pull your right leg even closer towards your chest and repeat points 4 and 5.

7. Repeat the test described above.

8. If there is improvement repeat points 2–7 once or twice, depending on the result.

9. After finishing the test, relax in a symmetrical position for a few breaths.

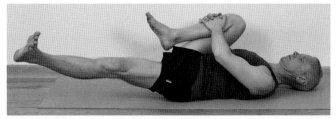

Figure 6.157

Hints

If you cannot feel any improvement continue working with exercises 7.2 and 7.3 instead.

If you are not using this exercise to correct pelvic torsion you can use it bilaterally to mobilize and strengthen your hips.

Exercise 7.7: Mobilizing the symphysis pubis

Aims: balanced activity of the adductor muscles, mobilizing the symphysis pubis.

1. Lie on your back; use a pillow for your head if you need it to relax your neck.

2. Bend your knees, keeping the soles of the feet on the floor; the feet are about one foot length away from the buttocks.

3. Put a brick or rolled blanket between your knees; adjust your feet to the distance of your knees (Figure 6.158).

4. Press the brick or blanket with one-third of your full strength, and feel your inner thighs; hold for 2–3 breaths, then release while you exhale, still holding the brick or blanket.

5. Perform point 4 3 times.

6. Remove the brick or blanket, bring your knees together, and stay calm for a few breaths, relaxing your abdomen and thighs.

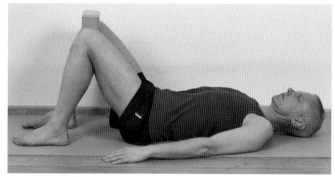

Figure 6.158

Seated variation

1. Sit on the floor with your knees bent; use a back support if you need it.

2. Keep your feet and knees in line and apart so that you can put your right elbow and hand between your knees.

3. If you are not using a back support, put your left hand on the floor to stabilize your trunk.

4. Lifting yourself up from your pelvic floor, push your knees towards the elbow and hand with one-third of your full strength (Figure 6.159).

5. Hold for 3 breaths; release as you exhale.

6. Rest both hands behind your buttocks for 1–2 breaths.

7. Put your left elbow and hand between your knees and repeat points 3–6.

8. Repeat points 2–7 once or twice.

9. To finish, sit upright with your legs crossed or straight and slightly apart for a few breaths.

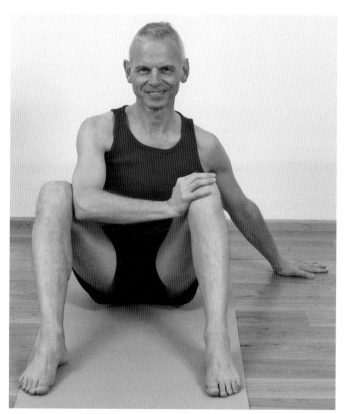

Figure 6.159

Exercise 7.8: Stabilizing the hips
(Figure 6.160)

Aims: balanced strengthening of the external rotators, stabilizing the hips and iliosacral joints.

1. Stand with your feet slightly apart and your knees slightly bent, maintaining a neutral lumbopelvic position.

2. Feel the bones on your outer thighs (trochanter major) with your hands.

3. Keeping your big toes on the floor, turn your knees slightly outwards until you start feeling these bones rotating backwards, then bring the knees to the starting position.

4. Perform point 3 up to 10 times, each movement for the length of one exhalation; on the last attempt hold for 3–5 breaths.

5. To finish release your hands, straighten your knees, and stand upright for a few breaths.

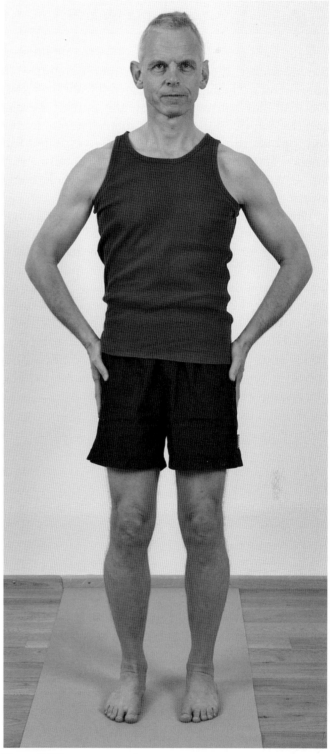

Figure 6.160

8. Basic exercises for the hips

The hip joint is formed by the head of the femur and the hip socket; the fused bones ilium, ischium, and pubis meet in the hip socket. Viewed from the front the joint lies halfway between the pubic tubercle and the anterior superior iliac spine. The hip joints and the axis through the hip joints are essential for balance and movements of the whole body. "The hip joint is a fulcrum upon which the whole body pivots" (Kingston 2001, p. 160).

The balance between mobility and stability through good cooperation of all the hip-moving muscles is crucial for the hip. It is particularly important to strengthen the abductor muscles and lengthen the iliopsoas and hamstrings. In standing posture the head of the femur does not fit ideally into the hip socket. This is best in 90° flexion with some abduction and external rotation. To balance the hip muscles and strengthen the abductor muscles the following points are particularly relevant:

- standing symmetrically

- making the hips narrow, as if squeezing them together

- lengthening around the hip joints before bending

- maintaining the position of the pelvis and keeping the line of the iliac crests horizontal while standing on one foot

- keeping the thigh perpendicular to the floor and the pelvis horizontal in the one-leg variations of four-point kneeling.

For precision of movement the following can be practiced:

- Hip flexion lying supine: Lie on your back; bend one leg, holding the shin bone with both hands. If the ilium stays unchanged, the movement is in the hip joint. If the ilium moves so that the sitting bone is moving away from the floor, the iliosacral joint is involved. If the knee is moved even closer so that the lumbar area becomes flatter, the lumbar spine is also involved.

- Hip extension standing: Stand on one foot, and raise the other leg backwards. Control the anterior superior iliac spine on the side of the raised leg with one hand, and the sacrum with the other hand. Move the leg backwards, so long as the iliac spine does not change – the movement is in the hip joint. If the iliac spine is moving forwards and downwards but the sacrum does not move, the movement is in the iliosacral joint. If the sacrum is tilting forwards, the movement is between the sacrum and the fifth lumbar vertebra, probably also further up into the lumbar spine, particularly in a hypermobile segment.

With all its multiple tasks the hip joint is vulnerable for degeneration with associated loss of mobility. Hypomobile hip joints often affect the lumbar spine, the knees, and the feet. In mild cases mobilization, particularly the rhythmic type, gives relief. "Restoration of even a small part of lost mobility can be very successful in relieving many of the symptoms of hip disorders, even if the progress of the degenerative state has not been changed at all" (Hartman 2001, p. 227). For more serious degenerative changes hip replacement surgery is now very successful, and has greatly improved patients' quality of life. Throughout our practical experience we have observed that patients who were already in the habit of exercising before the operation recovered quickly. They reported that their surgeons and rehabilitation therapists were very pleased.

Exercise 8.1: Rhythmic external and internal rotation

Aims: mobilizing the hip joints into external and internal rotation.

1. Sit on the floor with straight legs, the feet at least two foot lengths apart; either use a back support or support yourself with your hands behind your buttocks. Keeping your thighs relaxed, move your legs rhythmically, oscillating into external and internal rotation for 1–2 minutes (Figures 6.161 and 6.162).

2. To finish sit quietly for a few breaths.

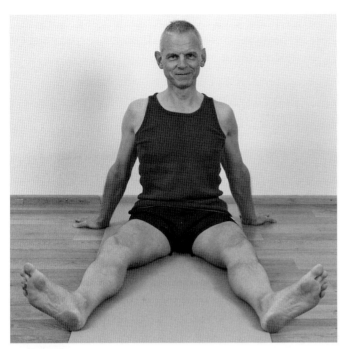

Figure 6.161

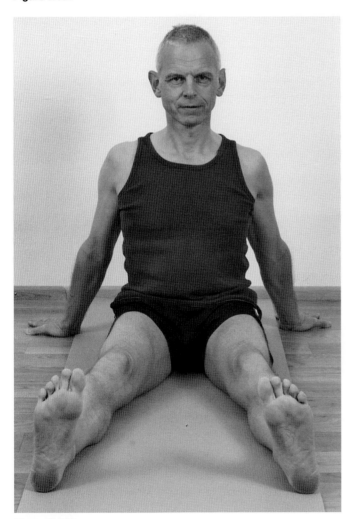

Figure 6.162

Variations for external and internal rotation in different planes

Sitting variation

1. Sit on a folded blanket.
2. Bend your knees so that the soles of your feet come together.
3. Hold your feet or ankles with your hands, with your elbows straight (Figure 6.163); if you need help in sitting upright, use a short belt loop around your feet, holding the belt with your hands (see Chapter 7, Baddha Koṇāsana).
4. Rhythmically oscillate your legs like the wings of a butterfly for 1–2 minutes.
5. Stay calm in the position for a few breaths.
6. Move your feet slightly away from the pelvis; bring your knees together, and straighten the legs, so that the kneecaps and the toes are pointing towards the ceiling.

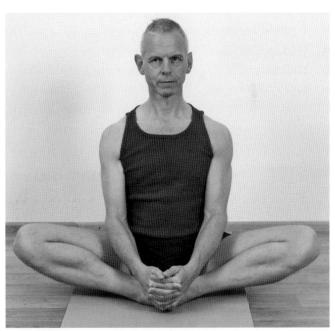

Figure 6.163

Supine variation

1. Lie on your back with straight legs, with your head comfortably supported.
2. The legs are to be apart, and the feet at least two foot lengths apart.

3. If you cannot lie comfortably with straight legs, use a suitable support underneath your knees.

4. Keeping your thighs relaxed, move your legs rhythmically, oscillating into internal and external rotation for 1–2 minutes. To make it easier to achieve the movement, initiate by pressing your hands rhythmically on your outer thighs.

5. To finish remain calm for a few breaths.

Exercise 8.2: Circumduction of hips

Aims: mobilizing the hip joints, coordination.

1. Lie on your back, comfortably supporting your head.

2. Bend your hips and knees; bring your knees towards your chest and spread them apart, keeping the back of your pelvis on the floor.

3. Hold your right knee with your right hand, and your left knee with your left hand (Figure 6.164).

4. Circumduct both hips contrarotating rhythmically, guiding the movement of the knees with your hands; let the movements be round and smooth:

   a. starting the circumduction left and right at the same time, for 5–10 breaths, change the direction in between.

   b. after half a circle of one side start the circumduction of the other side; continue for 5–10 breaths, changing the direction in between.

5. Hold your right knee with your left hand, your left knee with your right hand, so that the right arm is on top (Figure 6.165).

6. Repeat point 4b with this hand hold.

7. Change over the crossing of the arms and repeat point 4b.

8. To finish stay calm for a few breaths in any symmetrical position that you like.

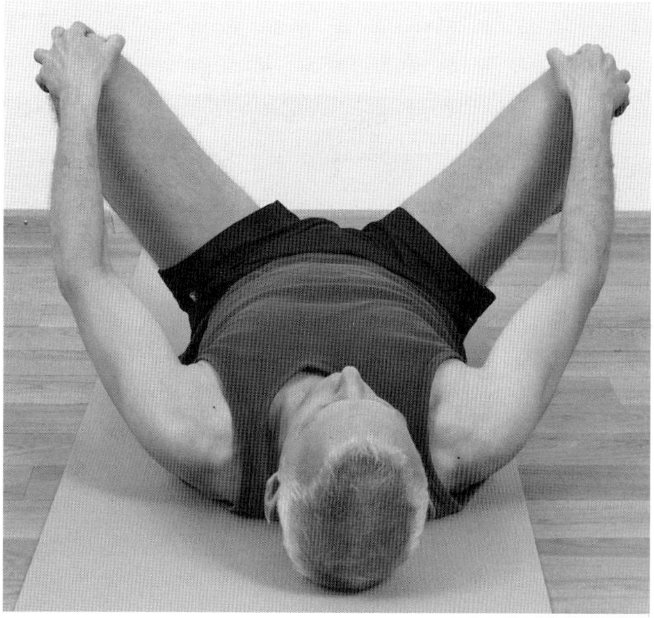

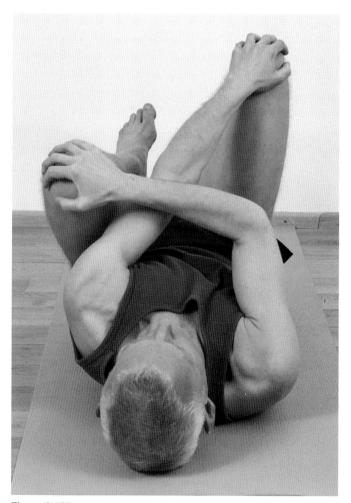

Figure 6.164

Figure 6.165

Exercise 8.3: Strong external and internal rotation

Aims: strengthening the external and internal rotators, balance, coordination.

1. Prepare a sufficiently soft support so that you can lie comfortably on one side.

2. Lie on your right side, with your head resting on your right hand. Put your left hand in front of your chest on the floor to stabilize your position.

3. Keeping your side-lying position, hold your left leg parallel to the floor, and bend it 90° at the hip joint, and 90° at the knee.

4. Continuing normal breathing, internally (Figure 6.166) and externally (Figure 6.167) rotate your left leg from your hip joint, about one movement per breath; the femur, the thighbone, is the axis of rotation; the knee stays at the same height; in external rotation your left big toe may touch the floor.

5. Perform point 4 3–5 times; with increasing practice you may wish to increase the number of repetitions.

6. Come back to a comfortable sidelying position for a few breaths.

7. Turn on your left side and repeat points 2–6 for the right leg.

8. To finish, lie comfortably on your back for a few breaths and relax your hips.

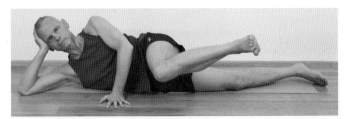

Figure 6.166

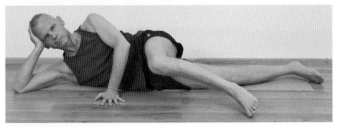

Figure 6.167

Variation: the sleeping tree

1. Lie on your right side, with your head resting on your outstretched right arm. Put your left hand in front of your chest on the floor to stabilize your position.

2. Keeping your side-lying position, bend your left knee, externally rotate from the hip to move the knee towards the ceiling, and rest the left foot on the inner side of your right thigh or lower leg.

3. Hold for 3–5 breaths, constantly finetuning the correct side-lying; keep a straight line from the right arm to the right heel.

4. To challenge the balance more, extend your left arm over your head, with the left palm facing the right one, and arms parallel (Figure 6.168).

5. If you need a support for balance, lie close to a wall to rest your back against the wall.

6. Repeat points 1–5 lying on your left side.

7. To finish lie on your back with bent knees; keep the soles of the feet on the floor, about one foot length away from the buttocks, hip width apart, knees together, or lie with straight legs, if comfortable; stay calm for a few breaths.

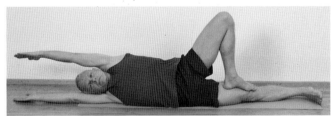

Figure 6.168

Exercise 8.4: Hip swing

Aims: stabilizing and mobilizing the hips, balance.

1. Stand with your left foot on a brick or book.

2. Maintain the stability of your left hip joint, keeping both hips at the same level.

3. Keeping your trunk upright and your arms loosely hanging, swing your right leg rhythmically for up to 5–10 breaths (Figures 6.169 and 6.170).

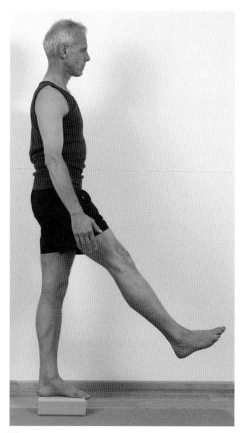

Figure 6.169

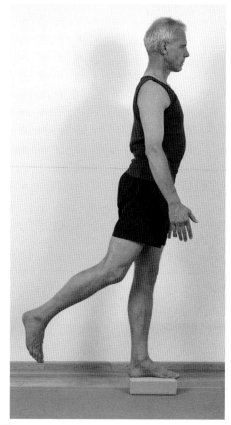

Figure 6.170

4. If you need a support for stability, stand sideways close to a wall or table so that you can hold on with your left hand; start practicing a few pendulum movements independently, then gradually increase.

5. Stand with your right foot on the brick or book; repeat points 2–4 for the left leg.

6. To finish stand with both feet on the floor for a few breaths; lift yourself from your pelvic floor and lower abdomen.

Exercise 8.5: Half-lotus variations

Aims: mobilizing the hip joints, coordination.

Variation a

1. Sit on the floor; with the help of your hands, bend your right hip and knee, as far as you feel comfortable; the sole of the foot is resting on the floor, close to the left leg.

2. Rest your hands on the floor to stabilize your trunk.

3. As you exhale release your bent leg to the right side (Figure 6.171).

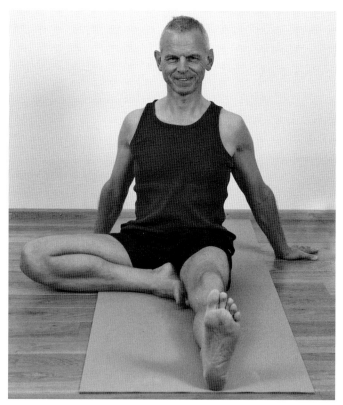

Figure 6.171

4. Exhaling, release it further towards the floor, 3–5 times.

5. To enhance the release, put your right hand on your thigh.

6. When you reach the limit bring the right knee a tiny bit higher, but resist this with your right hand; maintaining your upright centered sitting position, hold for 3 breaths; then release the leg again as you exhale.

7. Depending on the result you may wish to perform points 5 and 6 2–3 times.

8. Bring the right foot onto the floor; with the knee facing the ceiling, straighten the right leg.

9. Sit quietly for 1–2 breaths, supporting the position with the hands on the floor.

10. Repeat points 1–8 for the left leg.

11. To finish sit with straight legs for a few breaths, keeping your legs slightly internally rotated.

Variation b

From the starting position of variation a (Figure 6.171) slightly press the bent leg on the floor or on a firm pillow or rolled blanket if the leg is not on the floor. Hold for 3 breaths; after releasing, feel the relaxation of the bent leg.

Variation c

Bend your right hip and knee, with the foot resting on your left thigh (Figure 6.172); if this is uncomfortable, bring your right foot slightly over the left thigh and rest it on a support left of the thigh (Figure 6.173); the support is the same height as the thigh, and the right foot is relaxed.

Modify variation a, points 2–11, for this position.

Variation d

1. Sit on the floor, with both hands resting on the floor slightly behind the pelvis.

2. Perform the following steps as a slow, continuous movement.

3. Bend your right knee, then release it to the side as close as possible towards the floor; the foot is resting on the floor close to the left leg (Figure 6.174).

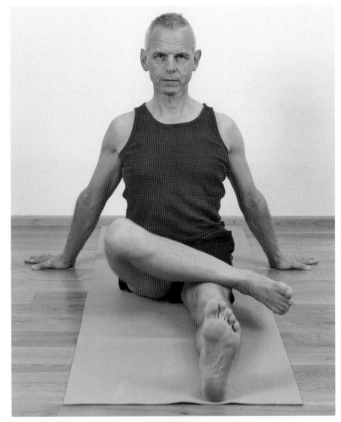

Figure 6.172

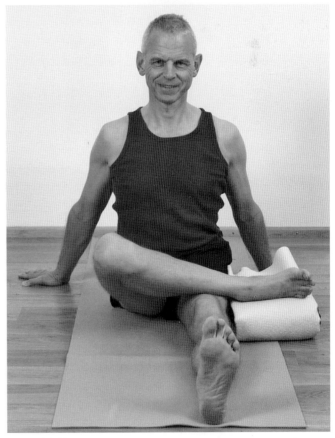

Figure 6.173

131

4. Move your straight left leg towards the right over the bent right leg (Figure 6.175).

5. Bend your left leg, and move it back to the central plane (Figure 6.176); bring the foot towards the floor and the knee to the left side as close as possible towards the floor, with the left sole of the foot touching the right sole (Figure 6.177).

6. Then straighten the right leg (corresponding to Figure 6.174), move it over the bent left leg to the left (corresponding to Figure 6.175).

7. Bend the right leg, move it back to the central plane (corresponding to Figure 6.176); bring the foot towards the floor and the knee to the left side as close as possible towards the floor, with the soles of the feet together (Figure 6.177).

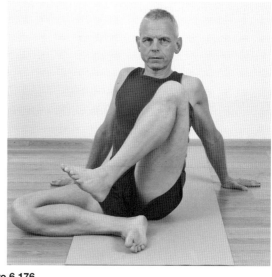

Figure 6.176

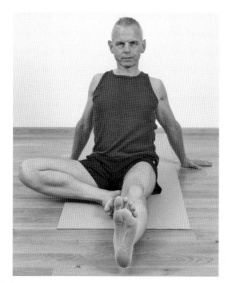

Figure 6.174

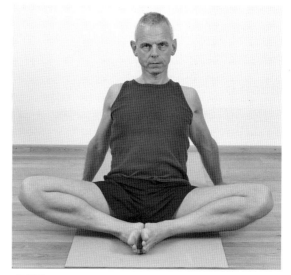

Figure 6.177

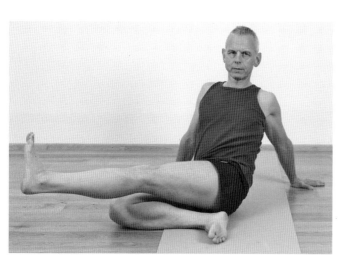

Figure 6.175

8. Straighten your left leg, and continue with point 4.

9. Perform 5–10 cycles in a continuous smooth movement.

10. To finish sit with both legs straight for a few breaths and be aware of your hips.

Hint

All variations can be practiced with your back resting against a wall.

Variations a, b, and c can also be performed sitting on a chair.

Exercise 8.6: Four-point kneeling

Aims: stabilizing the hips, balance.

1. Start from the four-point kneeling position; if necessary use a soft support for your knees; the knees are hip width apart, the thighs are perpendicular to the floor, and the lower legs parallel; put your hands on the floor, with the wrists underneath your shoulder joints.

2. Adjust the neutral lumbopelvic position.

3. Stretch your right leg backwards, as high as you can maintain the pelvis neutral, the foot is in dorsiflexion, the left thigh vertical (Figure 6.178).

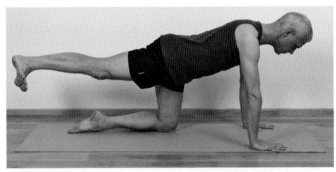

Figure 6.178

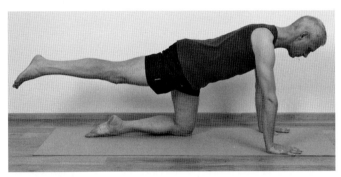

Figure 6.179

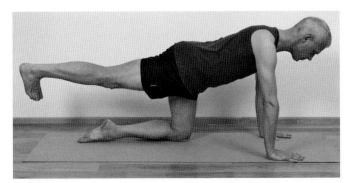

Figure 6.180

4. Hold for 2–3 breaths, constantly finetuning the lumbopelvic position.

5. Bring your right leg back to four-point kneeling; be centered in your position.

6. Repeat points 2–5 for the left leg.

7. Repeat points 2–6 with the following variations:
   a. foot in plantar flexion (Figure 6.179)
   b. foot in dorsiflexion, the leg externally rotated; the kneecap should indicate the rotation (Figure 6.178)
   c. foot in dorsiflexion, the leg internally rotated; the kneecap should indicate the rotation (Figure 6.180).

8. To train your balance more, lift your opposite arm at the same time as the leg.

9. To finish bring your buttocks as far as comfortable towards your heels, bend forwards, and rest for a few breaths (see Figure 6.16).

Exercise 8.7: Hip relaxation

Aims: gentle traction and relaxation for the hips.

1. Lie on your back, using sufficient support for your head, if necessary.

2. Rest your lower legs on a chair; adjust the distance from the chair so that the back of your pelvis stays on the floor and your legs are slightly pulled away from the hips to achieve gentle traction; the lower legs remain comfortably on the chair, knees and thighs relaxed (Figure 6.181).

3. Keep this position for 1–3 minutes in the beginning; with practice you may like to increase up to 10 minutes.

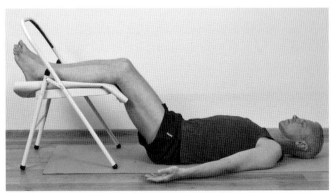

Figure 6.181

9. Basic exercises for the knees

The knee is probably the most complicated joint of the body. Among the synovial joints, those joints that are enclosed in a capsule, producing a lubricant fluid, it is the largest joint. Like the hip the knee also has to cope with weight-bearing from above and absorption of forces from below. The menisci increase the surface for these functions, improving stability. The ligaments and muscles are important for stability. The exercises should improve not only muscle power but also coordination and the balanced cooperation between the different groups of muscles. Alignment of the kneecaps and feet, of the knee joints and ankle joints, is essential for each exercise: good function is equally as important. For the best nutrition of the cartilages and menisci the full range of movement is essential (Roth 2009).

We have already mentioned stability. The primary movements are flexion and extension: the secondary movements are small ranges of internal and external rotation, abduction and adduction. There is a minor play of translation as well. Knee stability is increased by a small external rotation of the tibia when stretching the knee. A slight outwards movement of the tibial tuberosity can be seen and felt, or the lower leg can be kept stable and the thigh slightly turned inwards. Both movements lock the fully stretched knee.

There are exercises for improving both stability and movement. The effects are achieved not only through the actions themselves, but rather in the quality of the movements, which should be smooth. Finetuning, easing away slightly from the limit of movement, helps to stay within the physiological range and use the muscles in a balanced, coordinated way. For the fully stretched knee this means minimal flexion combined with extension. While bending the knees a minimal stretching action can be combined, like resisting the action of bending. These actions are particularly relevant for standing. In summary it is a balanced activity of the flexor and extensor muscles.

Knee problems are frequently related to the feet, ankles, and hips. Therefore posture and movement patterns need to be considered in a wider sense. Particular care in alignment is necessary if the muscles are hypertonic to protect instable knee joints. Furthermore the primary cause of knee problems may be in the hips, feet, and ankles, and the whole posture. A change in muscular forces due to wrong alignment and movement patterns contributes to degeneration and inflammatory processes of the structures of the knees. Muscular forces also change the shape of the bones (Raman 2008). From all this we understand the importance of exercising and particularly learning or relearning healthy positioning and movement. Also knee surgery is now the therapy of choice in serious cases of degeneration. As we have mentioned for hip replacement, these patients seem to recover well if they have exercised before the operation. It is strongly recommended to continue improving posture and movement patterns both before and after the operation.

Exercise 9.1: Rhythmic knee movement

Aims: mobilizing the knee joints, improving the movement of fluid.

1. Sit on a table.
2. Rhythmically oscillate the lower legs forwards and backwards for 1–3 minutes.
3. Relax the lower legs for a few breaths.
4. Rhythmically circumduct the lower legs for 1–3 minutes, so that the legs can dangle; change the direction in between.
5. Relax the lower legs for a few breaths.

Exercise 9.2: Finetuning the knee extension

Aims: full extension of knee joint, balance of flexor and extensor muscles.

1. Sit on the floor with straight legs, with the feet in dorsiflexion.
2. Use a back support if you need it, or put your hands behind your pelvis on the floor.
3. Hyperextend both knees, and alternate with a trace of flexion, 3–5 times.
4. Hold for 3–5 breaths the connection of knee extension with a trace of flexion, keeping the foot in dorsiflexion and the toes stretched.
5. Relax both legs and arms; stay calm for a few breaths.

Exercise 9.3: Mobile patella

Aims: mobilizing the kneecaps, coordination.

1. Sit on the floor with straight legs, and the feet in dorsiflexion; use a backrest if necessary; put your fingertips around the kneecaps to feel the movement.

2. Continuing normal breathing, rhythmically contract and relax your thigh muscles to move your kneecaps, 5–10 times, contracting both sides at precisely the same time, then alternating left and right 5–10 times.

3. Contract your thigh muscles; hold the contraction for 3–5 breaths; add a trace of flexion of your knee joints.

4. Slowly let go of the thighs; relax them for 1–2 breaths.

5. Perform points 3 and 4 3–5 times.

Variation

Perform points 2–5 while standing.

Exercise 9.4: Posterior knee

Aims: mobilizing the knee joints, relaxing the back of the knee.

1. Sit on the floor using a support for the pelvis that is high enough so that you can bend your right knee, with the toes pointing backwards and both buttocks resting equally on the support (Figure 6.182); the left toes are pointing towards the ceiling.

2. Slightly raise your right buttock until you can put the right palm and the flat fingers on the calf; the fingers are touching the back of the knee.

3. With your fingers very gently pull the calf muscle away from the back of the knee and sideways, while lowering your right buttock; then remove your right hand from the calf.

4. Sit evenly on both buttocks.

5. Put the right palm on your right thigh, the left palm on your left thigh; stay for 3–5 breaths.

6. Put the sole of your right foot on the floor, with the knee pointing towards the ceiling, and slide

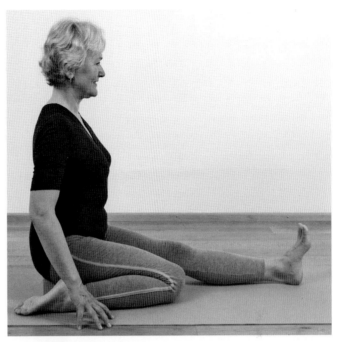

Figure 6.182

the right heel away to stretch the leg, keeping the back of the knee soft.

7. Repeat points 1–6 for the left leg.

8. To finish sit with both legs straight for a few breaths, with the kneecaps and toes pointing towards the ceiling.

Exercise 9.5: Rotation of the lower leg

Aims: mobilizing the knee joint into rotation and stabilizing it.

1. Sit on a chair, with the knees and feet more than hip width apart, and the shin bones perpendicular to the floor.

2. Bend forward so that you can rest your left elbow on your left thigh; put your left hand on your right thigh close to the knee; keep the fingers on the outside of the thigh; the right hand is around the top of the right shin bone.

3. Keeping your right heel as a pivot, turn your right foot inwards (Figure 6.183) and outwards (Figure 6.184), 5–10 times.

4. Your left hand is stabilizing the right thigh.

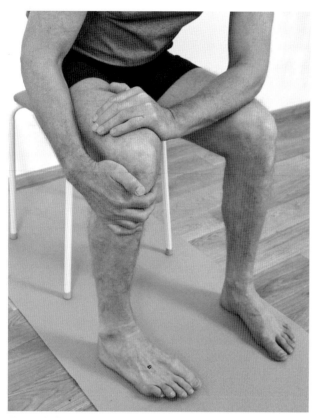

Figure 6.183

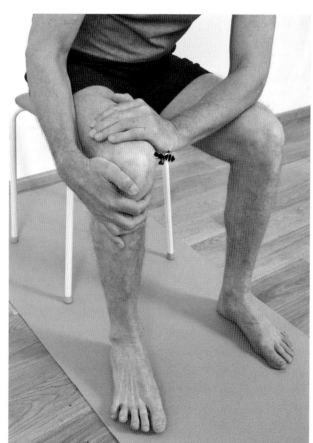

Figure 6.184

5. With your right hand you can feel the rotation movement of the lower leg on the tuberosity of the shin bone.

6. Continue stabilizing the right thigh with your left hand.

7. Repeat the movement of the right foot as described in point 3, resisting the rotation with the right hand.

8. Repeat points 2–7 for your left knee.

9. To finish sit straight for a few breaths, keeping your knees and feet parallel, slightly apart, correctly aligned.

Exercise 9.6: Stable knees

Aims: stabilizing the knee joints, connecting with pelvic stability.

1. Lie on your back, with your head comfortably supported, your legs straight, and feet relaxed.

2. Tilt your pelvis so that the lumbar spine moves closer to the floor; you can feel this movement with your hands on your front hip bones (Figure 6.185).

3. Tilt your pelvis further so that your knees just start bending.

4. Maintain the position of the pelvis; stretch your knees at the same time.

5. Hold for 1–2 breaths.

6. Slightly release the backwards tilt of the pelvis only as far as feels comfortable in the lumbar area and the back of the pelvis; relax your legs and feet.

7. Perform points 2–6 3–5 times.

8. Repeat points 2–7 with your feet in dorsiflexion.

9. Stay calm for a few breaths, feeling the contact of the back of your pelvis and the back of your legs on the floor.

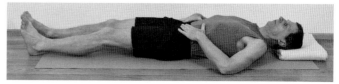

Figure 6.185

Variation: transferring the action into standing

Stand with your feet close together. Combine tilting your pelvis backwards with stretching your knees, 3–5 times. Slightly ease away from the full stretching of the knees when you release the backwards tilt of your pelvis in between. You can control the movement with your hands on your hips.

Exercise 9.7: Deep knee bend

Aims: balance of stability and mobility of the knees.

1. Stand facing a wall or a column with both feet parallel and one foot width apart; the toes are almost touching the wall or the column.

2. Slightly bend your right knee, and move the left foot two foot lengths backwards (Figure 6.186).

3. Keeping your trunk upright, slowly bend your knees, with the rear heel lifting off the floor; your right knee stays precisely in the plane of the right foot. The right kneecap and the right toes are facing exactly forwards. The left knee is moving close to the right inner ankle. The wall or column helps to control the angle of the right knee (Figure 6.187).

4. Maintaining the precise alignment straighten both knees.

5. Perform points 3 and 4 5–10 times, each movement for the length of one breath.

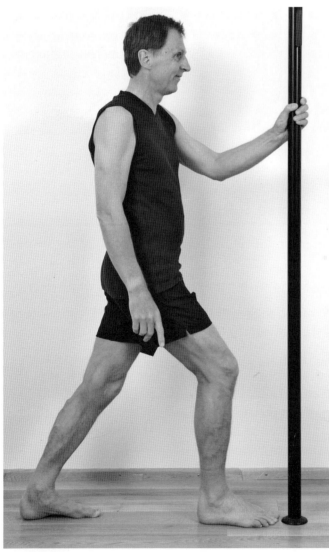

Figure 6.186

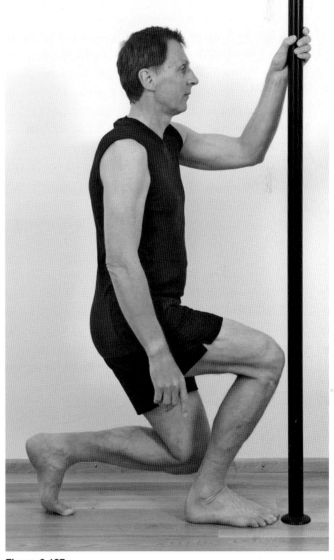

Figure 6.187

6. Repeat points 2–5 for the left leg in front.

7. To finish stand straight for a few breaths with your feet parallel, and your knees straight.

Exercise 9.8: Bent-leg knee stability

Aims: stabilizing and precisely aligning the bent knee joints.

1. Stand with your feet parallel, hip width apart.

2. Walk your feet one leg length apart; adjust the distance so that you feel stable and well stretched.

3. Hold your hips and your hands.

4. Keeping your trunk upright and in line turn your left foot on the heel 15° inwards, and your right leg 90° outwards as follows: lifting the front foot, turn 45° on the heel, put the whole foot on the floor, lifting the heel turn 45° on the ball of the foot; in this way the line of the right foot is crossing the center of the arch of the left foot.

5. Keeping your left leg firm and the outer edge of the left foot pressed to the floor, bend your right knee as you exhale until your right shin bone is perpendicular to the floor, the knee in line with the heel.

6. Keep your trunk upright.

7. Maintaining your right big toe firmly on the floor, gently lengthen your inner right thigh towards the knee (Figure 6.188).

8. Keeping your right heel firmly on the floor and maintaining the right knee exactly over the right heel, the shin bone perpendicular, move your right buttock slightly forwards.

9. Hold the position for 3–5 breaths.

10. Straighten your right knee, and bring your feet parallel.

11. Repeat points 4–10 for the left side.

12. Bring your feet together and stand calmly for a few breaths.

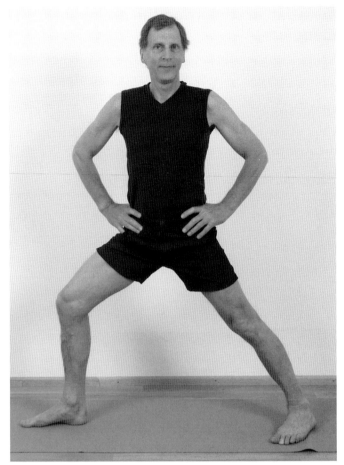

Figure 6.188

Exercise 9.9: Triangle

Aims: stability and correct alignment of the straight knees.

1. Stand with your feet parallel, hip width apart.

2. Walk your feet one leg length apart.

3. Hold your hips with your hands.

4. Turn the right foot and leg 90° outwards, the left foot and leg 45–60° inwards, and your pelvis and trunk 90° to the right; the left heel is in line with the right foot; in both legs the front of the thighs, the kneecaps and the toes are pointing in the same direction (Figure 6.189).

5. Keeping your left leg firm, press the outer edge of the foot on the floor.

6. Keep your right foot centered, with the big toe firmly on the floor.

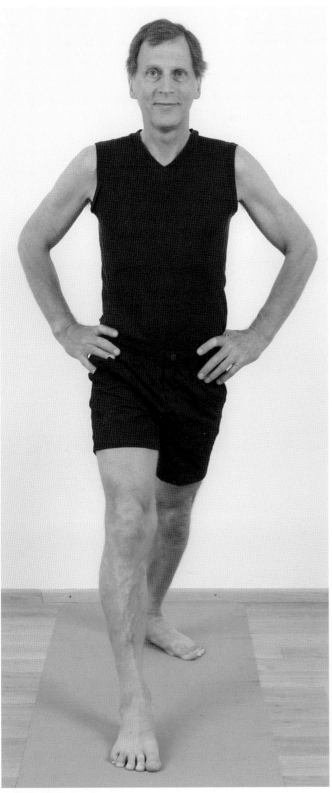

Figure 6.189

7. Using your thigh muscles, adjust your right kneecap so that it is pointing exactly the same way as the toes.

8. Slightly lift the right outer ankle when you turn the right thigh more outwards.

9. Relax slightly from the full extension of the right knee; continue refining the alignment of the kneecap for 3–5 breaths.

10. Turn back to the center; bring your feet parallel.

11. Repeat points 4–10 for the left side.

12. Bring your feet together and stay calm for a few breaths.

10. Basic exercises for the feet

The feet carry the whole weight of the body and are constantly adapting to different directions and floor shapes. The 26 bones in the foot, with numerous joint planes in different directions, are highly adaptable to these challenges. The feet are also the foundation for many other areas, such as ankles, knees, hips, pelvis, and vertebral column. They support the mechanics of the vertebral column from a postural point of view. They also send proprioceptive messages to the spinal muscles to keep the body upright. It is best to consider the feet in any neuromusculoskeletal problem.

Many patients have dropped and weak arches; the muscles for strengthening these arches are weak. Many people are not very aware of their feet. Therefore becoming conscious of the feet and their movements is an important start for foot exercises. The most commonly seen deviation is the hallux valgus. It is frequently associated with everted feet, flattened medial arches, and weak interosseous muscles between the metatarsals. Unless it is very far advanced, the problem can be improved or at least halted by strengthening the hypotonic muscles and correcting the posture. Orthotics are recommended for many patients. If they are used, the changes made should be small and gradual and a competent expert should be consulted. All standing exercises should be done barefoot.

Exercise 10.1: Awareness of the feet

Aim: developing awareness of the feet.

1. Sit on the floor or on a chair.
2. Touch and feel the different parts of your feet with your hands.
3. Rest the feet on the floor; be aware of the contact of your feet with the floor.

Exercise 10.2: Shake the foot

Aims: mobilizing and relaxing the whole foot.

1. Sit on the floor or on a chair; use a back support if you need it.

2. Maintaining the upright sitting position and your shoulders relaxed, hold your right lower leg just above the ankles with both hands (Figure 6.190).

3. Shake it rhythmically for 3–5 breaths.

4. Release the right leg, and sit in the starting position for 1–2 breaths.

5. Feel the difference in both feet; you may also stand for a few breaths to experience the difference.

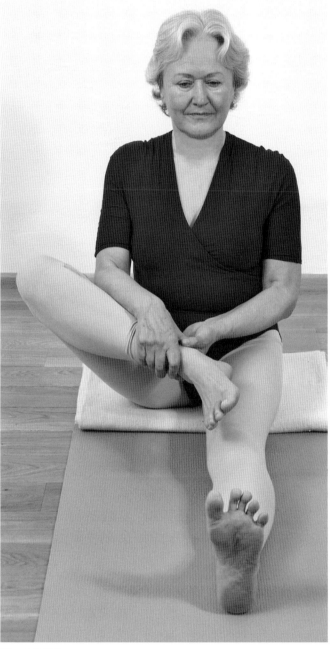

Figure 6.190

6. Repeat points 2–4 for the left foot.

7. Depending on the result you may like to perform points 2–6 2–3 times, varying the speed and amplitude of the oscillations.

8. To finish stand for a few breaths and feel the contact of your feet with the floor and the upwards movement of the arches of your feet.

Exercise 10.3: Active movements of feet without weight-bearing

Aims: understanding the active movements of the feet and toes, coordination.

Sit in any comfortable position from which you can move your feet.

Perform each movement 10 times, about one movement per breath or slightly faster:

1. Curl and stretch the toes; do this a few times alternating left and right, and a few times both feet simultaneously (Figure 6.191).

2. Move the straight toes towards the sole and towards the back of the feet; do this a few times alternating left and right, and a few times both feet simultaneously (Figure 6.192).

3. Move the straight toes rhythmically opposite to each other, like a wave moving from the big to the little toe (Figure 6.193).

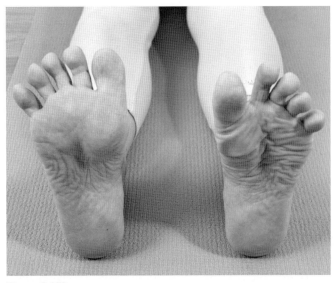

Figure 6.192

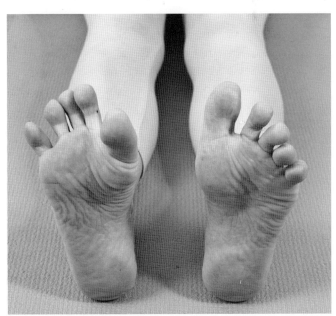

Figure 6.193

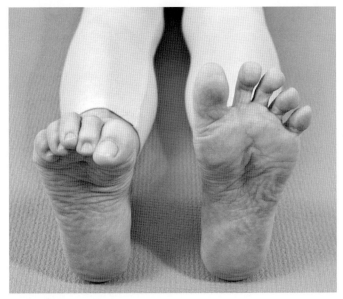

Figure 6.191

4. Move the whole foot:

    a. into plantar flexion and dorsiflexion, do this a few times alternating left and right, and a few times both feet simultaneously (Figure 6.194)

    b. into inversion (Figure 6.195) and eversion (Figure 6.196)

    c. into circumduction, clockwise and counterclockwise.

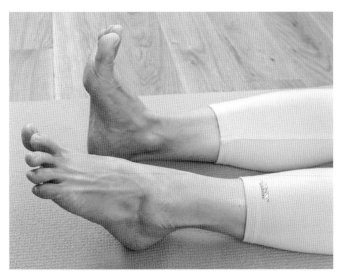

Figure 6.194

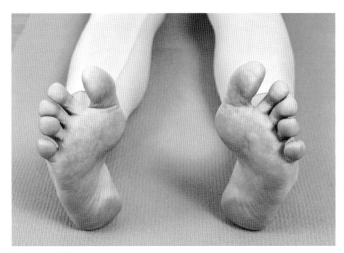

Figure 6.195

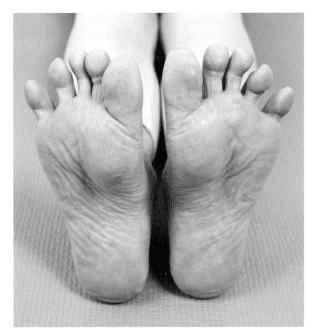

Figure 6.196

Exercise 10.4: Understanding the arches of the feet

Aim: developing awareness of the arches of the feet.

1. Sit on the floor or on a chair so that the soles of both feet are on the floor.

2. Bend down so that you can feel your feet with your hands.

3. Press all toes into the floor to lift the front transverse arch; feel with your fingers the back of the feet, hold up to the length of one breath, release; do this up to 10 times (Figure 6.197).

4. Press the big toes into the floor, lift the inner arch. Feel the inner arch with your fingers; hold up to one breath (Figure 6.198).

5. Press the little toes into the floor, lift the outer arch. Feel the outer arch with your fingers; hold up to one breath (Figure 6.199).

6. Perform points 4 and 5 alternating up to 10 times, feeling the whole foot with your hands.

7. Combine all the previous movements, feeling the whole foot with your hands.

Hint

For this series it is particularly important to keep the ankle joints stable, in order to reach the arches of the feet with the movements.

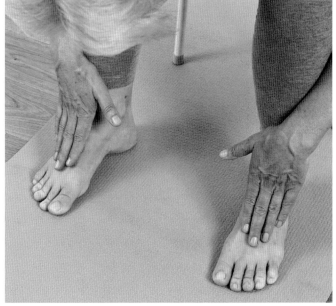

Figure 6.197

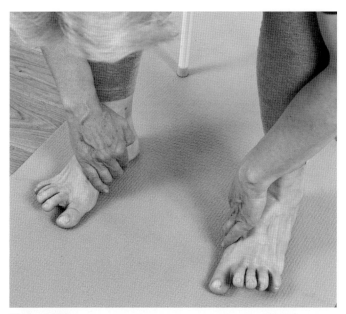

Figure 6.198

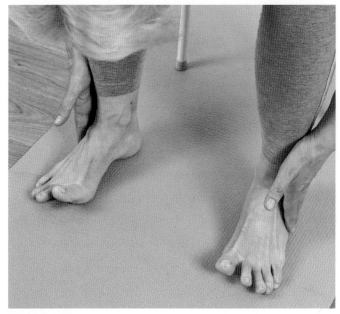

Figure 6.199

Exercise 10.5: Spreading the toes

Aims: spreading the toes in line with the metatarsals, mobilizing the joints between the toes and the metatarsals, subtle correction of hallux valgus.

1. Sit on the floor with straight legs or on a chair; if necessary use a back support.

2. Bend your right leg to rest your lower leg on the left thigh so that the ankle is laterally off the thigh.

3. Bring your left little finger between the right fourth and fifth toe, the ring finger between the third and fourth toe, the middle finger between the second and third toe, the index finger between the big and second toe, and the thumb around the big toe (Figure 6.200).

4. With your left hand gently move the toes into plantar flexion (Figure 6.201) and dorsiflexion (Figure 6.202), 5–10 times.

5. With your left hand gently move the toes and the midfoot into supination (Figure 6.203) and pronation (Figure 6.204), 5–10 times.

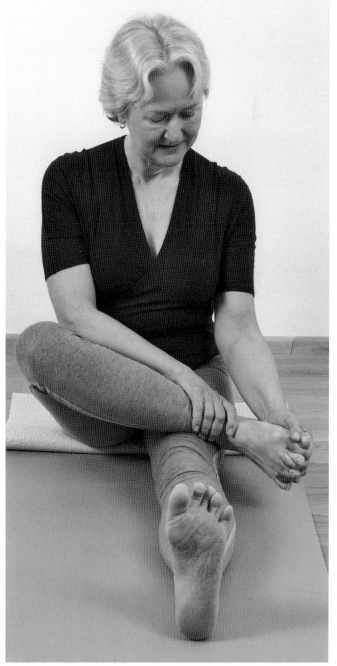

Figure 6.200

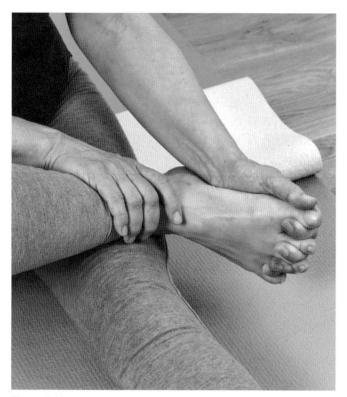

Figure 6.201

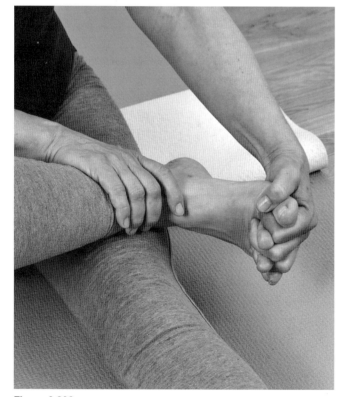

Figure 6.202

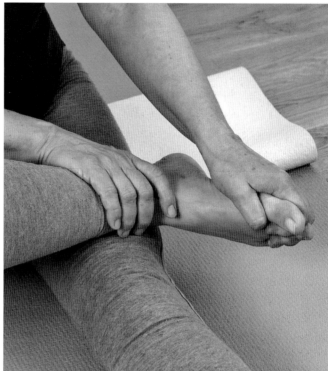

Figure 6.203

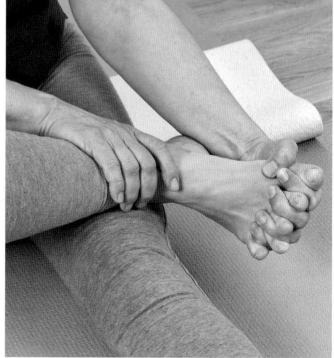

Figure 6.204

6. Release your left hand from the foot, bring the foot back to the starting position (point 1) for 1–2 breaths; feel the difference in both feet.

7. Repeat points 2–5 for the left foot.

8. Release your right hand from the foot; bring the foot back to the starting position (point 1) for 1–2 breaths.

9. To finish stand and feel the contact of your feet with the floor.

Exercise 10.6: Weight-bearing foot exercises

Aims: strengthening the arches of the feet, stabilizing the ankle joints.

1. Stand bent forwards so that you can see your feet, your hands resting on a chair or table (Figure 6.205).

2. Stretch your toes and put them on the floor; slide the straight toes about 1 cm towards the heels so that the whole foot is like a bridge (Figure 6.206).

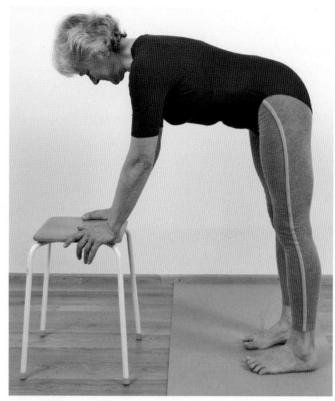

Figure 6.205

3. Perform point 2 up to 10 times, one movement lasting the length of one breath or faster.

4. Press the big toes on the floor; lift the inner arches and inner ankles (Figure 6.207).

5. Perform point 4 up to 10 times, one movement lasting the length of one breath or faster.

6. Press the little toes on the floor; lift the outer arches and outer ankles (Figure 6.208).

7. Perform point 6 up to 10 times, one movement lasting the length of one breath or faster.

8. Press all toes into the floor to lift your front transverse arch.

9. Perform point 8 up to 10 times, one movement lasting the length of one breath or faster.

10. Visualize your feet like a suction cup lifting the mat off the floor.

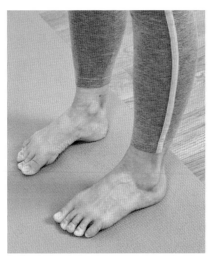

Figure 6.206

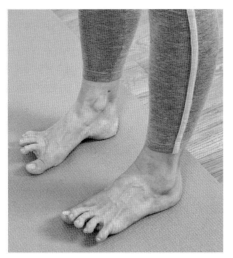

Figure 6.207

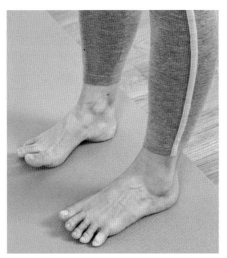

Figure 6.208

Refined work

Stand straight with your feet slightly apart; you cannot see your feet.

Perform points 2–10 without looking at your feet.

Be aware of your feet and the effect of each exercise on your whole posture.

Exercise 10.7: Rolling over the toes

Aims: mobilizing the ankle joints and metatarsophalangeal joints.

1. Stand with both feet parallel, one foot width apart.
2. Move the right foot two foot lengths backwards; keep the heel on the floor.
3. Slowly lift your right heel, keeping the toes straight on the floor (Figure 6.209).
4. Lift the heel further off the floor. Roll over the tips of the toes until the backs of the toes are on the floor (Figure 6.210).
5. Stretch the back of your foot.
6. Reverse the movement to bring the sole of your foot back to the floor.
7. Perform points 3–6 2–3 times, taking 1–2 breaths for one movement.
8. Perform these movements at increased speed 3–5 times.
9. Repeat points 2–8 for the left foot.
10. To finish stand straight for a few breaths.

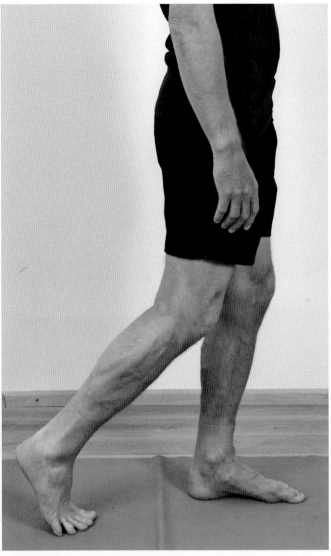

Figure 6.209

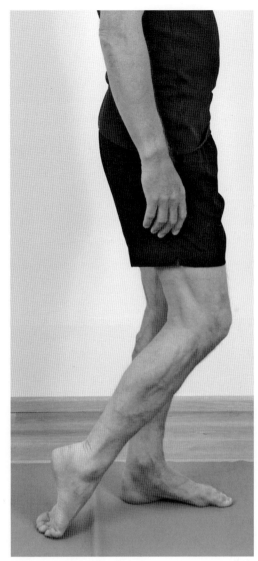

Figure 6.210

Exercise 10.8: Achilles tendon alignment

Aims: aligning the Achilles tendon, adjusting the subtalar joint, balance.

1. Sit on a chair with both feet parallel and one foot length apart.

2. Maintaining the knees stable with your hands, or alternatively with a brick between your knees,

tilt both heels into inversion (Figure 6.211) and eversion (Figure 6.212).

3. Start with slow movements, about one movement per breath, 5–10 times.

4. Gradually increase the speed up to oscillation. Reduce the amplitude of the movement until you reach the neutral position of the heel.

5. Slightly lift the heels from the floor and slowly bring them in a vertical line back to the floor.

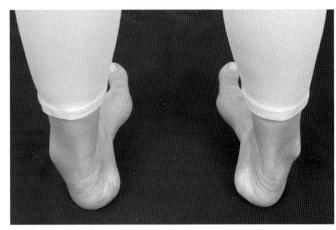

Figure 6.211

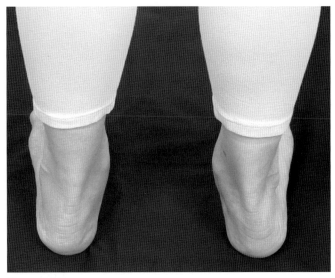

Figure 6.212

6. Perform point 5 5–10 times.

7. Stand for a few breaths and feel the contact of your heels with the floor.

Variation

Perform points 1–7 standing.

Refined work

Instead of tilting and moving the heels a subtle shift of weight is performed.

1. Sit on a chair or stand upright.

2. Maintaining the knees stable and the big toes firmly on the floor, shift the weight onto the outer heels.

3. Feel the change in the transverse and inner arches of your feet.

4. Maintaining the knees stable and the little toes firmly on the floor, shift the weight onto the inner heels.

5. Feel the change in the transverse and outer arches.

6. Perform points 2–5 5–10 times, about one movement per breath.

7. Maintaining the knees stable and the big toes firmly on the floor, shift the weight onto the outer heels.

8. Feel the effect on the inner ankles and the subtle upwards movement through the inner legs.

9. Hold points 7 and 8 for 3–5 breaths.

10. Maintaining the knees stable and the little toes firmly on the floor, shift the weight onto the inner heels.

11. Feel the effect on the outer ankles and the subtle upwards movement through the outer legs.

12. Hold points 10 and 11 for 3–5 breaths.

13. To finish stand upright for a few breaths; feel the toes and the centers of the heels on the floor and the lifting of the arches of the feet and the ankles.

Exercise 10.9: Foot seesaw

Aims: strengthening the foot and ankles, balance.

1. Stand facing a wall or holding a column with both feet parallel and one foot width apart. Stabilize yourself with one or both hands on the wall or column. Lift your left foot off the floor.

2. Raise your right heel until you are standing on the ball of your right foot, with the knee slightly bent (Figure 6.213).

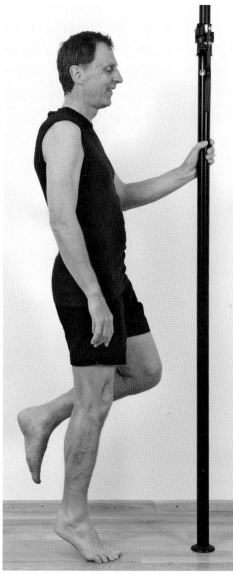

Figure 6.213

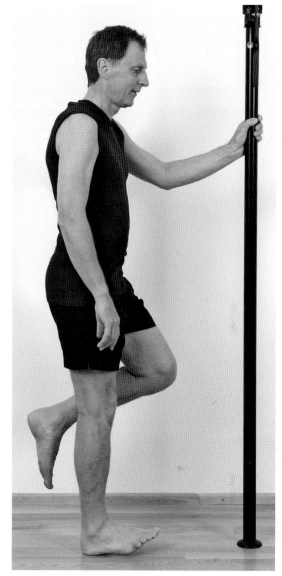

Figure 6.214

3. Lower your heel and lift your right forefoot to stand on your heel (Figure 6.214).

4. Repeat points 2 and 3 5–10 times, performing one movement for the length of one breath or shorter.

5. Repeat points 1–4 for the left foot.

6. To finish stand straight for a few breaths.

Variation

Practice independently without holding onto anything, on both feet and on one foot.

Exercise 10.10: Foot caterpillar

Aim: strengthening the longitudinal arches.

1. Stand with both feet parallel and one foot width apart.

2. Shift about two-thirds of your weight to the left foot.

3. Spread and lift your right toes (Figure 6.215).

4. Grasp the floor with the right toes so that you pull your right foot forward (Figure 6.216).

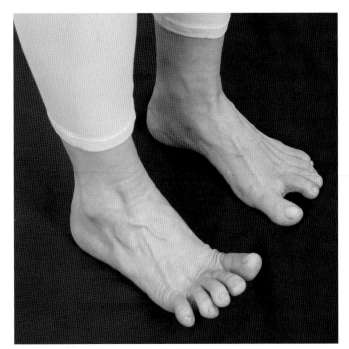

Figure 6.215

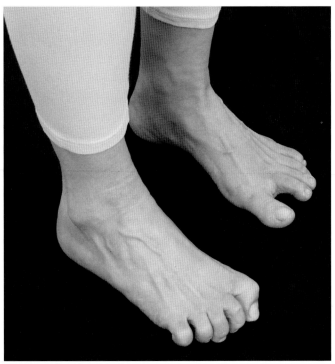

Figure 6.216

5. Perform points 3 and 4 3–5 times, then bring both feet to the starting position.

6. Shift about two-thirds of your weight to the right foot.

7. Spread and lift your left toes.

8. Grasp the floor with the left toes so that you pull your left foot forward.

9. Perform points 7 and 8 3–5 times.

10. Stand equally on both feet.

11. Spread and lift all toes; grasp the floor with the toes of both feet simultaneously and pull the whole body forwards.

12. Perform points 10 and 11 5–10 times.

13. To finish stand on both feet for a few breaths and feel the contact of your feet with the floor.

References

Feldenkrais, M., 1984. The Master Moves, second ed. Meta, Cupertino, CA.

Hartman, L., 2001. Handbook of Osteopathic Technique, third ed. Nelson Thornes, Cheltenham.

Kapandji, I.A., 2008. The Physiology of the Joints, vol. 3. The Trunk and the Vertebral Column, sixth ed. Churchill Livingstone, Edinburgh.

Kingston, B., 2001. Understanding Joints. Nelson Thornes, Cheltenham.

Lasater, J., 1995. Relax and Renew. Rodmell Press, Berkeley, CA.

Lederman, E., 2001. Harmonic Technique. Churchill Livingstone, Edinburgh.

Lederman, E., 2005. The Science and Practice of Manual Therapy. Elsevier, Edinburgh.

Magee, D.J., 1997. Orthopaedic Physical Assessment, third ed. Saunders, Philadelphia.

Norris, C., 2000. Back Stability. Human Kinetics, Champaign, IL.

Pullig Schatz, M., 1992. Back Care Basics: A Doctor's Gentle Yoga Program for Back and Neck Pain Relief. Rodmell, Berkeley, CA.

Raman, K., 2008. A Matter of Health. Integration of Yoga and Western Medicine for Prevention and Cure, second ed. EastWest, Madras.

Roth, L., 2009. Anatomie: Lehrbrief I. Fernlehrgang Yoga-Lehrer/in SKA. Sebastian Kneipp Akademie, Bad Wörishofen.

Stone, C., 1999. Science in the Art of Osteopathy. Stanley Thornes, Cheltenham.

Tanzberger, R., Kuhn, A., Möbs, G., 2004. Der Beckenboden – Funktion, Anpassung und Therapie. Elsevier, Munich.

Titze, M., Eschenröder, C.T., 2003. Therapeutischer Humor. Grundlagen und Anwendungen, fourth ed. Fischer Taschenbuch, Frankfurt am Main.

CHAPTER 30

Selected āsanas for integrating the aims and principles

Introduction

The basic exercises teach us mindfulness, awareness, precision of movement, and postures of the different areas of the body. They give many details on how to position and move in a healthy way. Each basic exercise helps to achieve one or more intended aims. This approach is also essential for performing the āsanas. The classical āsanas are very useful to integrate these basic details and aims into more complex, functional tasks. Performing the āsanas also goes deeper into mindful exercising and all stages of yoga. The other principles – variety, economical practice, precision, finetuning – are also followed during their practice. First the gross outer movements are learned, and then with increasing practice the inner, conscious movements are further refined.

As we saw in Chapter 1, a dedicated practice of āsanas can include all other stages of yoga, such as yama, niyama, āsana, prāṇāyāma, pratyāhāra, dhāraṇā, dhyāna, and samādhi. The ultimate aim of yoga is the union of the human with the divine, the individual soul with the universal soul. Health is a byproduct of practice, and a very important one (Iyengar 2002a). As described in Chapter 1, pratyāhāra, the fifth stage of the eightfold yoga path, is essential to prepare for the depth of practice of the āsanas. To achieve the inner movements during āsana practice, distractions of the senses, the organs of perception, must lessen and finally stop. The concentration and calmness needed to achieve this can be learned through breathing and listening (see Chapter 2) or the experience of subtle breathing (see Chapter 5). B K S Iyengar recommends cognitive action (Iyengar 2002a). This means that, while you are performing an āsana, the organs of perception – the eyes, ears, nose, tongue, and skin– are feeling what is happening in the body. This refined awareness must be integrated with willpower, intellectual and mental effort to move into the āsanas and to perform the instructions. When acting and awareness merge together the precision of the performance of the āsanas can be refined further: all layers of the body are penetrated, and body, mind, and soul become one. Learning the āsanas is a long and sometimes difficult process. There is a balance of activity and passivity, of strength and relaxation. Even if the body is fully stretched, there is relaxation at the same time.

With increasing practice hard work is transformed into inner strength, inner life, sensitivity. Each cell of the body is like an eye. What was effortful in the beginning becomes effortless (Iyengar 2005).

Practical steps to achieve calmness and relaxation are to let the throat, tongue, and back of the head become relaxed while practicing āsanas. Further a minimal distance can be created between the lower and upper teeth. Also with open eyes the relaxation of the eyes can be practiced, letting them sink towards the back of the head. This calms the mind, which improves the ability to learn. All this can be practiced in everyday situations as well.

As a demonstration of what can be achieved through practice, we show the āsanas in their final position. Not everyone can reach this final stage; however, we can all grasp the essence of the āsana, the finetuning of the body, and understand how to modify the āsanas appropriately.

The essence of each āsana can be divided into a frame and inner movements, learning which parts are stable, which parts are moving, and understanding healthy postures and movements. For therapeutic work the variations where props are used are particularly relevant. Using props also helps to achieve relaxation during effort. The props are simple objects or items of furniture found in most homes. In addition we recommend that you acquire a sticky mat, belt, and cork or foam brick. There is one example for each method, which can then be applied to many other āsanas. The possibilities for using props and modifying āsanas are countless. Careful observation, refined awareness, mindfulness, and the desire to experiment and continue learning

will help you to make the right decisions about how to use props and modify the āsanas. There are many ways of adjusting each method. The support can be made shorter or taller, harder or softer, and shifted to other areas of the body until it feels right. Precision is important when using props. They must be positioned correctly, and blankets must be carefully folded without creases. The floor should not be too hard or cold.

The description of each āsana has different sections:

- Meaning of the āsana and its name

- Getting into the posture

- Being in the posture. This section is divided into basic work and refined work. The basic work concerns the frame and the correct alignment of the āsana, physiological posture, and movement. The refined work leads to the inner work and awareness. Various suggestions are given; they are not meant to be included all at once. Choose an option depending on what you wish to emphasize, and gradually integrate the learned steps. Although the yoga postures may look static, there is a lot of inner movement and life.

- Finishing the posture. Getting out of the posture is as important as getting into the posture and the work in the posture. Good alignment and precision of movement when getting out of the posture contribute to the overall quality of the practice.

- Suggestions for modifications using props: refer to this if the patient cannot perform the āsana or there is instability. The props open up possibilities for modifications. Even when there are no restrictions, using props may make the basic and refined work more precise and help to understand the essence of the āsana. In the triangle poses, such as Utthita Trikoṇāsana and Parivṛtta Trikoṇāsana, putting the hand on the floor creates a wrong basic alignment for many people, and so fine adjustments are not possible. First of all the lower hand should get enough support, for example on a brick, and then the alignment can be corrected precisely.

- For some āsanas we have given variations as an alternative or to help get deeper into the āsana.

The descriptions of the asymmetrical āsanas start with the right side; for the left side reverse the instructions for left and right. In individual practice it helps to start with the easier side. Practical performance of the instructions is very individual and depends on experience and awareness. It is like a faceted crystal. When the crystal is turned in the sun, it shines differently depending on the angle, but stays the same crystal. An instruction is not a dogma. Recommendations for how long to hold the āsanas are average times, but may vary according to individual needs. Particularly for beginners it is helpful to hold for a shorter time and perform the āsanas twice to improve understanding.

While working in an āsana basic stability must be maintained; this relates to the calmness described above. In Yoga-Sūtra II.46 it is described as follows: "sthira sukham āsanam – āsana is perfect firmness of body, steadiness of intelligence and benevolence of spirit" (Iyengar 2002b, p. 157). As an example of basic stability, we used the neutral lumbopelvic position extensively in Chapter 6. This position is important and helps to protect the spine in many lifting, bending, and twisting actions in the āsanas. Depending on the posture it needs to be adjusted differently. Where there is lumbar lordosis, it is important to tilt the pelvis backwards and lengthen the back of the pelvis. Where there is a flatter lower back it may be necessary to tilt forward. Both cases also need countermovements to achieve the optimal balance. For different āsanas different areas are relevant for this basic stability; for example, the feet, hips, shoulder blades, or cervical spine. There are no āsanas for isolated work on a special area, for example the pelvic floor, although the pelvic floor is strengthened through the correct performance of each āsana. As there are so many āsanas and variations, this work integrates the pelvic floor in many different ways.

From all these considerations we can see that the following points are essential for yoga as therapeutic exercise:

- Selecting the program for practice according to the aims that need to be improved: mobility, strength, stamina, relaxation, balance, coordination, synchronization, and breathing.

- The quality of practice can be improved and adjusted in many individual conditions by applying the principles of mindfulness, variety of exercise approaches, economical practice, precision, and finetuning.

- Mindfulness particularly supports the therapeutic effects, as it allows patients to practice in an appropriate way.

- Certain exercises for certain pathologies are not prescribed in this approach.

- Programs are selected in order to achieve certain aims, keeping in mind the diagnosis and contraindications.

- The selected program not only improves the condition, but also helps patients to understand why their health problems have occurred and learn how to avoid these causes in the future. For example, common low-back pains may be relieved through exercises relaxing the area and building up a balanced activity of the trunk muscles. Mindful practice, improving awareness, leads to understanding and therefore avoiding the causes of the low-back pain.

In general the introductory āsanas or introductory versions have been selected from among all the āsanas. Abilities learned from the basic exercises are integrated into more complex tasks when practicing āsanas. A further criterion for selection is variety:

- to cover all positions: standing, sitting, lying, inverted, balanced

- to include activity and relaxation

- to cover firmness in a centered position, movements of bending forwards, backwards, side-bending, and rotation.

At the end of this chapter, after all the āsana descriptions, hints will be given on how to combine basic exercises and āsanas and how to sequence āsanas. The basic exercises 1.4, 1.11, 1.13, 1.15, 3.2, 3.3, 3.4, 4.6, 4.11 and 8.5 (see Chapter 6) are preparations or easier versions of classical āsanas not explained in this book. For the full āsana, see Iyengar (2001) and Mehta et al (1990).

When learning the āsanas we strongly recommend that you work under the guidance of a qualified yoga teacher. Personal learning from a teacher is the traditional approach. The oldest yoga textbooks, the Upaniṣads, were first learned by heart from a personal teacher (see Chapter 1). This book is for your own additional practice. Regular practice in addition to learning from a teacher is essential to improve ability. To practice the āsanas with this book, a good method is to work in small groups. One person reads the instructions, while the other practices. If there are three of you, the third can observe. Interchanging the roles is a very good learning process.

Selected āsanas

1. Tāḍāsana (Figures 7.1 and 7.2)

Meaning of the āsana and its name

Tāḍāsana is the mountain pose; it means being firm like a mountain, standing upright, concentrated, and still. You grow taller as a result of being firmly grounded. Tāḍāsana is one of the simplest and at the same time the most complex āsanas. It develops a good habit of standing; activity and calmness merge together.

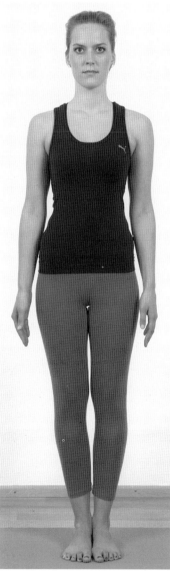

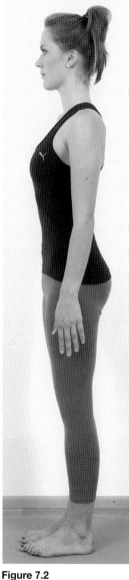

Figure 7.1   Figure 7.2

Getting into the posture

Stand upright with your feet as close together as possible, your arms at your sides, palms facing your outer thighs.

Being in the posture: basic work

1. Stretch your toes; rest your toes straight on the floor.
2. Balance between lifting the inner and outer ankles, keeping the base of the big and little toes on the floor.
3. Straighten your knees; ease off a tiny bit; make your quadriceps muscles firm and pull your kneecaps up.
4. Move the front of your thighs towards the back of your thighs, the groins slightly backwards; shift the weight slightly more into the heels.
5. Adjust your pelvis to the neutral position; lift from your lower abdomen.
6. Maintain the neutral pelvic position while you lift your thorax.
7. Relax your shoulders.
8. Let your arms hang naturally.
9. Maintaining the position of your chin, parallel to the floor, slightly move the back of your head backwards parallel to the floor and away from the neck.
10. Relax your face.
11. Breathe naturally.

Being in the posture: refined work

1. Distribute the weight evenly between the left and right foot, and the front and hind feet, slightly more into the heels.
2. Balance lifting the inner and outer arches of your feet; feel how this influences the upward movement through the lower legs.
3. Balance this lifting action of the arches while stretching the soles of the feet through the toes and through the heels.

4. Keeping your knees straight, balance a subtle forward movement of the back of the knees with sucking your kneecaps into the thighs.

5. Pull the thighs upwards.

6. Slightly bring your groins backwards and your tailbone and sacrum inwards and upwards. Feel the effect of this action on the position of your pelvis, the lifting of your spine and thorax.

7. Perform a subtle movement as if pulling the skin of the lower abdomen through the abdominal muscles, the abdominal cavity, towards the diaphragm and upper lumbar spine.

8. Maintaining the neutral lumbopelvic position and the abdomen soft, lift the center of your diaphragm.

9. Lift your lower sternum upwards and your upper sternum upwards and slightly forwards.

10. Gently turn your arms inwards; feel the space between the shoulder blades.

11. Gently turn your arms outwards; feel the space in your chest and the subtle stretch of the skin over your upper ribs and clavicles.

12. Keeping the arms vertical, move the upper arms away from the armpits to create space in this area.

13. Maintaining a balance of the sensations built up in points 8–11, relax your arms and hands naturally.

14. Move your upper thoracic vertebrae inwards; this is a slight back-bending action in this area and supports the lifting and forward movement of the upper sternum and upper ribs.

15. Balance your head; maintaining the position of the chin and the throat soft, slightly pull the back of the head away from the neck; feel the effect of this on the lifting of the upper ribs and sternum.

16. Balance your left and right ear.

17. Keeping the mouth closed, slightly lift the upper teeth and the palate away from the lower jaw.

18. Look horizontally; let your eyes be calm.

19. Relax your face as if smiling slightly.

Finishing the posture

Observe and feel how you are standing after finishing the fine adjustments.

Suggestions for modifications using props

- Rest the back of the pelvis and shoulder blades on a wall.

- Raise the heels on a brick or rolled mat.

- Raise the balls of the feet on a brick or rolled mat.

- Observe yourself in a mirror.

- Prepare two chairs with sufficient bricks or books on them. Stand in between the chairs. Adjust the bricks so that you can rest your left palm on the left chair and your right palm on the right chair; push yourself up from the palms. Alternatively you can adjust the height so that you can push yourself up from the fingertips. Integrate this pushing-up action without chairs, as if you are pushing the air down.

Variations

- Stand with the feet slightly apart.

- Lift the heels so that you are standing on the balls of your feet; raise your arms.

- Lift the front feet to stand on the heels.

- Stand with your feet hip width apart. Maintaining your trunk and head upright bend your knees over your toes. Maintaining the balance of the big and little toes, and the inner and outer arches, adjust your kneecaps precisely in the center between the big and little toes. Keeping your feet firmly on the floor, your pelvis neutral, and your trunk and head upright, straighten your knees.

In summary, Tāḍāsana teaches many aims and principles which apply to all other āsanas.

2. Vṛkṣāsana (Figure 7.3)

Meaning of the āsana and its name

Vṛkṣa means tree in Sanskrit. In all cultures, religions, and many fairy tales, the tree is a symbol of life. Vṛkṣāsana particularly teaches you to find your balance and stay concentrated even if you are moved around, and to combine stability and flexibility in growing from solid roots.

Getting into the posture

1. Stand in Tāḍāsana.
2. Lift your pelvis away from your legs.

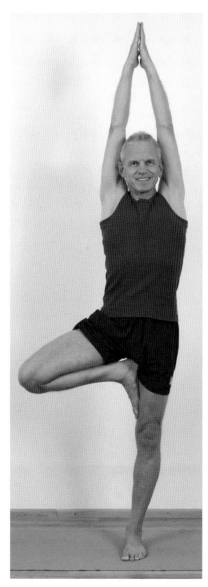

Figure 7.3

3. Shift more weight into the left foot and make the left leg firm.
4. Maintaining the lifting of the pelvis, bend your right knee, keeping the tips of your toes on the floor, and externally rotate your right leg as far as you can, keeping your left leg and pelvis in line.
5. Move your right foot up to the inside of your left thigh as high as possible; hold around the ankles with your right hand to move the foot higher on your inner left thigh.
6. Moving your lower abdomen inwards and upwards, lift your chest and raise your arms over your head so that the palms come together and the elbows are stretched.

Being in the posture: basic work

1. Lift from the arches of the left foot.
2. Keep your left knee firm.
3. Push the right foot into the left inner thigh, resisting with the left thigh.
4. Keep the pelvis lifted and neutral; move the right sitting bone slightly forwards.
5. Keep the thorax lifted and the arms extended.
6. Balance the head between the chin and the back of the head.
7. Breathe naturally.

Being in the posture: refined work

1. Keeping the right big toe and the ball of the foot firmly in contact with the left thigh, press the outer edge of the right foot more into the left thigh.
2. The inner right thigh moves away from the groin slightly.
3. Move the upper outer right thigh towards the right hip joint.
4. Keeping the hips at the same level, slightly move the lower abdomen inwards and upwards; feel the effect of this action on the lifting of the spine.
5. Lift the side ribs.

6. Suck the shoulder blades into the thorax; feel how this helps to raise your front upper ribs.

7. Move the upper thoracic vertebrae inwards; feel how this connects to the lifting of the upper sternum.

8. Move the arms slightly more backwards.

9. Slightly turn your upper arms outwards to create more freedom for the neck without losing height.

10. Relax your face.

11. Breathe naturally.

Finishing the posture

Stay in the posture for 5–10 breaths, then release according to one of the following methods:

1. Bring your right foot and your arms down as you exhale to come back to Tāḍāsana.

2. Lower your right foot as you exhale; with a further exhalation lower your folded hands to the sternum; hold them in front of the sternum for 2 breaths; with another exhalation release your hands to stand in Tāḍāsana.

Repeat "getting into the posture" and "being in the posture" for the left leg.

Suggestions for modifications using props

• Stand with your back close to a wall; let your hips rest against the wall, the thumbs slightly touching the wall when the arms are elevated.

• Practice in front of a mirror to check your alignment.

Variations (Figure 7.4)

• If there is less mobility of the bent knee or you cannot balance, adjust the height of the foot starting with the toes on the floor; gradually move the foot higher.

• If you cannot stretch your elbows with the palms together, keep the hands apart at shoulder width.

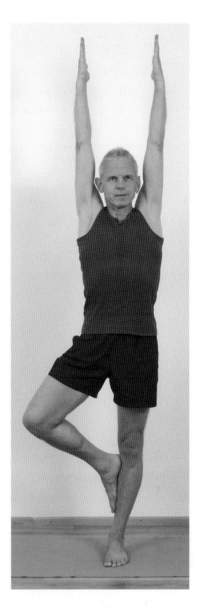

Figure 7.4

3. Utthita Trikoṇāsana (Figure 7.5)

Meaning of the āsana and its name

Utthita means extended, and trikoṇa means triangle. The number 3 and the triangle are fundamental in nature and in many philosophical and religious systems to describe the secret of life.

Utthita Trikoṇāsana trains awareness of position in space; it particularly refines precision.

Getting into the posture

1. Stand in Tāḍāsana.

2. Walk your feet one leg length apart.

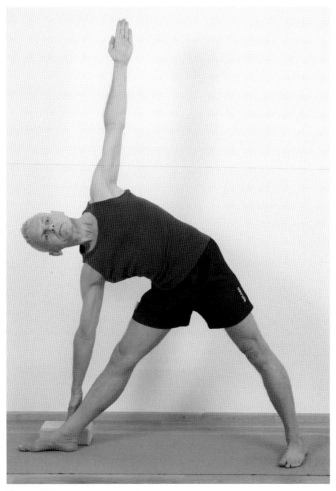

Figure 7.5

3. Maintaining the neutral pelvic position lift your chest and raise your arms horizontally in line with your shoulder girdle, with the palms facing the floor.

4. Keeping your trunk upright and in line turn your left foot on its heel 15° inwards, and your right leg 90° outwards: lifting the front foot, turn it 45° on its heel, lifting the heel, turn it 45° on the ball of the foot; in this way the line of the right foot is crossing the center of the arch of the left foot.

5. Stretch your left leg firmly; keeping the big toe on the floor, press the outer edge of the foot on the floor.

6. Move the front of the left thigh backwards.

7. Keeping the right big toe on the floor, and the right outer ankle lifted, move your right thigh upwards and turn it out until its center, the right kneecap, and the toes are pointing in the same direction.

8. Moving the outer side of your upper right thigh into the hip socket, the right hip to the left and forwards, and lengthening your right trunk side, and turning the right side ribs slightly forwards, bend your trunk sideways to the right as you exhale.

9. Hold your right hand above the ankle; only if you can maintain the correct alignment, bring the fingertips or the palm to the floor beside your outer heel.

10. Stretch the left arm up in line with the shoulder girdle, with the palm facing forwards.

11. The shoulder blades move away from the head slightly.

12. Keep your head in line with your spine; keep your neck and throat comfortable.

Being in the posture: basic work

1. Lift your left inner arch and ankle.

2. Keep your right big toe on the floor when you lift your inner arch and ankle.

3. Lift your outer ankle when you turn your right thigh further out to maintain the center of the thigh, the kneecap, and the toes in the same direction.

4. If your right knee is hyperextended, slightly relax from full extension.

5. Maintaining the right upper thigh and hip towards the left and forwards and your spine lengthened, lift your left hip, and turn your abdomen and chest to the left; the trunk and head are in the plane of the legs.

6. Lift your shoulder girdle away from the right arm, your left shoulder away from the sternum and the thoracic spine, and the left arm away from the left shoulder.

7. Both arms are in line with the shoulder girdle; the head is in line with the spine so that the throat and neck are comfortable.

8. Breathe naturally.

Being in the posture: refined work

1. Shift some more weight into the right heel to enhance the movement of the right upper thigh into the hip joint.

2. Balance the inner and outer ankle and the right inner and outer arch; lengthen from the center of your right arch into the toes; the toes remain on the floor.

3. Balance between hyperextension and minimal flexion of your right knee.

4. Lift your right outer ankle; turn the right thigh outwards, to move your right upper outer thigh forwards, and your left front thigh backward.

5. Move your tailbone and middle buttocks inwards.

6. Very gently pull your lower abdomen inward; feel how this initiates the lengthening of your spine.

7. Slightly rotate one vertebra after the other, like an inner spiral movement.

8. Move your shoulder blades into the thorax and and shift your head backwards.

9. Keeping the head in line with your spine turn the head towards the ceiling as long as the neck and throat are comfortable.

10. Stretch your left arm up further; keep it firm and calm.

11. With your right eye look at your left thumb.

Finishing the posture

Stay in the posture for 5–10 breaths.

Be strong in your left leg; press the outer edge of your left foot onto the floor; move the right knee and thigh upwards, extending the left arm away from the shoulder girdle, keeping the right middle ribs slightly turned forwards, the arms in line with the shoulders; come back as you inhale. Bring your feet parallel and repeat on the left side. After finishing both sides come back to Tāḍāsana; stay calm for a few breaths.

Suggestions for modifications using props

- Practice with your back close to a wall to check the alignment; the hip of the externally rotated leg touches the wall.

- Rest your lower hand on a brick, chair, or table depending on your flexibility. If you are less flexible, this enables you to grasp the essence of the āsana, and to perform it correctly. For flexible individuals it may improve their performance of the āsana, if they lose correct alignment when they put their lower hand on the floor (Figure 7.6).

- Raise the forefoot of the externally rotated leg; rest it on a brick or a rolled mat or towel (Figure 7.6).

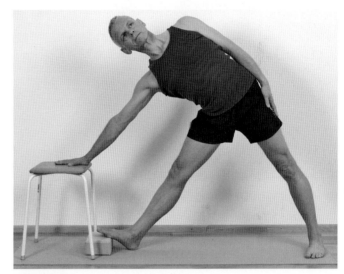

Figure 7.6

4. Vīrabhadrāsana II (Figure 7.7)

Meaning of the āsana and its name

Vīrabhadra was a powerful hero in ancient Indian mythology. This āsana is the second of a series of three āsanas dedicated to him (Vīrabhadrāsana I, II, and III). It is performed with strength and at the same time is relaxed.

Getting into the posture

1. Stand in Tāḍāsana.

2. Walk your feet one leg length plus one foot length apart; adjust the distance so that you feel stable and well stretched.

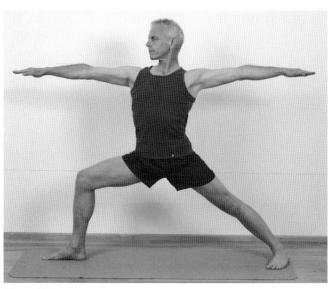

Figure 7.7

3. Raise your arms to the sides; stretch them in line with your shoulder girdle

4. Fully extend your wrists so that the palms are at right angles to the lower arms, and the fingers and thumbs are pointing towards the ceiling (Figure 7.8).

5. Extend through your wrists first.

6. Maintain the extension of the arms; bring the hands in line with the arms; lengthen the backs of the wrists; keep the fingers together.

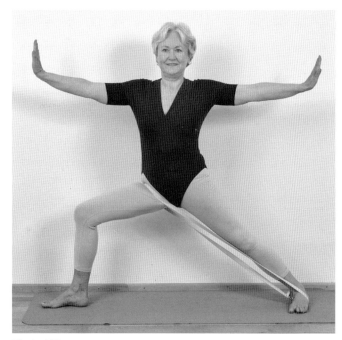

Figure 7.8

7. Keeping your trunk upright and in line, turn your left foot on its heel 15° inwards, and your right leg 90° outwards: lifting the front foot, turn it 45° on its heel; lifting the heel, turn it 45° on the ball of the foot; in this way the line of the right foot is crossing the center of the arch of the left foot.

8. Keeping your left leg firm, the outer edge of the left foot pressed to the floor, and the trunk vertical, and moving the right upper outer thigh into the hip joint, bend your right knee as you exhale until your right shin bone is perpendicular to the floor and the knee is in line with the heel.

9. Lift your right hip away from the right upper thigh; bring your left hip down so that it "sits" on the head of the left thigh bone.

10. Keep your trunk upright, and the pelvis, thorax, shoulders, and arms in line.

11. Lift from your lower abdomen to your upper sternum.

12. Stretch your arms more to the sides, particularly the left one.

13. Keeping your head in line with your spine, gently turn it to the right and look towards your right hand.

Being in the posture: basic work

1. To keep your left leg strong, press the outer edge of your left foot to the floor; keep your left knee firm, the upper outer thigh slightly down.

2. To keep your right knee correctly aligned, bring more weight onto the outer edge of your right foot and your right heel; the big toe stays on the floor.

3. Move the upper thighs slightly downwards, the right buttock forwards, and the left hip away from the middle lower abdomen.

4. Move the right side of your chest forwards, and the left ribs backwards.

5. Lift from your lower abdomen to your upper sternum; feel the length of your spine.

6. Slightly move your shoulders down; keep your arms horizontal and well extended, particularly the left arm.

7. Breathe naturally.

Being in the posture: refined work

1. Lift your left inner ankle and the left outer ankle slightly.

2. Keeping your left big toe on the floor, lift your left inner knee and thigh.

3. Bring your left sitting bone down, and the right sitting bone forwards.

4. Balance your right inner and outer ankle, your right inner and outer knee.

5. Keeping the right big toe and the inner heel on the floor, shift more weight onto the right outer foot.

6. Move your sacrum and tailbone in.

7. Maintaining the neutral lumbopelvic position, lift your side ribs and your sternum; move the shoulder blades inwards.

8. From your upper sternum extend your arms to your thumbs, from the inner shoulder blades to your little fingers.

9. Extend both arms through the middle fingers, the left more than the right.

10. Slightly shift the head on the upper cervical spine backwards; relax your throat and neck, to get the optimum balance for the head, and length for the spine.

11. Relax your face and look at your right hand with an inner smile and your eyes relaxed.

Finishing the posture

Hold the posture for 5–10 breaths. With an inhalation straighten your right knee and turn your feet parallel; if necessary, relax your arms. Repeat on the left side. After finishing both sides come back to Tāḍasana, and stay calm for a few breaths.

Suggestions for modifications using props

- Stand with your back against a table. Rest your hands on the table while you build up the posture (Figure 7.9). At the end extend your arms horizontally in line with the shoulder girdle.

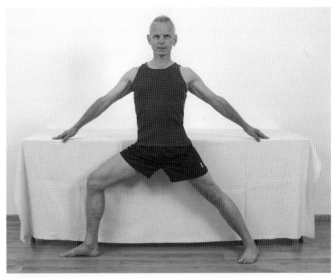

Figure 7.9

- Stand close to a wall or a column on your right side. To help control the stability of the bent knee, hold a brick between the upper right shin and the wall or column, as shown for Vīrabhadrāsana I (see Figure 7.24). Repeat on the left side.

- Have a long belt around the left foot and the upper right thigh (Figure 7.10); perform both sides.

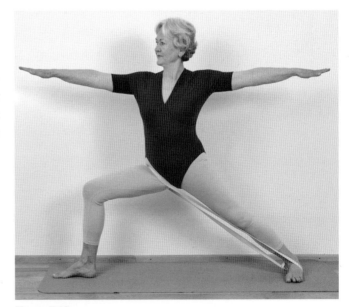

Figure 7.10

5. Utthita Pārśvakoṇāsana (Figure 7.11)

Meaning of the āsana and its name

Utthita means extended, pārśva is the side, and koṇa means angle. In Utthita Pārśvakoṇāsana one leg is bent at a right angle, the trunk is stretched over it to the side; the straight leg, the upper side of the trunk, and the upper arm are in one line. There is an intensive stretch from the toes to the fingertips. Precise alignment, particularly from the deep structures of the body, is vital for this āsana.

Getting into the posture

1. Stand in Tāḍāsana.

2. Walk your feet one leg length plus one foot length apart; adjust the distance so that you feel stable and well stretched.

3. Raise your arms to the sides, and stretch them in line with your shoulder girdle, palms facing the floor.

4. Keeping your trunk upright and in line turn your left foot on its heel 15° inwards, your right leg 90° outwards: lifting the front foot, turn it 45° on its heel; lifting the heel, turn it 45° on the ball of the foot; in this way the line of the right foot is crossing the center of the arch of the left foot.

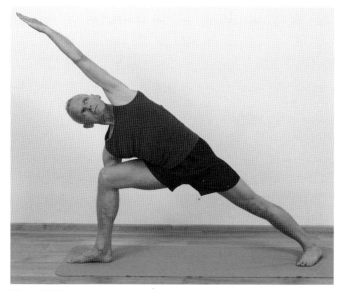

Figure 7.11

5. Keep your left leg firm, and the outer edge of the left foot pressed to the floor, with the big toe on the floor; bend your right knee as you exhale until your right shin bone is vertical, and the knee is in line with the heel.

6. Keeping the pelvis, thorax, shoulders, and arms in line, be in Vīrabhadrāsana II for a moment.

7. With an inhalation lengthen your spine and the left leg.

8. Keeping the right big toe on the floor, press the right heel and the outer edge of the left foot into the floor, lengthening the right side of your trunk.

9. With an exhalation bend your trunk sideways to the right, and place your right palm or fingertips beside your right outer heel on the floor.

10. Keep the right shin bone vertical and the right knee in contact with the right arm.

11. Place your left hand on your left hip; lift your left hip.

12. Place your left hand on your left costal arch, and lift the costal arch and turn it back.

13. Place your left fingers on your left shoulder; lift your left shoulder away from the center of the chest.

14. Maintaining this posture for the legs and the trunk, stretch your left arm over the head, in line with the left trunk side; turn the arm from the shoulder joint so that the palm is facing the floor; create space from the neck to the upper arm.

15. Keep your head in line with the spine; throat and neck comfortable.

Being in the posture: basic work

1. Press the outer edge of the left foot to the floor.

2. Keep the left knee well stretched, with the inner left leg lifting towards the outer leg, the front left thigh moving backwards.

3. Move the right sitting bone forwards, the right upper outer thigh towards the hip joint, and the right side of your chest forwards.

4. Keeping the back of the pelvis long, slightly lift the left hip.

5. Move the left ribs backwards.

6. Slightly turn your left arm from the shoulder joint so that the little finger is getting closer to the floor.

7. Keep the hand in line with the lower arm and the fingers together.

8. Feel the continuous stretch from the left outer heel to the left fingertips.

9. Keep your head in line with your spine; shift it slightly backwards.

10. Slightly move the back of your head away from the neck and be aware of the line between the back of the head and the sacrum.

11. Breathe naturally.

Being in the posture: refined work

1. Keeping the outer edge of the left foot on the floor, slightly lift the inner and outer ankle.

2. Lift your left inner knee towards the outer knee.

3. Keep more weight in the right heel than in the forefoot.

4. Feel how the position of the right knee is stabilized when you shift the weight more to the outer edge of the foot, also keeping the right big toe on the floor.

5. Keeping the right big toe on the floor, lengthen from the inner ankle to the big toe.

6. Slightly move your lower abdomen inwards; feel the length in your lumbar spine.

7. Keep your abdomen soft.

8. Move your right upper thigh slightly down and forwards, and the right buttock forwards; maintain this when you lift your left hip.

9. The right inner thigh moves towards the knee, and the outer thigh towards the hip.

10. Move your right sitting bone forwards so that you can feel the lengthening of the back of your pelvis away from the lumbar area.

11. Feel the length of your spine.

12. Move your shoulder blades as if sucking them into your upper back.

13. Move your upper thoracic spine inwards; feel how this combines with lifting and widening in your upper sternum and upper front ribs.

14. Keep your left arm slightly rotated so that the little finger is getting closer to the floor and move it backwards more behind the ear; feel the lengthening of your armpit, particularly the posterior edge.

15. Fully stretch your left elbow; lengthen the wrist, the palm and the palmar side of your fingers.

16. Slightly shift your head backwards; starting from your upper thoracic vertebrae turn it to the left as long as the throat and neck are comfortable.

17. Look upwards in front of the left arm.

Finishing the posture

Stay in the posture for 5–10 breaths. Make your left leg very firm; press the outer edge of your left foot on the floor. With an inhalation stretch your right knee, and come up until your trunk is upright and your arms are horizontal. If necessary relax your arms for a moment. Turn your feet parallel and repeat on the left side. After finishing both sides come back to Tāḍāsana and stay calm for a few breaths.

Suggestions for modifications using props

- Be with your back against a wall. The buttock of the bent leg and the shoulder and arm of this side are touching the wall. The other areas are slightly away from the wall; the wall helps the correct alignment.

- As shown for Utthita Trikoṇāsana (see Figure 7.6) you can put the ball of the foot and the toes on a brick or rolled mat, and the lower hand on a support such as a brick or chair.

Variation (Figure 7.12)

Instead of resting the lower hand on the floor or on a support you can rest your lower arm on the thigh

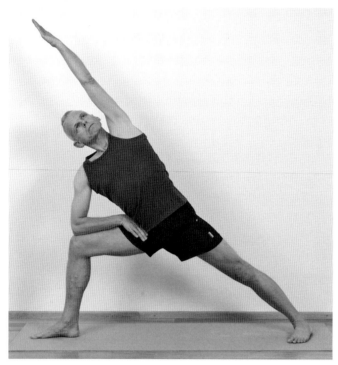

Figure 7.12

with the thumb and index finger on the groin of the bent leg. This helps to stabilize the bent knee and improve awareness of the movement of the upper thigh and hip.

6. Ardha Candrāsana (Figure 7.13)

Meaning of the āsana and its name

Ardha means half, and candra is the moon. The different positions while going from Utthita Trikoṇāsana to Ardha Candrāsana are reminiscent of different shapes of the moon. Practicing this is good training in staying stable and calm during changes. Ardha Candrāsana develops stability during moving, and harmony between what we feel and what we are doing. It teaches coordination and synchronization between the actions of the legs and arms.

Getting into the posture

1. Stand in Tāḍāsana.
2. Go into Utthita Trikoṇāsana to the right.

3. Bending your right knee in the plane of your right little toe, place your right hand on the floor or on a brick in line with the right little toe one foot length away; the left heel is lifting and the foot is sliding closer to the right foot.

4. Rest your left arm on your left trunk side; look towards the floor.

5. As you exhale straighten your right leg while lifting your left one; move your right sitting bone forwards.

6. Keep the weight in the right heel and the right big toe; the toes, the middle of the kneecap, and the middle of the right thigh are facing exactly the same way; keeping the right knee firm and moving the thigh muscles upwards, turn your pelvis to the left, turn your thorax to the left, and lift your left shoulder so that the shoulder girdle is in line with the right arm.

7. Keep your head in line with your spine; feel a continuous stretch from your left foot to the crown of your head.

8. If you can keep your balance, stretch your left arm up in line with the shoulder girdle.

9. If you can still keep your balance, turn your head to look up at your left hand.

Being in the posture: basic work

1. Keep the weight in the front of your right heel and in the big toe.

2. Pull the right kneecap upwards.

3. Move the outer upper right thigh towards the inner upper right thigh.

4. Maintaining this action of the right thigh, lift your left hip, turn the lower abdomen, the ribs, and the shoulders to the left.

5. Feel the length of your spine and the continuous stretch from the left heel to the crown of your head.

6. Have a continuous stretch through your arms and shoulder girdle.

7. If you cannot balance, turn your head to look towards the floor; you can also rest your left arm on the left side of your trunk.

8. Breathe naturally.

Being in the posture: refined work

1. Lift from your inner and outer ankle when you turn your pelvis to the left.

2. Coordinate the external rotation of your right thigh and the rotation of the lower abdomen.

3. Coordinate the stretching of the right and left leg.

4. Keep your trunk long between the pelvis and the shoulder girdle.

5. Lift your shoulder girdle away from your right arm.

6. Lengthen from your upper sternum through your left clavicle into your left arm, wrist, palm, and fingers; keep the fingers together.

7. Adjust your head in line with your spine, and slightly shift it backwards, keeping the neck and throat comfortable.

8. Maintain awareness of your legs and arms and the line of your spine when you turn your head to look upwards towards the thumb.

9. Breathe naturally.

Finishing the posture

In the beginning staying for 2–3 breaths may be enough; with practice you may increase up to 10 breaths. Exhale, bend your right knee exactly in line with the right foot, come back to Utthita Trikoṇāsana, and then to a standing position with the legs apart and the feet parallel. Repeat on the other side. After finishing both sides stay calmly in Tāḍāsana for a few breaths.

Suggestions for modifications using props

- Perform with your back against a wall.

- Support your lower hand on a brick or on a chair depending on your flexibility (Figures 7.13 and 7.14).

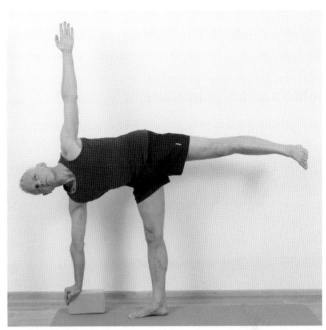

Figure 7.13

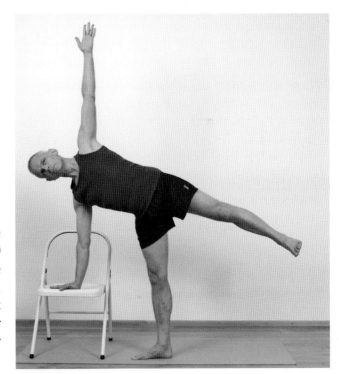

Figure 7.14

7. Parīghāsana (Figure 7.18)

Meaning of the āsana and its name

Parīgha is an oblique beam closing a gate. This posture resembles a gate with an oblique beam. The straight leg is the beam, the trunk is an arch, the top of the gate, and the core of the arch is the spine in side-bending.

Getting into the posture

1. Prepare a folded blanket if you need a support for your lower legs and a brick on your right side.

2. Kneel with your knees and feet close together; press your shin bones and metatarsals into the blanket (Figure 7.15).

3. Keeping your pelvis in the center, lift your right leg, turn it 90° outwards, with the knee and the foot exactly pointing to the right side (Figure 7.16).

4. Adjust your right, bent leg exactly in line with the left thigh and the pelvis.

5. Keeping your left thigh vertical, and your right sitting bone forwards, stretch your right leg to the side in the plane of the left thigh and the trunk (Figure 7.17).

6. Turn it out from the hip socket so that the center of the thigh, the kneecap, and the toes are facing towards the ceiling; rest the ball of the right foot on the brick; control the movement so that the left thigh stays vertical.

7. Put your right palm on your right leg; slightly turn your thorax to the left, so that your abdomen and your chest are exactly facing forwards.

8. Keeping your left hip stable and sliding your right palm down on the right leg, bend to the right as you exhale as long as your trunk stays in the plane of the right leg: moving your right groin down, bend from the pelvis first, then from your waist, then your thorax, and finally the head.

9. To avoid too much compression of the right trunk side, slightly lengthen it while you push yourself off the right shin bone to turn your trunk.

10. Extend your left arm over your left ear, with the palm facing the floor (Figure 7.18).

Being in the posture: basic work

1. Press the back of your left foot and the left shin bone into the blanket.

2. Keep your left thigh strong, the back of the upper right thigh towards the hip joint.

3. Keep the right knee firm.

4. Slightly turn your abdomen and thorax to the left and lift your shoulder girdle off the right arm.

5. Breathe naturally; feel the lengthening of your left side ribs during inhalation.

Being in the posture: refined work

1. Suck your right kneecap into the right thigh.

2. If your knee is overextended slightly relax from the full extension.

3. Very gently move your lower abdomen inwards and upwards.

4. Refine the lengthening of the left side during exhalation by extending your left arm even more as you exhale.

5. Be aware of the side-bending of your head to the right; combine it with turning it to the left as long as your neck and throat are comfortable.

Finishing the posture

Stay in the posture for 5–10 breaths. Move your right foot off the brick into dorsiflexion, pull your right kneecap and thigh upwards, inhale, bring your trunk upright (Figure 7.17). Bend your right knee and kneel on both knees. Repeat on the left side.

Suggestions for modifications using props

• Try different heights for the support of the foot of the straight leg.

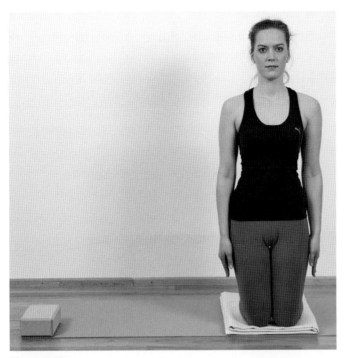

Figure 7.15

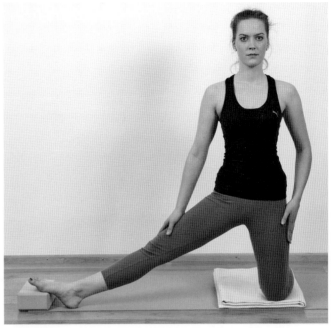

Figure 7.17

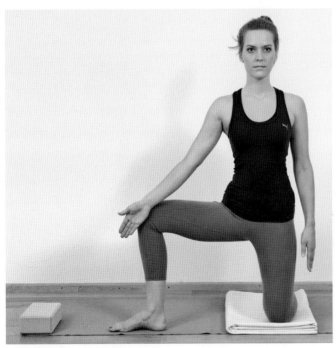

Figure 7.16

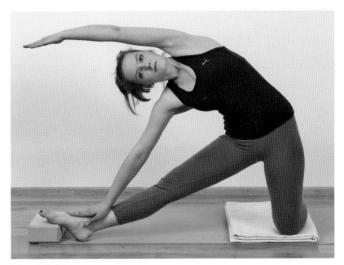

Figure 7.18

- Put the ball of your right foot on a wall or column, rest the right hand on that wall, with the right arm nearly horizontal. If the left fingertips can reach the wall, you can use the left arm as a lever to turn (Figure 7.19).

Variations

- If your shoulder can take it, turn your upper arm so that the palm is facing the ceiling to get a stronger stretch for the upper side of your trunk.

- If possible you can rest the foot of the straight leg flat on the floor.

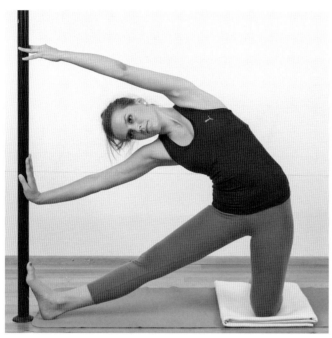

Figure 7.19

8. Pārśvottānāsana (Figures 7.20 and 7.21)

Meaning of the āsana and its name

Pārśva is side, uttāna means extending intensively. Pārśvottānāsana is an intensive stretch, particularly of the sides of the thorax, but also of the whole body, while being firmly on the feet.

Getting into the posture

1. Stand in Tāḍāsana.

2. Turn your arms inwards and move them backwards; join your palms behind your back, with the fingers pointing towards the floor first.

3. Turn your hands, with the fingers towards the back first, then pointing upwards.

4. Maintaining a neutral lumbopelvic position, move your shoulders and elbows back and the little fingers upwards along the spine to the level of the shoulder blades as high as you can.

5. Feel the stretch from your sternum to your upper ribs, clavicles, and upper arms.

6. Walk your feet one leg length apart.

7. Turn the right foot and leg 90° outwards, the left foot and leg 75° inwards; the left heel is in line with the right foot; turn your pelvis and trunk

90° to the right; in both legs the center of the thighs, the kneecaps, and the toes are pointing in the same direction.

8. Maintaining the neutral lumbopelvic position lift from your lower abdomen and lift your chest, the upper thoracic vertebrae inwards and the upper sternum upwards and slightly forwards.

9. Lengthen gently from your upper neck to the back of your head; extend your head backwards as far as comfortable and look upwards (Figure 7.20).

10. Stay there for 2–3 breaths.

11. Bring your head in line with your spine.

12. Be firm in your left leg; the outer edge of the foot is pressing on the floor.

13. Keeping your right big toe on the floor and moving the right outer thigh towards the right inner thigh, bend over the right knee as you exhale (Figure 7.21).

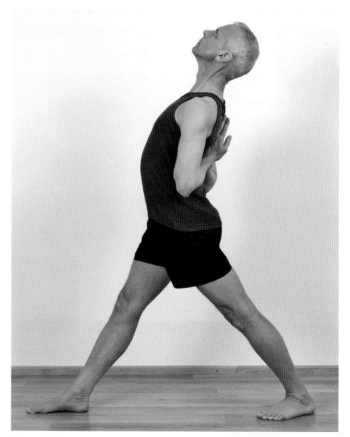

Figure 7.20

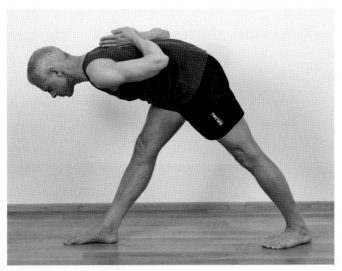

Figure 7.21

Being in the posture: basic work

1. Shift the weight on the outer left foot and right heel.

2. Move the left hip forwards and the right hip backwards.

3. Gently play with the rotation of your pelvis until the central line of your trunk is exactly in line with the front leg.

4. Lengthen from your lower abdomen to your sternum.

5. Move your elbows backwards and upwards, towards the ceiling.

6. Lengthen your spine and the back of your head.

7. Breathe naturally.

Being in the posture: refined work

1. Lift the inner arch of your left foot; resist from the outer ankle to keep the ankle joint stable.

2. Pull the left kneecap into the left upper thigh and move the left inner thigh backwards.

3. Keep your right big toe stretched and firmly on the floor; keep the right ankles stable, the right kneecap pulled upwards; slightly externally rotate the right thigh.

4. Slightly turn your abdomen towards the right thigh.

5. Inhaling, lengthen your thorax and the front of your spine; exhaling, bend further down and lengthen the back of your spine.

6. Relax from your neck to the back of your head.

Finishing the posture

With an inhalation lift your trunk upright, turn your feet parallel, and turn your pelvis and trunk to the center. If necessary relax your arms. Perform to the left side. After finishing both sides come back to Tāḍāsana, and stay calm for a few breaths.

Suggestions for modifications using props

- To help the alignment put a belt on the floor; have the front foot close to the belt on one side and the rear foot close to the belt on the other side.

- Rest your hands on bricks or on a higher support if you need it (Figure 7.22).

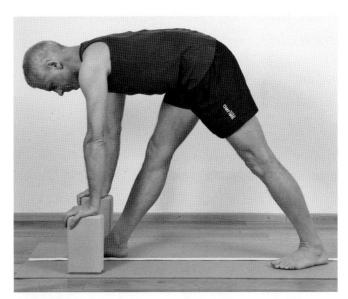

Figure 7.22

Variations

If it is not possible to fold your palms on your back, you can practice Pārśvottānāsana:

- with the hands holding your elbows on your back

- with the back of your hands together, the fingers pointing upwards.

169

9. Vīrabhadrāsana I (Figure 7.23)

Meaning of the āsana and its name

Vīrabhadrāsana I is the first of the three āsanas dedicated to the powerful hero Vīrabhadra of ancient Indian mythology. It is performed with strength while at the same time being relaxed.

Getting into the posture

1. Stand in Tāḍāsana.

2. Walk your feet one leg length plus one foot length apart; feet are parallel, the arches of the feet are active.

3. Slightly lift from your lower abdomen, raise your arms to the sides in line with the shoulder girdle, and turn the arms from the shoulder joints so that the palms are facing the ceiling.

4. Maintaining a neutral lumbopelvic position, elevate your arms vertically and keep them parallel.

5. Turn the right foot and leg 90° outwards, the left foot and leg 45–60° inwards, and your pelvis and trunk 90° to the right; the left heel is in line

with the right foot; in both legs the center of the thighs, the kneecaps, and the toes are pointing in the same direction.

6. The central front line of the trunk and the tip of the nose are facing exactly forwards.

7. Be firm in your back leg and maintain the alignment, exhale and bend your right knee until the shin bone is vertical.

8. Adjust your pelvis, thorax, and elevated arms so that you are comfortable throughout the spine.

9. Join your palms, if you can keep your elbows straight.

10. Gently lengthen from the upper neck to the back of your head; extend your head backwards as far as comfortable, but you may like to keep your head upright.

Being in the posture: basic work

1. Press the outer edge of the left foot towards the floor.

2. Keep the left knee straight.

3. Keeping the right big toe on the floor and the weight in the right heel, move the right knee towards the plane of the right little toe.

4. Maintain the rotation of the pelvis; move your sacrum down and in, the lower abdomen slightly inwards and upwards.

5. Lift your thorax up and the upper part slightly forwards to stay comfortable in the lumbar area, and to have a continuous stretch through your spine.

6. Move your shoulder blades into the thorax to widen the upper chest from there.

7. Elevate your arms further to lift the side ribs more.

8. Breathe naturally.

Being in the posture: refined work

1. Lift from your left inner arch throughout your left inner leg, move the front and inner left thigh backwards, and slightly turn your left hip forwards.

2. Move your sacrum down and inwards.

3. Move your right groin in and down, keep it soft.

4. Slightly turn your right hip backwards.

5. Lift the front hip bones away from the thighs.

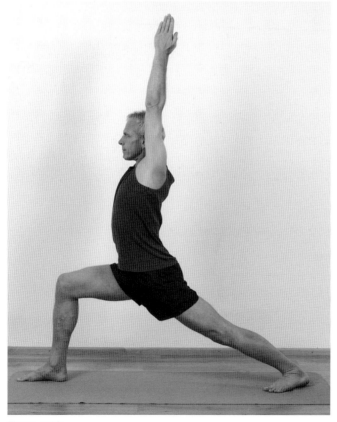

Figure 7.23

6. Gently pull the area below your navel inwards and towards your upper lumbar spine; feel the effect of this on your lumbar spine.

7. Move your upper thoracic vertebrae inwards to lift your sternum and upper front ribs.

8. If you have moved your head backwards, relax the head extension a tiny bit by moving the back of the head slightly away from the neck.

9. Relax your face.

10. Breathe naturally and subtly.

Finishing the posture

Hold the posture for 2–3 breaths in the beginning; increase to 5–10 breaths with practice.

Bring your head in line with your spine. With an inhalation straighten your right knee, and turn your pelvis and trunk to the center, feet parallel. If necessary, relax your arms.

Repeat on the left side. After finishing both sides come back to Tāḍāsana, and stay calm for a few breaths.

Suggestions for modifications using props

• Hold a brick between your upper shin bone and a wall or pillar; this keeps your bent knee well aligned throughout all adjustments. Hold your hands on your hips and your thumbs on your middle sacrum to encourage the slight inwards and downwards movement of the sacrum (Figure 7.24).

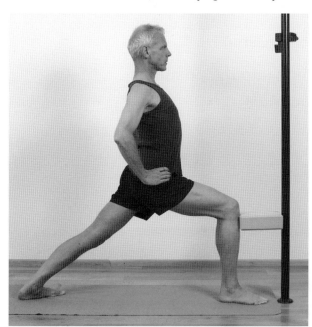

Figure 7.24

• If you cannot bring the rear heel onto the floor, rest it on a rolled mat; gradually decrease the height of the roll.

Variations

• Keep your head in line with your spine.

• Hold your hands on your hips, with your thumbs on your middle sacrum (Figure 7.24).

• Use less distance for your feet, about one leg length.

10. Vīrabhadrāsana III (Figure 7.25)

Meaning of the āsana and its name

Vīrabhadrāsana III is the third of the three āsanas dedicated to the powerful hero Vīrabhadra of ancient Indian mythology. It is performed with strength while at the same time being centered and relaxed. Vīrabhadrāsana III develops strength and balance while moving. It teaches coordination and the synchronization of movements and calms the mind.

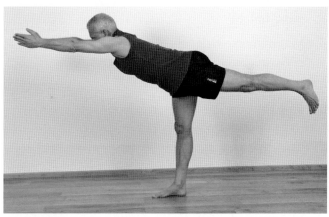

Figure 7.25

Getting into the posture

1. Stand in Tāḍāsana.

2. Go into Vīrabhadrāsana I to the right.

3. With an exhalation, bend forwards to bring your trunk close to the right thigh; move the upper right thigh into the hip joint.

4. Turn your left leg further inwards so that the heel is coming off the floor and the middle of the thigh, the kneecap, and the toes are facing the floor.

5. Keep your right foot balanced between inner and outer ankle, the right knee bent towards the right little toe.

6. Feel the center of gravity inside your pelvis.

7. From this center lengthen backwards into the left leg and to the front into the arms; at the same time shift your weight forwards, lift your left foot off the floor, and straighten your right leg, so that you stay balanced in this center.

8. Lift the right inner and outer ankle, stretch the right leg, pull the kneecap upwards; the inner and outer thigh are equally active.

9. Lift your inner left thigh higher.

10. Adjust your pelvis horizontally; bring your left leg, trunk, and arms in a horizontal line; raise your head as long as the neck is comfortable.

Being in the posture: basic work

1. Maintain the balance between the right inner and outer ankle.

2. Keep the right leg firm; both hips are at the same height.

3. Maintain the balanced stretch of the left leg backwards and the trunk and arms forwards.

4. Adjust your head so that the neck is gently stretched.

5. Feel the continuous stretch from your left heel to the fingertips.

6. Breathe naturally.

Being in the posture: refined work

1. Move your shoulder blades in; turn your arms in your shoulder joints to bring your little fingers slightly closer together; this helps to move the arms higher.

2. Maintaining a subtle length from the upper neck to the back of the head, raise your head to look towards your thumbs.

3. Slightly pulling your lower abdomen inwards, move the front of your left thigh towards the back; the left toes remain pointing towards the floor.

4. Move your left leg away from the hip and slightly higher.

5. Turn your left hip away from the sacrum; move your left inner upper thigh upwards.

Finishing the posture

With an exhalation bend your right knee, come back to Vīrabhadrāsana I, straighten the right leg, and turn to the center. Relax your arms if necessary. Repeat on the left side. After finishing both sides come back to Tāḍasana; stay there calmly for a few breaths.

Suggestions for modifications using props

Rest your hands or your hands and your lifted foot on a support. This helps to get the alignment and the adjustments with greater precision.

Variations

- Four-point kneeling with one arm and one leg lifted is a very helpful preparation for Vīrabhadrāsana III (see Chapter 6, exercise 1.14).

- Holding the arms to the sides in line with the shoulder girdle helps you to balance.

- If you cannot stretch the leg on which you are standing, slightly bend the knee. Maintain the correct alignment, with the kneecap pointing in exactly the same direction as the toes and moving upwards.

11. Parivṛtta Trikoṇāsana (Figure 7.26)

Meaning of the āsana and its name

Parivṛtta means turned around, trikoṇa is the triangle. In this āsana the trunk is turned on a solid, triangle-shaped base. The core is the rotation of the spine in a clear alignment.

Getting into the posture

1. Stand in Tāḍasana.

2. Walk your feet one leg length apart.

3. Stretch your arms to the sides in line with the shoulder girdle.

4. Turn the right foot and leg 90° outwards, the left foot and leg 45–60° inwards, and your pelvis and trunk 90° to the right; the left heel is in line with the right foot; in both legs the front of the thighs, the kneecaps, and the toes are pointing into the same direction.

5. Keep your left leg firm; press the outer edge of the foot on the floor.

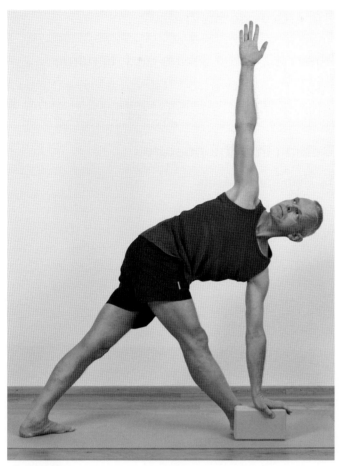

Figure 7.26

4. Feel the length of your spine.

5. Keep your head in line with your spine; shift it slightly backwards.

6. Turn your head, and look towards your right thumb.

7. Breathe naturally.

Being in the posture: refined work

1. Lift your left inner arch; from there lift and strengthen the whole left leg.

2. Suck the left kneecap into the left thigh; move the front and inner left thigh backwards.

3. Lengthen and turn one segment of your spine after the other; this is supported by moving the hips closer together and the left upper outer thigh inwards.

4. Lengthen the front of your trunk.

5. Gently turn your abdomen and your diaphragm.

6. Move your left shoulder blade away from your spine; this may be supported by moving the left hand on the floor or with the brick to the right, several centimeters away from the right foot, then move this shoulder blade inwards.

7. Extend your right arm further up as if starting the stretch from your upper sternum through your right upper ribs and clavicle.

8. Feel the turning of your head starting from your upper thoracic vertebrae, maintaining a subtle length into the back of your head.

9. Let your breath be subtle and steady.

Finishing the posture

With an inhalation come up with your trunk, with the arms to the sides in line with your shoulder girdle. Turn to the center and keep your feet parallel. If necessary relax your arms for a moment. Repeat on the left side. After finishing both sides come back to Tāḍāsana, and stay there calmly for a few breaths.

6. With an exhalation bend forwards from your hips and turn your trunk from your hips to bring your left hand beside the right outer heel on the floor or on a brick or on the lower leg above the outer ankle.

7. The left arm, the shoulder girdle, and the right arm are in one line, together with the head in the plane of the front leg.

8. Turn your spine from the bottom to the top.

Being in the posture: basic work

1. If the left leg is not turned inwards enough, slightly lift your left heel and move it outwards as far as necessary, then bring it back to the floor.

2. Keep the left leg firm, press the outer edge of the foot on the floor, and keep the knee straight.

3. As long as you can maintain this firmness in the left leg, turn from your pelvis; turn your ribs and your shoulders to the right, so that your left ear is in line with your right big toe.

Suggestions for modifications using props

- Rest the lower hand on a brick or chair, with the upper hand on the lower back.

- Stand close to a table with your back towards the table. Build up the twist to face the table (Figure 7.27).

- Stand close to a table, facing the table first. Build up the twist so that your back is towards the table, your hands or arms are resting on the table (Figure 7.28).

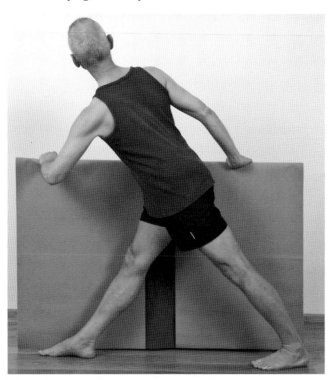

Figure 7.27

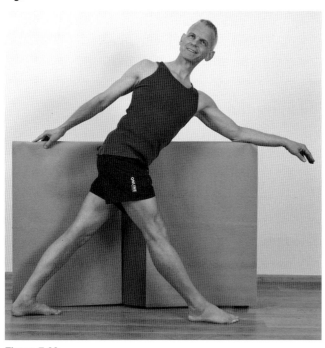

Figure 7.28

12. Utkaṭāsana (Figure 7.29)

Meaning of the āsana and its name

Utkaṭa means powerful. Utkaṭāsana is like sitting on a high chair. It is strengthening the ankle and knee joints. It teaches lifting the spine, thorax, and arms against gravity.

Getting into the posture

1. Stand in Tāḍāsana.

2. Elevate your arms.

3. Join the palms if this is possible with straight arms; otherwise leave the arms parallel, with the palms facing each other.

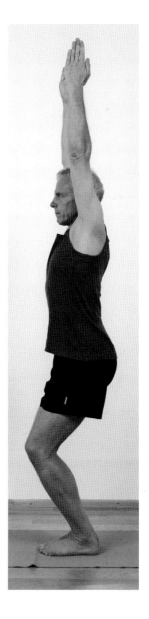

Figure 7.29

4. Keeping the arches of your feet strong and the inner and outer ankles at the same level, bend your knees as long as the heels stay on the floor and the trunk and arms remain lifted.

Being in the posture: basic work

1. Have slightly more weight on the heels than on the forefoot.

2. Adjust the angle of the knees so that the knees are comfortable.

3. Maintaining a neutral lumbopelvic position, gently move your lower abdomen inwards and upwards, your shoulder blades and your upper thoracic spine in and up.

4. Balance your head so that the neck and throat are comfortable.

5. Breathe naturally.

Being in the posture: refined work

1. Stretch your toes; keep the arches of your feet strong; the shin bones active, moving away from the back of the feet; the weight shifting more into your heels; bend your knees a little more as long as the Achilles tendons are well aligned and the calf muscles are giving more stretch.

2. Lift the hip bones and the abdomen slightly upwards and backwards.

3. Balance the leaning forwards of the trunk with moving the abdomen, the costal arches, and the arms backwards.

4. Maintaining the position of the chin, slightly shift the head backwards.

5. Relax your face and eyes; breathe naturally.

Finishing the posture

Stay in the posture for 5–10 breaths. With an inhalation straighten your legs, relax your arms, and stay calmly in Tāḍāsana for a few breaths.

Suggestions for modifications using props

Keep your arms parallel, the palms facing forwards, resting them on a wall (Figure 7.30).

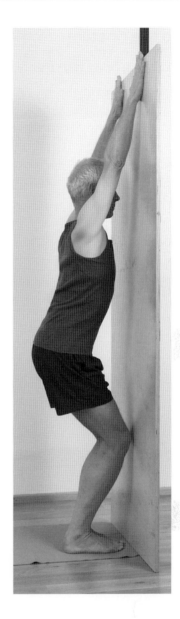

Figure 7.30

13. Uttānāsana (Figure 7.31)

Meaning of the āsana and its name

Uttāna is an intensive stretch. This posture gives an intensive lengthening from the feet through the legs, from the pelvis through the trunk into the head and arms, all while standing firm on both feet. In his book *Light on Yoga* (Iyengar 2001) B K S Iyengar also mentions the meaning "deliberation" of "ut."

If the posture is held for at least 2 minutes, it helps to calm the mind and aids recovery.

Getting into the posture

1. Stand in Tāḍāsana; bring your feet hip width apart.

2. Keeping your knees straight, elevate your arms, palms facing forwards, exhale and tilt your pelvis forwards to bend forwards; place your hands in front or to the left and right of your feet on the floor (Figure 7.31) or each hand on a brick if you need it.

3. Lengthen the front of your trunk, raise the head starting from your upper thoracic vertebrae, and make the back concave; stay there for 2 breaths.

4. Keeping the heels firmly on the floor, shift more weight into the front feet, until your legs are vertical; move the front of your pelvis and your abdomen towards your thighs.

5. Maintaining the length of your front trunk gently lengthen from the tailbone throughout the back of your spine to the back of your head.

6. Move your hands further back.

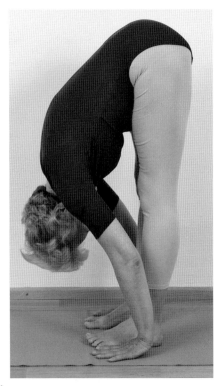

Figure 7.31

Being in the posture: basic work

1. Keep your toes stretched.

2. Balance your inner and outer ankles.

3. Balance the weight between the back of the balls of the feet and the front of the heels.

4. Keep your knees straight; pull your kneecaps up with a very gentle, smooth movement.

5. Move your sitting bones upwards from the middle of the back of your thighs.

6. Move your front and side ribs towards the floor.

7. Relax your abdomen and throat.

8. Breathe naturally.

Being in the posture: refined work

1. Lift your inner and outer arches, at the same time lengthening the soles of the feet into the toes and the heels.

2. Lengthen from your inner ankles to the big toes; keep the big toes on the floor.

3. Feel the inner length from your feet through the legs to the hips, from the tailbone through the whole spine.

4. Combine the upwards movement of the thigh muscles and the kneecaps with easing from the knee extension very slightly to get a well-balanced stretch of your knees.

5. Broaden the back of your knee.

6. Lengthen and broaden the back of your thighs.

7. Relax your abdomen.

8. Let your diaphragm move towards the floor – during exhalation this comes naturally.

9. Let your side and front ribs move further towards the floor – this is a natural action with inhalation.

10. Adjust the head so that your neck and throat are relaxed.

11. Finetune your breath to a subtle flow.

Finishing the posture

Inhale, lengthen the front of your trunk, lift your head accordingly; keeping your knees straight, pull your front thigh muscles upwards, inhale and lift your trunk with elevated arms with strength in your outer upper thighs and front hip bones, lifting these hip bones away from the thighs. With an exhalation relax your arms and stay calm in Tāḍāsana for a few breaths. Alternatively you can rest your hands on your hips to come back.

Suggestions for modifications using props

- Rest your hands on a chair or on a table (Figure 7.34).
- Rest your folded arms on a chair or on a table (Figure 7.35).

Variations

- Practice with your feet one foot length apart and your arms folded (Figures 7.32 and 7.33).
- Keeping the feet 1½–2 foot lengths apart gives more mobility in the area of the sacrum.
- Side-bending variation (Figure 7.36):
  - Stay firmly on your feet; maintain the position of your legs and pelvis.
  - Walk your fingertips to the right side to side-bend your spine to the right and stretch your left side from the hip to the hand.

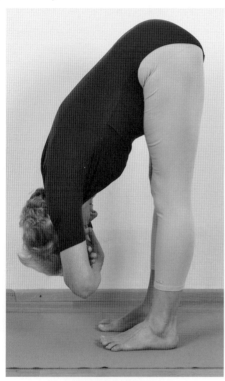

Figure 7.32

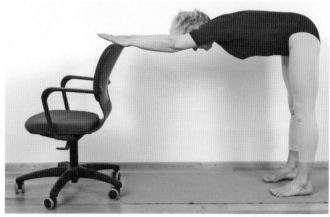

Figure 7.34

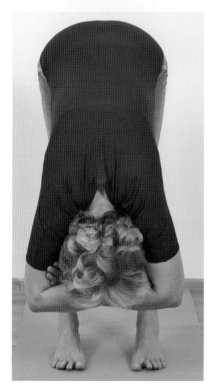

Figure 7.33

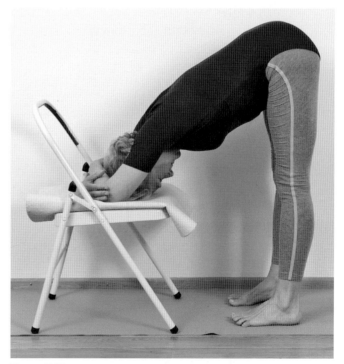

Figure 7.35

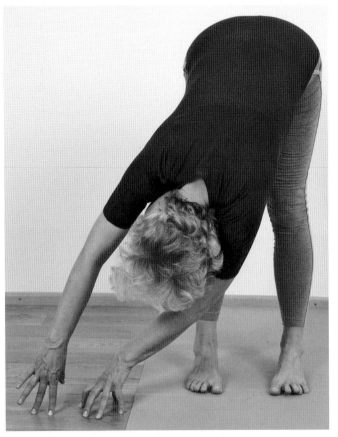

Figure 7.36

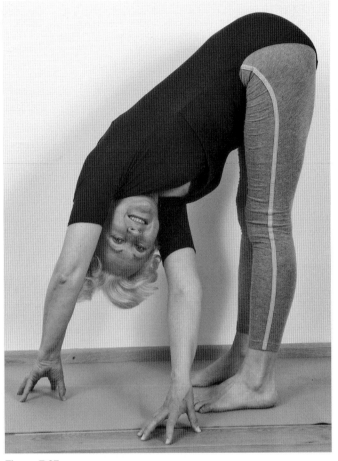

Figure 7.37

- If you need a brick or a chair, adjust the props so that you can rest your hands on the support to side-bend accordingly.

- Hold for two breaths.

- Repeat the side-bending to the left.

- Perform both sides 2–3 times.

- Rotation variation (Figures 7.37 and 7.38):

  - Place your right hand in front and left of the left foot; move your left arm over the right and place the fingers approximately in front of the right foot.

  - Turn your head, shoulder girdle, and spine to the left; go as far as you can while breathing naturally.

  - Stay there for 2–3 breaths.

  - Swap your hands and arms; repeat the rotation to the other side.

  - Perform both sides 2–3 times.

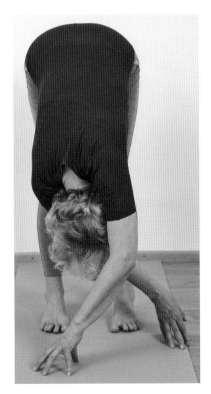

Figure 7.38

14. Adho Mukha Śvānāsana

Meaning of the āsana and its name

Downward-facing dog (Figure 7.39)

This posture is generally mobilizing and strengthening; it improves coordination and stamina. The lumbar spine is getting more forward-bending, the thoracic spine more back-bending; therefore the dorsolumbar junction is particularly mobilized. Adho Mukha Śvānāsana is a very good substitute for inversions for those who are not able to do them. It helps to improve awareness of the whole body and calms the heart.

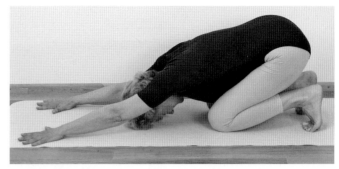
Figure 7.40

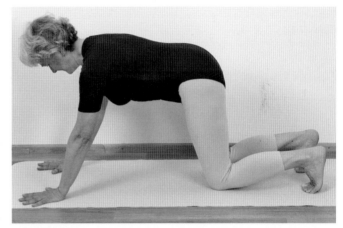
Figure 7.41

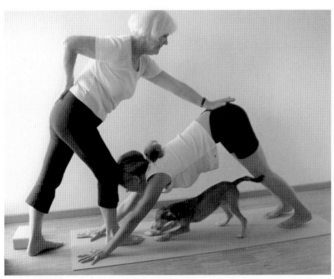
Figure 7.39

Getting into the posture

1. Start in a four-point kneeling position; use a folded blanket underneath your knees if you need it; the knees and feet are hip width apart; place your feet perpendicular to the floor, the toes pointing towards the hands, the arms at shoulder width and parallel.

2. To adjust the distance of the hands from the feet move your pelvis backwards as far as possible towards your heels; stretch your arms forwards from your ribs, maintaining the distance of the hands (Figure 7.40).

3. Keeping the feet, knees, and hands in position, come back to four-point kneeling; the hands will be more forward now than the shoulders (Figure 7.41).

4. Slightly adjust the hands so that the index fingers are parallel, the fingers are well spread, all fingers are at the same distance, while the thumbs are spread further away from the index fingers. To get a slightly different, stronger action in your arms and shoulders turn your middle fingers parallel for the second go.

5. Lift your head to move your upper thoracic vertebrae inwards; move your shoulder blades inwards.

6. Keep your palms and fingers in contact with the floor, particularly the thumbs and index fingers and the area in between; push yourself up into the pose, using the strength of your legs (Figure 7.42).

7. The heels can be lifted in the beginning, with the shin bones and the front of the thighs moving backwards.

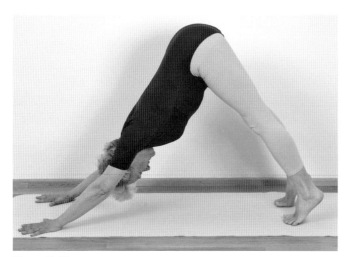

Figure 7.42

Being in the posture: basic work

1. Be strong in your legs; the shin bones and the front of the thighs are moving backwards.

2. Push yourself up from your palms and fingers, particularly the thumbs and index fingers; feel the lifting against gravity up to your hips.

3. Keep your head in line with your spine, between your upper arms; keep your neck and throat comfortable.

4. Move your chest towards your thighs.

5. Maintaining the lifting from the hands to the hips, move your heels as close as possible towards the floor, keeping the feet parallel and the arches of the feet active (Figure 7.43).

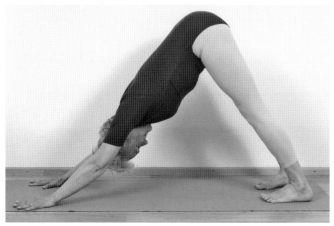

Figure 7.43

6. If the feet have reached their final position, lift your shin bones away from the feet and move the front of your thighs towards the back of your thighs.

7. Breathe naturally.

8. Stay for 5–10 breaths.

Being in the posture: refined work

1. Move the front of your thighs towards the back of your thighs, and the inner thighs backwards as well; counterbalance this action with a slight external rotation of the thighs and a slight movement of the lower abdomen towards the back of the pelvis.

2. Keep the shin bones moving backwards and the kneecaps sucked into the lower thighs; let the back of the knees move a tiny fraction towards the front, keeping the back of the knees broad.

3. Refine pushing up from the thumbs, from the index fingers, from the middle fingers, from the ring fingers, from the little fingers; feel the different effects on the stretching of the arms, the movement of the shoulder blades, and the lifting of the trunk, the inner movement against gravity.

4. Slightly press the fingers into the floor to get some isometric action in your palms and fingers; slightly lift the wrists off the floor, play with hollowing the carpal tunnels and stretching them again; feel the effect on lifting the lower arms and the elbows.

5. Balance your elbows between hyperextension and a tiny flexion; be firm above the elbows.

6. Maintaining the lifting from the hands, particularly from the thumbs and index fingers, slightly turn your upper arms away from the shoulders; feel the release and the space this creates for your neck and between your shoulder blades.

7. Vary the position of your head gently; slightly lift it from the area between your shoulder blades to encourage the back-bending action of the thoracic spine.

8. Combine the movement of the upper sternum towards your hands and the costal arches slightly

inwards; feel the release in the upper lumbar and lower thoracic area.

9. The heels are moving more and more towards the floor, inner arches and inner ankles lifted, outer arches and outer ankles lifted; toes are well stretched.

10. If the heels are on the floor, balance the weight between the back part of the balls of the feet and the front part of the heels.

11. With practice you can increase the time you stay in the posture.

Finishing the posture

With an exhalation come down to four-point kneeling; put the back of the feet on the floor, the toes pointing backwards. Bring your pelvis as close as is comfortable for the knees towards your heels. Bend forwards, and rest your forehead on the floor or on your hands or lower arms (see Chapter 6, Figure 6.16). Stay calm for a few breaths.

Suggestions for modifications using props

- Hands on bricks (Figure 7.44): grip a brick with each hand, preferably with the thumbs around the inner border, index and middle fingers around the front, ring and little fingers around the outer border of the bricks. The pushing off the floor is achieved by gripping the bricks and pushing them into the floor. All other previous instructions can be followed.

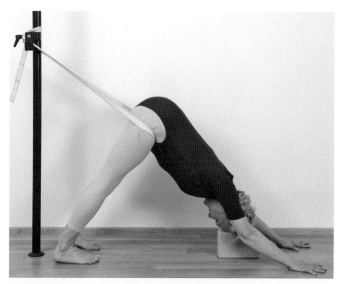

Figure 7.45

- Hanging in a rope or belt (Figure 7.45): fix a rope or a belt on a handle of an open door, using both sides of the handle; the handle must be higher than your pelvis. Adjust the length of the rope so that it fits your angle of your dog pose. Put the rope exactly into your groins. You can perform any instruction given for the work in the posture and relax and be calm at the same time. Resting the head on a brick or firm pillow makes the posture even more calming.

Variations

Side-bending (Figures 7.46 and 7.47)

1. Perform dog pose with heels on the floor or on a support, according to how far you can stretch the backs of the legs.

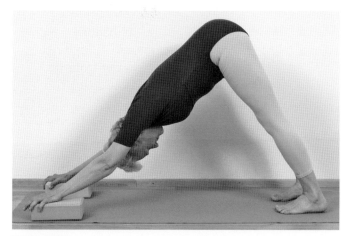

Figure 7.44

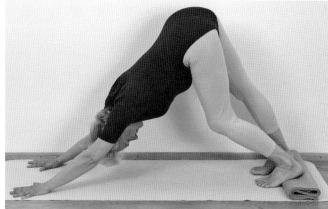

Figure 7.46

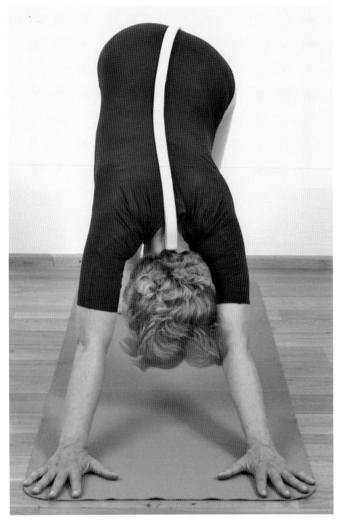

Figure 7.47

2. Bend both knees slightly.

3. Keeping the heels on the support, fully stretch the right knee to lift the right hip for a side-bending action to the left.

4. To get a stronger side-bending, side-bend your head towards the left arm.

5. Hold for 3 breaths.

6. Come back to the center by bending the right knee again and repeat on the other side.

7. Perform both sides 2–3 times.

8. Come back to the posture shown in Figure 7.40, but put the back of the feet on the floor.

Rotation (Figure 7.48)

1. Perform the dog pose with the heels on the floor or on a support.

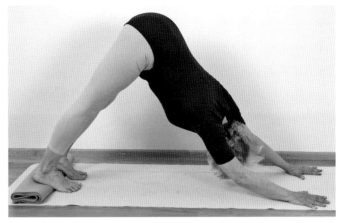

Figure 7.48

2. Keep your legs and hips firm; the hips are at the same height throughout the exercise.

3. Bend your right elbow one-third towards the floor and turn your head to the left until you have reached the optimal rotation.

4. Hold for 3 breaths.

5. Stretch your right arm and repeat on the other side.

6. Practice both sides 2–3 times.

7. Come back to the posture shown in Figure 7.40, but put the back of the feet on the floor.

15. Bakāsana (Figure 7.49)

Meaning of the āsana and its name

Baka is a crane. The posture balancing on the hands is reminiscent of a bird supported on its legs.

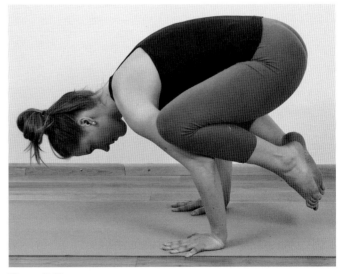

Figure 7.49

This posture particularly strengthens the wrists and hands, and mobilizes the spine into forward bending. It teaches balance, moving and holding against gravity, and a stable center and strength of the abdomen. Enjoying practice is an essential aspect of the posture.

Getting into the posture

1. Go into squatting position, the feet together and on the floor; if necessary slightly lift the heels.
2. The pelvis is off the floor.
3. Stretch your arms parallel, horizontally forwards.
4. Move your knees apart and your trunk in between your thighs.
5. Raise your heels.
6. Bend your elbows; move them underneath your shin bones backwards; put your palms on the floor and press your shin bones onto your upper arms, as close as possible to the armpits.
7. Shift your trunk forwards to find the optimum balance in this posture; stay there for 2–3 breaths.
8. Constantly adjusting your balance and moving your knees towards your armpits, straighten your arms more to lift your feet off the floor; you may lift one foot first, then the other one.

Being in the posture: basic work

1. Move your feet towards your buttocks, particularly from the inner arches.
2. Push your knees towards your shoulders.
3. Move your abdomen towards your back, and round your back.
4. To raise further, stretch your arms more; keep your pelvis at the same level.
5. Breathe naturally.

Being in the posture: refined work

1. Play with the point of balance.

2. Make the arms firmer and firmer, the trunk and legs lighter and lighter.
3. Feel the lifting of your legs in the arches of your feet.
4. Make your inner thighs strong.
5. Feel the length of the back of your spine in the round back.
6. Adjust the position of your head so that your neck and throat are comfortable.

Finishing the posture

Stay for 2–5 breaths. Exhale, bend your elbows to get your feet down, straighten your knees to go into Uttānāsana; stay calm for a few breaths. Repeat Bakāsana two or three times.

Suggestions for modifications using props

- Support your heels with a rolled towel or mat in the squatting position.
- Rest your buttocks on a brick or low stool in the squatting position.
- Support your buttocks and backs of the thighs with a chair; place your hands on bricks to learn the posture supported first (Figure 7.50).

Variation

Start with very short periods of balancing, like hopping.

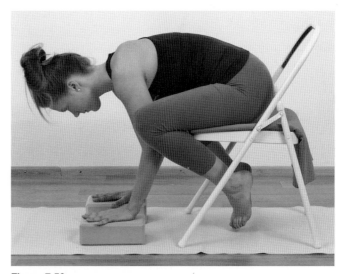

Figure 7.50

16. Sukhāsana (Figure 7.51)

Meaning of the āsana and its name

Sukha means easy; sukhāsana is an easy cross-legged sitting position. It improves mobility of the hip joints, and combines sitting upright with being relaxed and calm.

Getting into the posture

1. Sit with straight legs on a brick or a folded blanket.
2. Bring your right foot underneath your left knee, your left lower leg in front of the right shin bone, and the left foot underneath the right knee; the crossing of your lower legs is in line with the center of your body.
3. Place your hands or fingertips beside your hips; without moving your pelvis push yourself up from the fingertips to lift your spine and thorax.
4. Maintaining your trunk lifted, rest your hands on your knees (Figure 7.51).

Being in the posture: basic work

1. Adjust your pelvis in the neutral position.
2. Keep your lower abdomen slightly inwards and upwards while you lift your chest more.
3. Relax your shoulders and upper arms.
4. Keep your head in line with your spine.
5. Breathe naturally.

Being in the posture: refined work

1. Lift yourself as if pushing up from the sitting bones; raise your side and front ribs, move your middle thoracic vertebrae inwards; these actions come naturally as you inhale.
2. Lift the center of your thorax and the center of your pelvic floor; this comes naturally with exhalation.
3. Without tucking in your chin slightly lengthen the back of your head away from the neck; feel how this also lifts your front upper ribs.
4. Turn your arms so that the palms are facing the ceiling; feel the effect on your upper chest.
5. Breathe naturally.

Finishing the posture

Stay in the posture for 5–10 breaths. Put your hands on the floor beside your hips; bring your knees towards each other; place the soles of your feet hip width on the floor; the knees are pointing upwards; straighten your knees. Repeat the posture with the right lower leg in front.

After finishing both sides keep the soles of your feet on the floor and the knees pointing upwards for a few breaths; straighten your legs; the toes and kneecaps are pointing towards the ceiling.

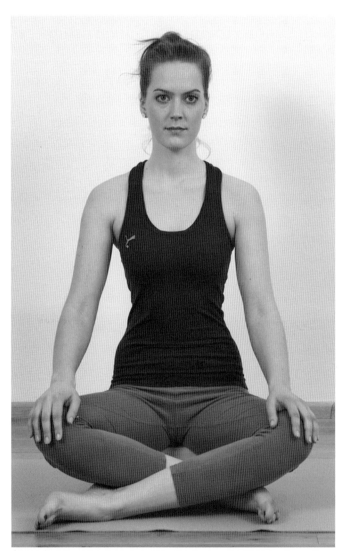

Figure 7.51

Suggestions for modifications using props

- Put a belt around your thighs (Figure 7.52).
- Support your thighs with a rolled blanket (Figure 7.53).
- Rest the back of your pelvis and the shoulder blades against a wall.

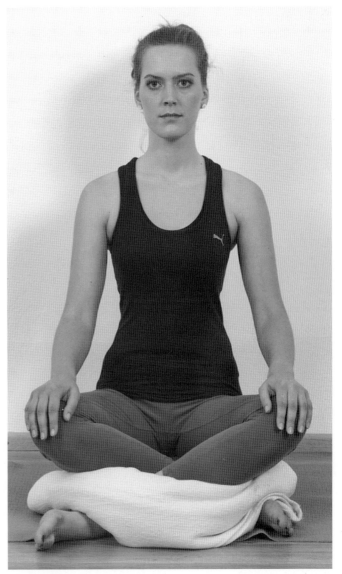

Figure 7.53

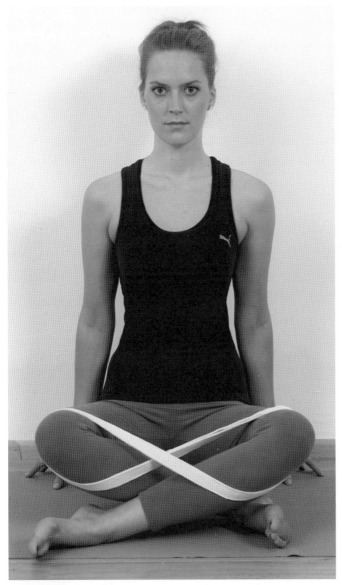

Figure 7.52

Variations

For Sukhāsana we show a series of variations. Most of these can also be performed with different leg positions such as Vīrāsana and Baddha Koṇāsana.

Parvatāsana in Sukhāsana

1. Sit in Sukhāsana, with the left lower leg in front.
2. Interlock your fingers, straighten your arms forwards, bend your wrists, with the tips of your thumbs touching.
3. Maintain the neutral lumbopelvic position; stretch your arms upwards while lifting your ribs and your sternum (Figure 7.54).
4. Stay for 3–5 breaths.
5. Bring your arms down horizontally.

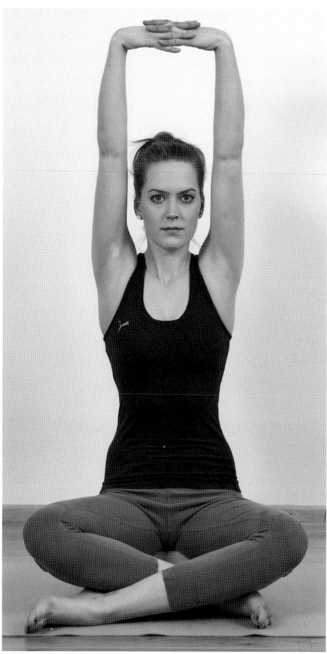

Figure 7.54

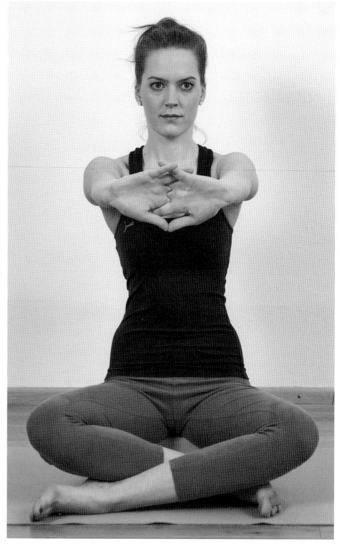

Figure 7.55

6. Internally rotate your arms so that your palms are turning out, the tips of the thumbs are touching, and the thumbs are well stretched in the plane of the palms (Figure 7.55).

7. Maintain the neutral lumbopelvic position; stretch your arms upwards while lifting your ribs and your sternum (Figure 7.56).

8. Keep your costal arches neutral and broad.

9. Stay there for 3–5 breaths.

10. Release your arms.

11. Change the crossing of your legs and the interlocking of your fingers so that the other thumb and the other fingers are on top, and repeat points 2–10.

Variation

To get a stronger stretch for the armpits start with the interlocked fingers behind your head to stretch your arms.

Supta Sukhāsana

Supta means lying on your back, resting.

1. Prepare a bolster with a folded blanket for the head.

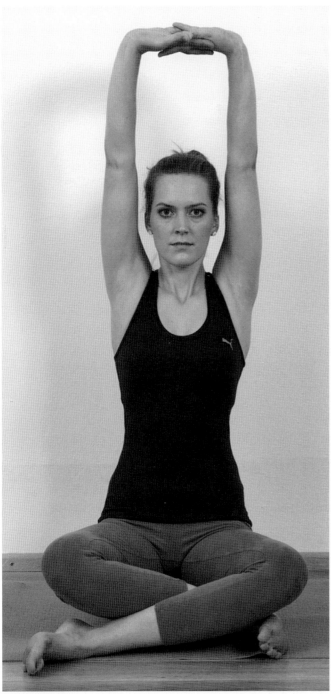

Figure 7.56

4. Maintaining a subtle lengthening of the back of your spine, lower your back and your head onto the bolster.

5. Adjust the blanket so that the head and neck are well supported and the neck and throat are relaxed.

6. Adjust the pelvis, maybe sliding slightly away from the bolster so that you are relaxed in your abdomen and lower back.

7. If your lumbar spine is curved too much or the bolster is irritating your back, start anew further away from the bolster or resting your buttocks on a folded blanket.

8. Rest your arms at your sides; feel the widening from your sternum into your upper ribs (Figure 7.57).

9. Stay there for 5–10 breaths.

10. Hold your elbows; keeping the pelvis neutral and the abdomen relaxed, move your arms over your head; feel the lengthening through the side ribs (Figure 7.58).

11. Stay there for 5–10 breaths; in the middle, change the hold on your elbows.

12. Release your arms, place them on your sides on the floor, swap the crossing of your legs, and repeat points 8–11.

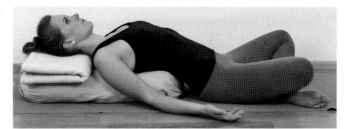

Figure 7.57

2. Sit in front of the bolster in Sukhāsana with your left shin in front.

3. Place your hands behind you, next to the front of the bolster; tilt your pelvis backwards so that you are relaxed in your groin, abdomen, and lower back.

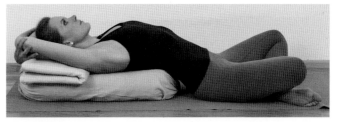

Figure 7.58

13. If you want to practice deep relaxation, stay up to 10 minutes; close your eyes, breathe evenly and quietly, be aware of your chest and your abdomen; if necessary adjust the support so that you can relax these areas.

14. For this version you may like to support each leg with an extra pillow.

15. Breathe evenly and quietly.

16. To come back, slowly open your eyes, bring your thighs parallel, the soles of your feet on the floor, slightly adjust your pelvis to be relaxed in the abdomen and lower back.

17. Turn to one side, whichever you prefer; from there come up to sitting; straighten your legs so that the backs of your knees stay soft; stay calm for a few breaths.

Adho Mukha Sukhāsana

1. Sit in Sukhāsana, the left lower leg in front first.

2. Keeping your buttocks on the floor, and maintaining enough length of your abdomen and front chest, walk your hands forwards to reach a comfortable forward-bending position; for deeper relaxation use a support for your head (Figure 7.59).

3. Stay for 5–10 breaths, feeling the relaxation in your back.

4. From there move the trunk over your right leg for 5–10 breaths, then over your left leg for 5–10 breaths; feel the relaxation particularly in your middle back.

5. Come back to the center; support yourself by walking your hands back to sit upright in Sukhāsana.

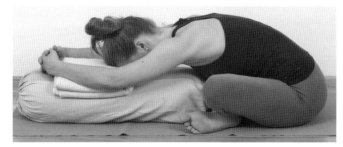

Figure 7.59

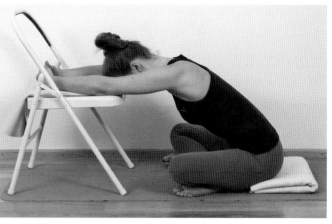

Figure 7.60

6. Change your crossed legs; repeat points 2–5.

7. If you need more support, use one or two bolsters underneath your abdomen and chest, an additional folded blanket underneath the forehead, one or two folded blankets underneath your buttocks, or rest your forehead and folded arms on a chair (Figure 7.60).

17. Vīrāsana (Figure 7.61)

Meaning of the āsana and its name

Vīra is a hero. Vīrāsana is sitting upright on a firm, solid basis. It develops flexibility in stability, concentration, and calmness.

Getting into the posture

1. Kneel with the thighs perpendicular, knees together, feet the width of your pelvis apart, the toes pointing backwards.

2. Slightly bend forwards; place your flat fingers on your calves, the fingertips touching the back of your knees.

3. Gently pull the calves away from the knees and outwards while lowering your pelvis on the floor between your feet.

4. Remove your hands from the calves.

5. Place your hands on your thighs; sit upright (Figure 7.61).

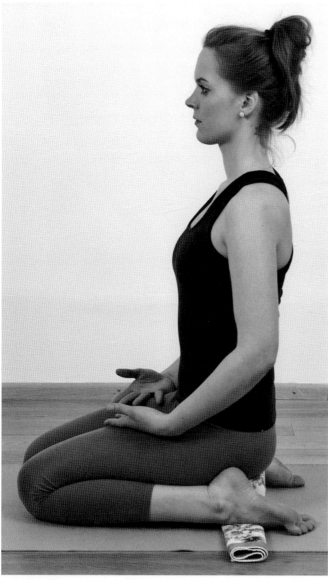

Figure 7.61

Being in the posture: basic work

1. Keep your knees together.
2. Balance your pelvis in the neutral position.
3. Slightly pull your lower abdomen inwards and upwards while you lift your chest.
4. Rest your hands on your thighs so that your shoulders are relaxed; lift and broaden your upper chest.
5. Maintaining the position of your chin, slightly lift the back of your head away from the neck.
6. Breathe naturally.

Being in the posture: refined work

1. Press the back of your toes into the floor; slightly lift your lower shin bones.
2. Let your upper thighs and groins move slightly downwards.
3. Feeling your sitting bones on the floor, adjust the pelvis in a neutral position.
4. Lifting yourself from the pelvic floor and the lower abdomen, feel the upwards movement through your spine.
5. Lift the center of your chest; this is also the movement of the diaphragm while exhaling.
6. Maintaining the neutral lumbopelvic position move your upper thoracic vertebrae inwards to lift your upper sternum and move it slightly forwards.
7. Adjust the position of your head so that the throat and neck are relaxed.
8. Feel the lifting of your upper ribs while lengthening the back of your head slightly away from the neck.

Finishing the posture

Stay in the posture for 5–10 breaths or longer. To release, lean forwards to place your palms on the floor for four-point kneeling.

Stretch your right leg backwards, then your left leg, holding each for a few breaths.

Alternatively you can practice Adho Mukha Śvānāsana to finish Vīrāsana.

Suggestions for modifications using props

- Support the buttocks with a brick, a folded blanket, or both if you need more height.
- Put a folded towel or blanket at the backs of your knees between the thighs and calves (Figure 7.62).
- Put a rolled towel underneath the ankle joints (Figure 7.61). Adjust the height as necessary.

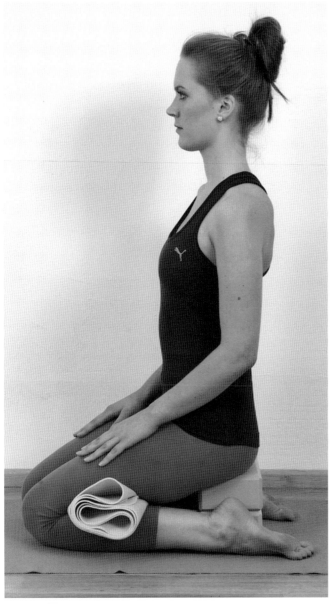

Figure 7.62

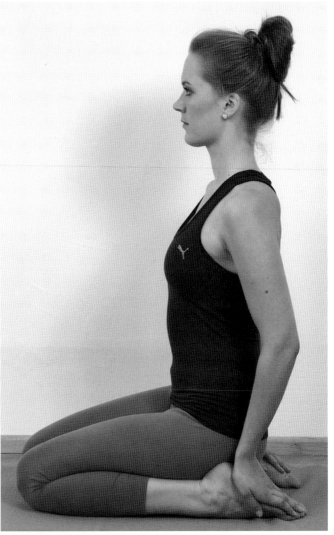

Figure 7.63

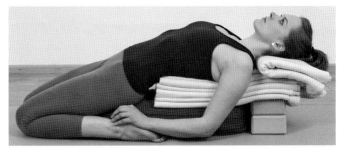

Figure 7.64

Variations

- Turn your arms so that the fingers are pointing backwards. Rest your palms on the soles of your feet. Slightly pull your lower abdomen inwards and upwards and lift your chest (Figure 7.63).

- Parvatāsana in Vīrāsana (see Parvatāsana in Sukhāsana).

- Supta Vīrāsana (Figure 7.64). Use any amount of support so that you are comfortable and relaxed in the position.

18. Triaṅg Mukhaikapāda Paścimottānāsana (Figure 7.67)

Meaning of the āsana and its name

Triaṅg means three parts: the foot, the knee, and the buttock. Mukhaikapāda means the face facing or touching one leg. Paścimottānāsana is an intense stretch of the back of the body.

The posture develops mobility and teaches relaxation while stretching intensively. It is an asymmetrical posture, and teaches finding the center in an asymmetrical position.

Getting into the posture

1. Sit with straight legs.

2. Keep your left leg still; bend your right leg into Vīrāsana, the heel close to the hip, the toes facing backwards.

3. Slightly lift your right buttock, place your flat fingers on the right calf muscles, the tips of the fingers in the back of the knee.

4. Gently pull the calf away from the knee and outwards.

5. Lower your right buttock at the same level as the left buttock.

6. Remove the right hand from the right calf.

7. Let the outer right thigh sink towards the floor.

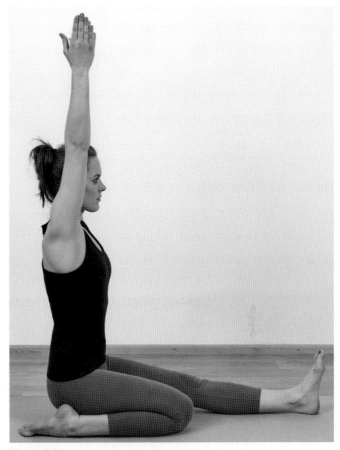

Figure 7.65

8. Keeping your weight evenly on both buttocks and both legs and maintaining the neutral lumbopelvic position, raise both arms, feeling a continuous stretch from the hips to the fingertips (Figure 7.65).

9. Maintaining this lifting in your trunk, lower your arms, tilt your pelvis forwards, put the tips of your fingers beside the buttocks on the floor to give an impulse for lifting your trunk from your fingertips (Figure 7.66).

10. Maintaining the length of your front trunk and both buttocks evenly on the floor, and the legs together, tilt your pelvis forwards and walk your hands forwards beside the left leg, if possible beyond the foot, as you exhale (Figure 7.67).

11. Continue point 10 as long as there is room for stretching your back and the back of your left leg.

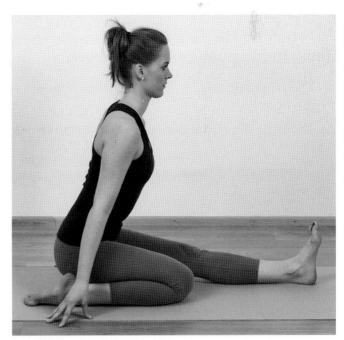

Figure 7.66

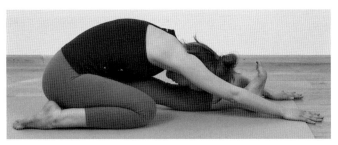

Figure 7.67

Being in the posture: basic work

1. Keep the left foot perpendicular, the left toes pointing towards the ceiling.

2. Keeping your left calf on the floor, slightly internally rotate the left leg; this helps to keep the weight centered.

3. Keep both buttocks evenly on the floor.

4. To bring the central line of your trunk in line with the left leg, slightly turn your abdomen towards your left.

5. With inhalation lengthen from your groin to your upper ribs.

6. With exhalation release forwards further, both arms stretched forwards evenly.

7. Breathe naturally.

Being in the posture: refined work

1. The inner left thigh is slightly moving towards the floor.

2. The right sitting bone is moving towards the floor.

3. Slightly move your abdomen inwards and lengthen it gently.

4. Lengthen both sides of your chest evenly with inhalation.

5. Lengthen the central line of your chest with exhalation.

6. Adjust the position of your hands according to this lengthening.

7. The sternum is resting on your left thigh, sliding a little further towards the foot.

8. Rest your forehead on the shin bone so that the neck is relaxed.

Finishing the posture

Stay 5–10 breaths. Lengthen the front of your trunk; raise your head. With an inhalation raise your trunk; if necessary, take support from your hands on the floor. Bring your right foot forwards, the sole of the foot on the floor beside the left knee, the right knee facing towards the ceiling. Straighten your right leg so that the kneecap and the toes are facing towards the ceiling. Repeat with the left leg bent.

Suggestions for modifications using props

• Place a thin folded blanket underneath the buttock of the straight leg side.

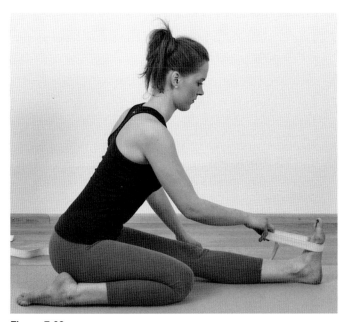

Figure 7.68

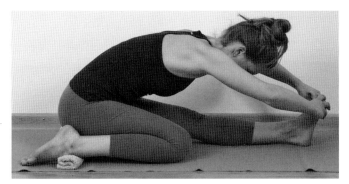

Figure 7.69

- Place a thicker folded blanket or a brick or if necessary the blanket on top of the brick underneath both buttocks.
- Use a belt around the foot of the straight leg (Figure 7.68).
- Place a rolled towel underneath the lower shin bone of the bent leg (Figure 7.69).

19. Baddha Koṇāsana (Figure 7.70)

Meaning of the āsana and its name

Baddha means bound, held. Koṇa is an angle. In this posture the angle of the knees is as small as possible, the hands are holding the feet. In India shoe-makers spend most of their time in this position. The posture develops mobility, it teaches you to lift the spine and trunk, and awareness of symmetry.

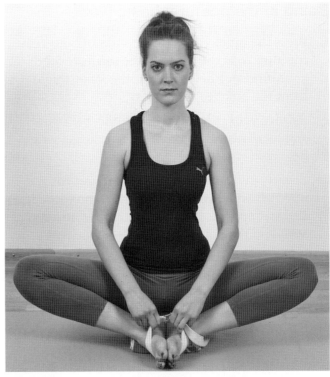

Figure 7.70

Getting into the posture

1. Sit on the floor with straight legs.
2. Bend your knees and move your feet as close as possible towards the pelvis without using the hands, to learn how far your knees can bend on their own.
3. Bring the soles of your feet together and let the knees sink towards the floor.
4. Holding your ankles with your hands, move the feet towards the pelvis as far as possible without straining the knees.
5. The soles of the feet are together in the central plane of the body; the outer edges of the feet are on the floor.
6. Hold the feet with your hands close to the toes; if you cannot lift well with this hand position, hold a short belt loop around your feet (Figure 7.70), or hold your ankles with your hands (Figure 7.71).

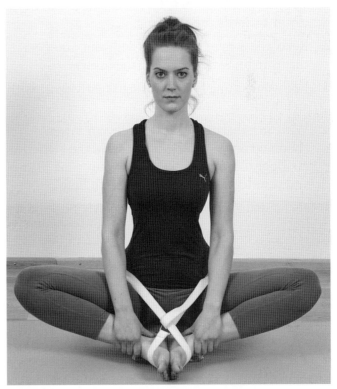

Figure 7.71

Being in the posture: basic work

1. Press the outer edges of the soles of your feet together to activate the outer thighs towards your hips; this helps release the inner thighs from the groin to the knees.

2. Balance your pelvis between tilting backwards and forwards so that your spine is lifting with ease.

3. Slightly pull your lower abdomen inwards and upwards while you lift your chest and move it slightly forwards between your arms; adjust the arms and the hold of the hands on the feet so that this is possible.

4. Relax your shoulders.

5. Bring your head in line with your spine.

6. Breathe naturally.

Being in the posture: refined work

1. Slightly move the centers of your inner arches away from each other; feel your knees coming closer towards the floor.

2. Relax the area of your groin and your inner thighs to bring the knees further down.

3. Feel your sitting bones moving slightly apart with an inhalation.

4. With an exhalation slightly pull your lower abdomen inwards and upwards and the center of your pelvic floor upwards; feel your trunk lifting and your legs letting go towards the floor.

5. Maintaining the neutral lumbopelvic position lift your upper chest while moving your shoulder blades into the back of the thorax.

Finishing the posture

Stay for 5–10 breaths in the posture. With increasing practice you can stay up to several minutes; this is a very beneficial posture for the whole pelvic area.

To come back, move both feet one foot length forwards; bring your knees together, slide your heels away to straighten your legs, the heels touching the floor exactly in the center, the feet pointing towards the ceiling. Stay there calmly for a few breaths.

Suggestions for modifications using props

- Sit on a folded blanket or on a brick, to gain enough height so that the neutral pelvic position is easier to adjust and to maintain.

- Sit close to a wall; put a long pillow or a rolled blanket or mat between your spine and the wall; the back of your pelvis and the area between your shoulder blades is touching the pillow (Figure 7.72).

- Support the bent legs with folded blankets or pillows (Figure 7.72).

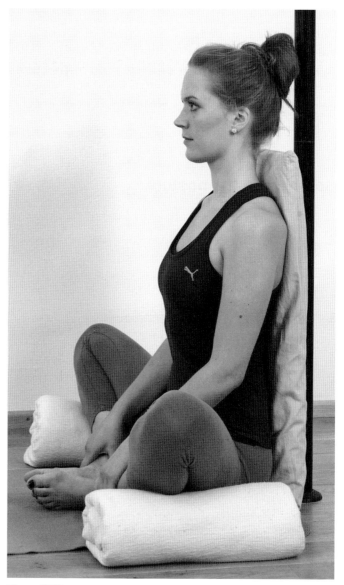

Figure 7.72

- Put a belt around the back of your pelvis, the groin, and the feet (Figure 7.71).
- For setting up Supta Baddha Koṇāsana, the supine position with the Baddha Koṇāsana legs, see Supta Sukhāsana (variation of Sukhāsana).

20. Jānu Śīrṣāsana (Figure 7.75)

Meaning of the āsana and its name

Jānu means knee, and śīrṣa head. One knee is straight, the other one is bent: the head is approaching the straight knee or lying on the shin. This posture particularly develops mobility and teaches relaxation while stretching intensively. It is an asymmetrical posture, and teaches you to find the center in an asymmetrical position.

Getting into the posture

1. Sit with both legs straight.
2. Move your right foot towards the buttock as long as you can bend your right knee comfortably.
3. Lower your right knee to the floor and move it backwards as much as possible.
4. Stretch your trunk and your arms upwards, the palms facing each other (Figure 7.73).
5. Keep your trunk lifted from your hips; tilt your pelvis forwards; lower your arms; place your fingertips on the floor behind the hips; the fingertips give the impulse to lift your trunk (Figure 7.74).
6. Keep your left and right leg on the floor, the left foot perpendicular; turn your pelvis and abdomen towards the left leg and place the fingertips of both hands on the floor left of the left thigh.
7. Further turning and tilting your pelvis forwards and with your left hip moving backwards, walk your fingers forwards along the left side.
8. Bring the center of your trunk in line with the left leg.
9. Hold your left foot with both hands (Figure 7.75).

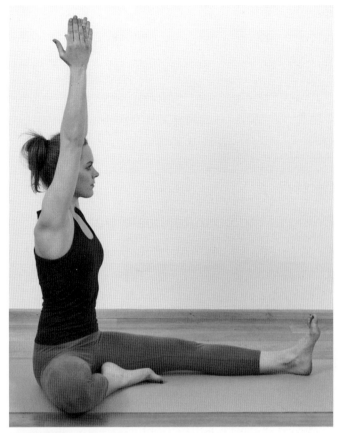
Figure 7.73

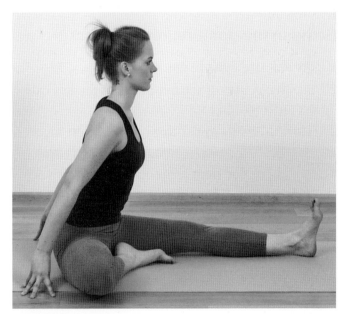
Figure 7.74

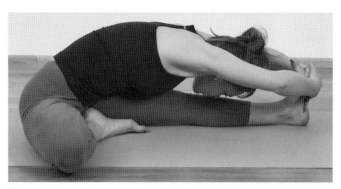

Figure 7.75

Being in the posture: basic work

1. Keep your left leg straight, the foot perpendicular.

2. Keep the right knee on the floor, press it onto the floor or on a rolled blanket, if it is not coming down on the floor; this helps to move the outer thigh into the hip joint and relax the right groin and the right inner thigh.

3. Lengthen the front of your trunk; maintaining this length, also lengthen the back.

4. Bend more forwards by tilting your pelvis forwards and bending and lifting your elbows, as you exhale.

5. Keep the head in line with the spine, the neck, and throat comfortable.

6. Breathe naturally.

Being in the posture: refined work

1. Stretch the sole of your left foot.

2. Feel the center of the left heel and the left calf on the floor.

3. Move your left upper thigh into the left hip socket.

4. Lengthen your front spine and your back spine; release your back spine as you exhale, broaden the muscles beside the spine.

5. Maintaining the right knee on the floor, move your right hip forwards and away from your right thigh.

6. Slightly turn your abdomen and your front ribs to the left.

7. Slightly pull your abdomen inwards and upwards.

8. Lengthen your front ribs, side ribs, and back ribs; move your back ribs inwards, where your back has the biggest curve.

9. Lengthen through your armpits into your arms.

10. If one part of your back is particularly round, lengthen the corresponding area in front.

11. Stretch both sides of your trunk equally.

12. To improve the stretch of the sides of the trunk, bend both elbows a little more, and slightly lift them; extend them forwards in line with the sides of the trunk.

Finishing the posture

Stay for 5–10 breaths. Release the hands from the foot. With an inhalation lengthen the front of your trunk, lift your trunk and head. Bring your right knee up facing the ceiling, and slide the right foot away to stretch the right knee, the kneecap, and toes in the same direction, both facing the ceiling.

Repeat the posture with the left leg bent.

Suggestions for modifications and using props

- Sit with both buttocks on a folded blanket.

- Use a belt around the ball of the foot of the straight leg (Figure 7.76).

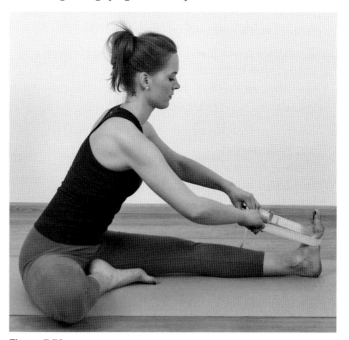

Figure 7.76

- Rest the bent leg and knee on a rolled blanket or pillow (see Baddha Koṇāsana).
- To make it a resting pose, rest your head on a folded blanket or on a chair so that the neck is relaxed; stay for 2 minutes on each side (see Sukhāsana, variations).
- Move the bent leg backwards only as far as the pelvis and the straight leg are at right angles.

21. Marīcyāsana III (Figure 7.77)

Meaning of the āsana and its name

Marīci was a sage of ancient Indian mythology. He was the son of Brahma, the creator of the universe, and the grandfather of Surya, the sun god. A series of four āsanas is dedicated to Marīci. We are choosing number III, as its leg position is basic, and the āsana is intensive and effective. It mobilizes the ribs, and teaches you to lift and turn the spine, and to breathe naturally, even with external compression.

Getting into the posture

1. Sit on a folded blanket or on a brick, both legs straight.
2. Bend your right knee, keeping the right calf as close as possible to the thigh; the right foot is parallel to the left leg.

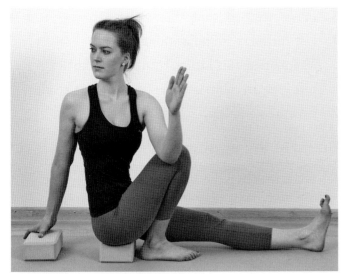

Figure 7.77

3. Keep your left leg straight, the kneecap and the toes facing the ceiling.
4. Put your right hand on the floor or if necessary on a brick, behind your right buttock.
5. Lift and turn your trunk to the right, stretch your left arm upwards, then put your left upper arm and elbow on the outside of your right thigh, the left lower arm and hand are vertical.
6. Press your right foot on the floor.
7. Turn your trunk more to the right.

Being in the posture: basic work

1. Keep your left leg straight, the left foot perpendicular, and the left front thigh moving towards the back thigh.
2. Push yourself up from the right heel and the right hand.
3. Inhaling, lift from your sacrum; exhaling, turn further while maintaining the lift.
4. Keeping the eyes relaxed, turn your head to the right, and hold for 3–5 breaths.
5. Keeping the eyes relaxed, and your right shoulder back, turn your head to the left, and hold for 3–5 breaths.
6. Breathe naturally.

Being in the posture: refined work

1. Refine the basic work so that you can breathe easily.
2. While lifting your trunk, particularly lift your sternum and the back of your head.
3. Feel the turning of your head to the right from your upper thoracic spine, and the gentle turning to the left from your lower cervical spine.
4. Very slightly move your right knee to the right; feel the left arm as a lever giving the left ribs more rotation.
5. Push your left upper arm into your outer right thigh to lift and turn more.
6. Move your shoulder blades inwards to lift your upper chest.
7. Sligthly move both shoulders away from the neck.

Finishing the posture

Stay for 5–10 breaths. Maintain the lifting; bring your head to the center; release the arms; with an inhalation release the rotation. Straighten your right leg, the kneecap and the toes facing towards the ceiling. Repeat with the left leg bent. After finishing both sides sit upright with both legs straight for a few breaths.

22. Utthita Marīcyāsana (Figure 7.78)

Meaning of the āsana and its name

This is a variation of Marīcyāsana III, explained above. It helps to lift the spine, if this is difficult

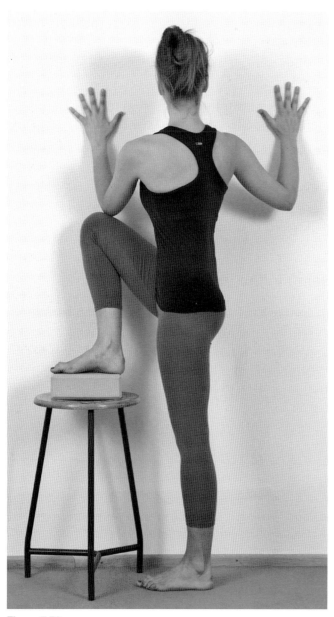

Figure 7.78

in the sitting variation. As this posture is standing, the base is particularly firm and strong. The hands on the wall make the arms a strong lever for turning the spine and ribs.

Getting into the posture

1. Place a stool at mid-thigh height against a wall.
2. If necessary adjust the height with a brick or book on the stool or stand on the item if the stool is too high.
3. Stand in Tāḍāsana facing the stool, with the wall on your right side.
4. Keeping your left leg vertical and firm, put your right foot on the stool, with the foot parallel to the wall.
5. Turn to the right, towards the wall.
6. Bend your left elbow, and put it on your right outer thigh.
7. Put both palms on the wall.
8. Press your right hand into the wall to rotate your trunk to the right.

Being in the posture: basic work

1. Keep your left leg straight and firm; press your right heel into the stool, to lift your spine further.
2. Your left elbow is resisting the right thigh.
3. Press your hands into the wall.
4. Lift further with inhalation.
5. Maintaining this lifting, turn as you exhale.
6. Lift your sternum and the back of your head.
7. Breathe naturally.

Being in the posture: refined work

1. Slightly lifting the back of your head further, feel the lifting of your upper chest.
2. Relax your neck and throat.
3. Turn your head to the right as long as the neck and throat are relaxed; hold for 3–5 breaths.
4. Turn your head to the left as long as the neck and throat are relaxed; hold for 3–5 breaths.

Finishing the posture

Bring your head to the center. Release your arms; with an inhalation release the rotation. Bring your right foot down on the floor. Repeat on the left side.

23. Bharadvājāsana I (Figure 7.79)

Meaning of the āsana and its name

Bharadvāja is a sage of ancient Indian mythology; this āsana is dedicated to him.

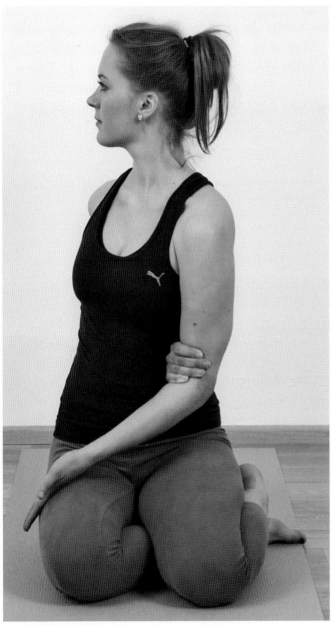

Figure 7.79

The essence of this āsana is an upwards spiral movement. It combines staying clearly in the central line with free space and lightness.

Getting into the posture

1. Sit on a brick or a folded blanket with both legs straight.
2. Keeping the legs together, bend both knees; both feet move to the left side.
3. The feet are just left of the left hip; the lower left shin bone is resting in the arch of the right foot.
4. Keep both sitting bones at the same level.
5. Bring your right arm around your back and catch the left upper arm with your right hand.
6. Lift your spine vertically and keep your head in line with your spine.
7. Keeping both sitting bones level, turn your trunk to the right as you exhale; the back of the left hand is on the right thigh.
8. Turn your head to the right, keeping your neck and throat relaxed.

Being in the posture: basic work

1. Keep your knees as close as possible together, your left hip and thigh down.
2. Keep the central line of your trunk straight.
3. Keep your shoulder girdle horizontally.
4. With the impulse from pressing the back of your left hand on your right thigh, move your right shoulder backwards and the left one forwards, more and more in line with the right thigh.
5. Breathe naturally.

Being in the posture: refined work

1. Move your left upper outer thigh down; turn from your hips.
2. To lift your spine more, press your right shin bone into the floor.
3. Drop your left groin.
4. Move your lower abdomen slightly inwards and upwards.

5. Move both shoulder blades inwards.

6. Move the upper thoracic vertebrae inwards.

7. Feel the spiral movement throughout your spine around its axis, from the bottom to the top.

8. Keeping your sternum and the back of your head lifted, turn your head to the left for a few breaths; keep your eyes soft; feel the effect of this counterrotation on your spine and ribs.

Finishing the posture

Hold the posture for 5–10 breaths. Stay well lifted; bring your head to the center first; with an exhalation turn back to the center. Release the arms; straighten your legs. Repeat on the left side.

Suggestions for modifications using props

• Put a belt loop around the left upper arm; hold the belt with your right hand.

• Tie a belt around the middle of your bent legs to help holding the knees together.

• Sit on a chair (see Chapter 6, exercise 2.8).

24. Ūrdhva Mukha Śvānāsana
(Figure 7.80)

Meaning of the āsana and its name

Ūrdhva means upwards, mukha is the face or mouth, and śvāna is a dog. The posture is evocative of a dog

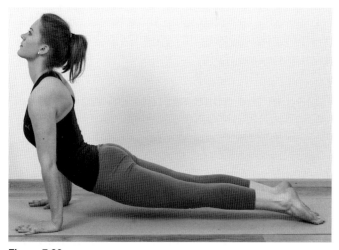

Figure 7.80

stretching itself with its head upwards. It is a balanced back-bending of the whole spine; the lumbar lordosis has to be controlled; the thoracic spine is moved inwards; and the feet and arms are strengthened.

Getting into the posture

1. Start in the four-point kneeling position, the feet pointing backwards, the thighs and arms perpendicular, the hands shoulder width apart, and the knees and feet hip width apart.

2. Move the hands about one hand's length forwards, depending on your proportions.

3. Keep your head in line with your spine; breathe normally.

4. Adjust the neutral lumbopelvic position; pull your lower abdomen inwards and upwards.

5. Maintaining the action of point 4, lift your knees off the floor to straighten your legs, contracting your buttocks; at the same time move your chest forwards in between your arms; synchronize the movement of your chest and your legs.

6. Externally rotate your arms; slightly relax from full extension of the elbows; lift your side and upper ribs.

7. Have only the palms and the backs of the feet and toes on the floor.

8. Lengthen from your neck into the back of your head; further lifting your upper ribs and upper sternum, bend your head backwards as far as the throat and neck are comfortable.

9. Look upwards.

Being in the posture: basic work

1. Keep your feet firm, with the ankles, shin bones, and thighs lifted.

2. Contract the buttocks; pull your lower abdomen inwards and upwards to lengthen and strengthen the lumbar spine.

3. Move your shoulder blades inwards and down.

4. Lift your side and front upper ribs and your sternum.

5. Adjust your head so that the neck and throat are comfortable.

6. Breathe naturally.

Being in the posture: refined work

1. Keep your feet and legs strong; keeping the heels centered, lift them slightly; this gives a subtle lengthening of the Achilles tendons.

2. Coordinate the inward movement of the lower abdomen with lengthening between your lower lumbar spine and sacrum.

3. Slightly internally rotate your thighs so that the outer thighs are moving towards the floor.

4. Synchronize the actions of points 2 and 3 with adjusting your head on the upper cervical spine so that the whole spine is a continuous arch.

5. Slightly relax from the full stretch of your elbows to be active in all flexor and extensor muscles; maintain the external rotation of your arms to get a backwards and downwards action of your shoulders.

6. Maintaining the action of point 2, move your upper thoracic vertebrae inwards to lift your upper sternum and upper front ribs further.

7. Slightly lengthen the back of your head away from your upper neck.

8. Feel the continuous, strong and flexible arch from your toes to the crown of your head.

Finishing the posture

Hold for 5–10 breaths. Keeping the buttocks firm, bring your knees onto the floor, release your feet. With an exhalation move the front of your body towards the back and come back to four-point kneeling.

Alternatively you can bend your elbows and lie on your front; rest there for a few breaths.

Suggestions for modifications using props

• Support the back of the feet and the ankle joints with a rolled mat (Figure 7.81).

• Support the groin with a bolster.

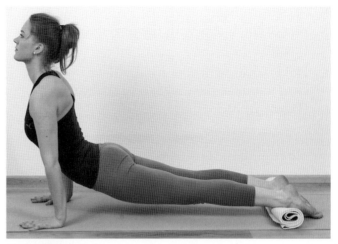

Figure 7.81

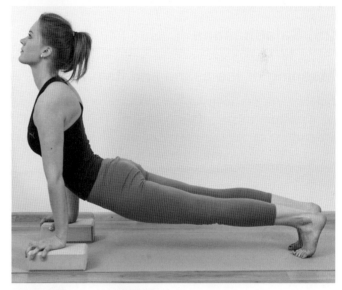

Figure 7.82

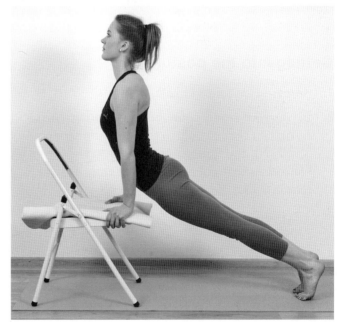

Figure 7.83

201

- Place each hand on a brick, gripping the front part of the bricks with the fingers and thumbs (Figure 7.82).
- Hold a chair with your hands. Make sure the chair is against the wall or on a sticky mat (Figure 7.83).

Variations

- Go into the posture from Adho Mukha Śvānāsana.
- Combine Adho Mukha Śvānāsana and Ūrdhva Mukha Śvānāsana several times to form a sequence in motion, keeping the legs firm.

25. Śalabhāsana (Figure 7.84)

Meaning of the āsana and its name

Śalabha means locust. The posture is reminiscent of a resting locust. The back-bending action only extends as far as the posterior muscles can hold it; there is no force applied from outside.

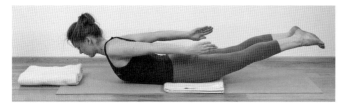

Figure 7.84

Getting into the posture

1. Prepare two folded blankets.
2. Lie on your front; your abdomen and groin are resting on the blanket so that the lumbar area is relaxed; the forehead is resting on the other blanket so that your nose is free and the neck is relaxed.
3. The arms are lying beside the trunk, with the palms facing the ceiling.
4. Move one leg after the other away from the hip as if the legs are being slightly pulled backwards.

5. With an inhalation lift your head, chest, arms, and straight legs; let the groin sink towards the floor. Lift as far as you can, slightly pull the lower abdomen inwards, and maintain the length between your lower lumbar spine and sacrum. As long as you are comfortable between your neck and the back of your head, look forwards.

Being in the posture: basic work

1. Contract the buttocks.
2. Keep the legs straight and together.
3. Pull your lower abdomen inwards and upwards to lengthen between your lower lumbar spine and your sacrum.
4. Moving your shoulders back, lift your arms further.
5. Adjust the position of your head for an optimum comfort of the neck and throat.
6. Breathe naturally.

Being in the posture: refined work

1. Inner thighs, calves, inner ankles, and big toes are together.
2. First, pull the toes towards your knees, then stretch the toes backwards; feel the difference for the stretch of your legs and your hips.
3. Pull your lower abdomen towards your lumbar area and the diaphragm; feel the lengthening of your lumbar spine.
4. Turn your arms so that the palms are facing each other, then lift them slightly more; move the shoulders backwards; feel the effect on the shoulder blades, upper sternum, and upper ribs.
5. Turn your arms so that the palms are facing the floor; feel the effect on the upper sternum and upper ribs.
6. Finely adjust your head on your upper cervical spine to lengthen your upper spine and widen your upper thorax and the area of your clavicles even further.

Finishing the posture

Stay for 3–5 breaths or longer if you can maintain the basic corrections and breathe naturally. Exhaling, lower your legs, chest, arms (palms facing the ceiling), and head back to the floor. Rest your forehead on the folded blanket to relax your head, throat, and neck; from there relax the whole spine.

Suggestions for modifications using props

Support the upper thighs with a rolled blanket (Figure 7.85).

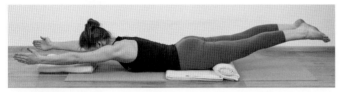

Figure 7.85

Variations

- Bend your elbows, interlock your fingers at the back of your head, and lift the elbows towards the ceiling.
- Stretch your arms forwards beside your head (Figure 7.85).
- Bend your knees, keeping the shin bones perpendicular (see Chapter 6, exercise 1.12).

26. Uṣṭrāsana (Figure 7.86)

Meaning of the āsana and its name

Uṣṭra is a camel. The body is bent backwards, reminiscent of a camel kneeling on the front legs when getting up; during this movement it is arching its thorax and extending the head back. The backbending in Uṣṭrāsana is built up slowly so that the spine can accept the change.

Getting into the posture

1. Kneel on a folded blanket, with your knees and feet hip width apart, the toes pointing backwards.

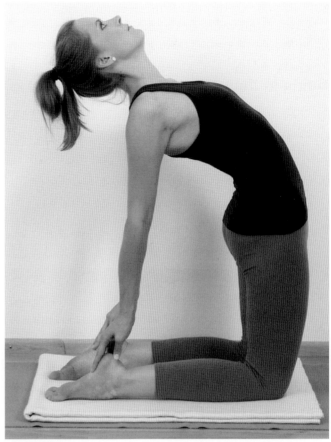

Figure 7.86

2. Moving your arms backwards, place the thumbs on your middle sacrum, your fingers flat on the hips; the elbows and shoulders are moving backwards.

3. Push your shin bones into the blanket, slightly move your upper thighs forwards, your sacrum down, lift from your lower abdomen upwards, lift your sternum and upper ribs, and keep your head in line with your spine.

4. Maintaining the actions of point 3, walk your hands further down the back of your thighs.

5. Further maintaining these actions, and permanently lengthening your spine, and lifting your sternum and upper ribs, move your shoulders backwards; straighten your arms; turn them out till the palms are facing forwards; contracting your buttocks, lengthen more from the lumbar area to the back of your pelvis downwards; put one hand on the corresponding heel, then the other hand on the other heel.

6. Lift your sternum further, lengthen your head away from your neck and bend it backwards as long as it its comfortable for your neck and throat.

Being in the posture: basic work

1. The arches of the feet are active, the heels slightly outwards.
2. Push your shin bones into the blanket.
3. Move your upper thighs slightly forwards; contract your buttocks, move your middle buttocks in and down, your sacrum and tailbone forwards and down; lift from your lower abdomen upwards.
4. Lift and move your middle and upper thoracic spine inwards; lift your sternum.
5. Move your middle back ribs inwards and up.
6. Move your shoulders back.
7. Keep your arms straight.
8. Adjust the position of the head so that the neck and throat are comfortable.
9. Breathe naturally.

Being in the posture: refined work

1. Push your lower shin bones into the blanket to lift yourself further.
2. Press your hands on your heels to lift your chest further.
3. Coordinate the forwards movement of your middle buttocks and the lifting of the lower abdomen, widening the chest and the adjustment of the head to get a continuous arch for your spine.
4. Lengthen between your pelvis and diaphragm.
5. Move your shoulder blades, particularly the medial aspect, inwards and upwards.
6. Coordinate the back-bending of your head with lifting your sternum.

Finishing the posture

Stay for 3–5 breaths. Slightly move your upper thighs and buttocks forwards; with an inhalation lift from your pelvis to your lower chest, then upwards; the arms and head come up easily. Sit on your heels for a few breaths.

Suggestions for modifications using props

- Rest your hands on a chair (Figure 7.87).
- Face a wall, keeping the front of your thighs against the wall.

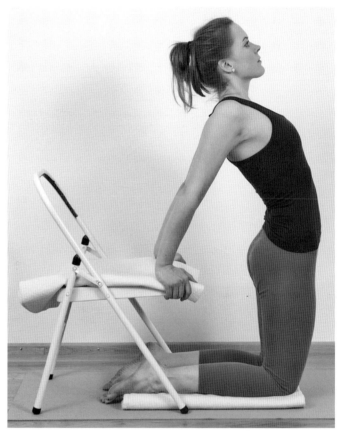

Figure 7.87

27. Naṭarājāsana (Figure 7.88)

Meaning of the āsana and its name

Naṭa means dance, and Rāja is a king. Naṭarāja is the king of dance, to whom this beautiful āsana is dedicated. The arch from the foot through the spine, head, and arms is balanced on one leg. We have chosen an easy variation, an approach that can be practiced by most people and developed further with increasing practice. For the full āsana see Iyengar (2001).

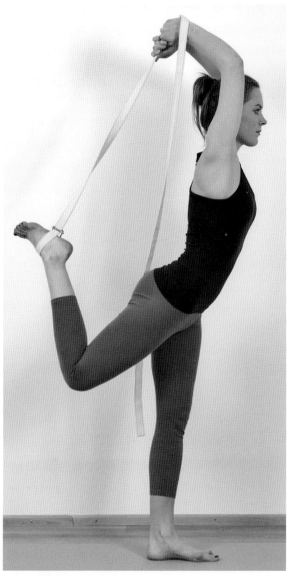

Figure 7.88

Getting into the posture

1. Stand in Tāḍāsana.

2. Tie a belt around the right foot so that the buckle is in the middle of the sole of the foot; hold the other end of the belt with both hands.

3. Stand on your left foot, with your toes pointing forwards, the left leg straight.

4. The right foot is one foot length back, the toes flat on the floor, the heel off the floor.

5. Elevate both arms above the head, the elbows shoulder width and bent; both hands are holding the belt.

6. Maintaining a neutral lumbopelvic position and both hips in the same plane, lift your right foot off the floor, bending the right knee.

7. As long as you can maintain this pelvic position, your thorax lifted and an even arch of your spine, gradually bring your right leg more backwards, your right foot higher; "climb" with your hands on the belt downwards to make it shorter.

Being in the posture: basic work

1. Balance on the left foot, keeping the leg straight.

2. Maintain sufficient length between the lumbar area and the back of the pelvis, and move the lower abdomen slightly inwards and upwards.

3. Lift your chest.

4. As long as you can maintain the length between the lumbar area and the pelvis and you are comfortable in the lumbar area, climb with your hands further down the belt, move your right leg higher and your foot slightly further backwards.

5. Breathe naturally.

Being in the posture: refined work

1. Slightly tilt your pelvis forwards, and move your trunk forwards so that you can maintain the length between the lower lumbar spine and the sacrum.

2. Keeping the hips in one plane, further lift your right leg and move the right foot further backwards.

3. Gently pull your lower abdomen inwards and upwards so that the back of your spine gets a good lengthening.

4. As long as your pelvis is not rotating and your whole back is smooth and comfortable, climb with your hands down the belt and lift your right leg higher.

5. Feel the lifting of your front and side ribs as you inhale, and the lifting of your central chest as you exhale.

6. Move your upper thoracic vertebrae inwards to lift your sternum further.

7. Adjust the position of your head to the position of optimum comfort for your throat and neck.

Finishing the posture

Hold for 3–5 breaths. Release the belt to bring your right foot to the floor slowly. Drop the belt, and move your arms down to the sides of your body. Change the belt to the left foot and repeat, standing on your right foot.

Suggestions for modifications using props

Hold the belt only with the hand of the lifted leg side; stretch the other arm forwards horizontally; and put the hand on a wall to stabilize yourself.

28. Adho Mukha Vṛkṣāsana (Figure 7.89)

Meaning of the āsana and its name

Adho means downwards, mukha means face, vṛkṣa is the tree. Adho Mukha Vṛkṣāsana is the downward-facing tree, the full arm balance. Before starting to practice it the arms and shoulders must be strong enough. Once this is achieved, the posture builds up strength and energy. To build up this strength Adho Mukha Śvānāsana with all the variations and Ūrdhva Mukha Śvānāsana are recommended.

Getting into the posture

1. Stand in Tāḍāsana about three foot lengths away from the wall.

2. Bend down to place the hands shoulder width apart on the floor, half a foot length away from the wall.

3. Push yourself up from the hands; keep your arms completely stretched and your shoulders exactly above the wrists; move your shoulder blades actively away from the neck and into the thorax.

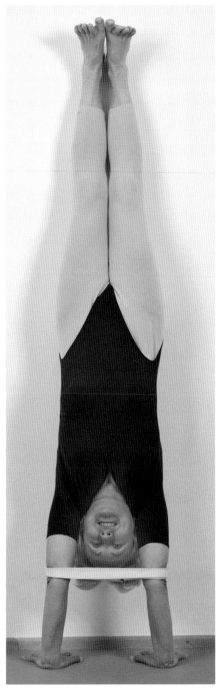

Figure 7.89

4. Walk your feet towards the hands in order to tilt the pelvis as far as possible. This position gives stability for the correct alignment and at the same time lightness for jumping up with the legs.

5. Maintaining your arms straight and firm, lifting your sitting bones, with an exhalation swing one leg upwards, keeping it straight – it is sensible to start with your easier side.

6. Let the second leg follow easily and quickly.

7. Stretch your elbows and your legs, the heels touching the wall and moving upwards on the wall.

Being in the posture: basic work

1. Press your palms into the floor; stretch your thumbs and fingers.

2. Keep your elbows strong.

3. Keep your head in line with your spine.

4. Lift your tailbone towards your heels; slightly move your costal arches inwards.

5. Maintaining the actions of point 4, lift your shoulders and move them slightly away from the wall.

6. Stretch both sides of your body upwards equally.

7. Breathe naturally.

Being in the posture: refined work

1. Press the pads of your fingers slightly more into the floor.

2. If your elbows are hyperextended, slightly relax from full extension.

3. Move your costal arches closer towards the wall and your shoulders away from the wall.

4. Adjust your pelvis into the neutral position and stretch your legs upwards to get a continuous stretch from your hands to your feet.

5. Have your feet in between dorsiflexion and plantar flexion.

Finishing the posture

Stay for 3–5 breaths or longer if you are breathing well. Keep your arms straight and the hips upwards; keep the legs straight; bring one leg down, then the other one as you exhale. If you want to repeat the posture, jump with the other leg first. At the end, stay calmly in Uttānāsana for a few breaths.

Suggestions for modifications using props

- Rest your back on one side of a door frame, the feet on the other side. Keep the hands on sandbags or a rolled mat; put a long, thin pillow or rolled blanket between your upper thoracic spine and the wall.

- Both feet can stay on the door frame or one leg stretched up alternatively (Figures 7.90 and 7.91).

- Put a belt around the elbows to stabilize the arms.

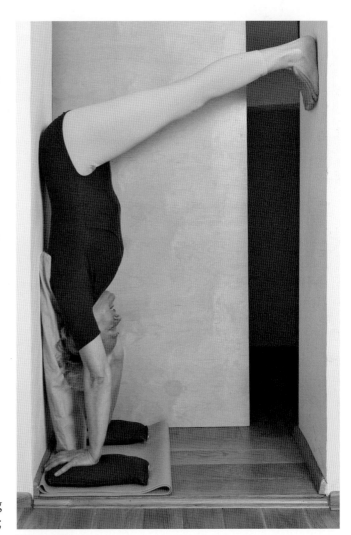

Figure 7.90

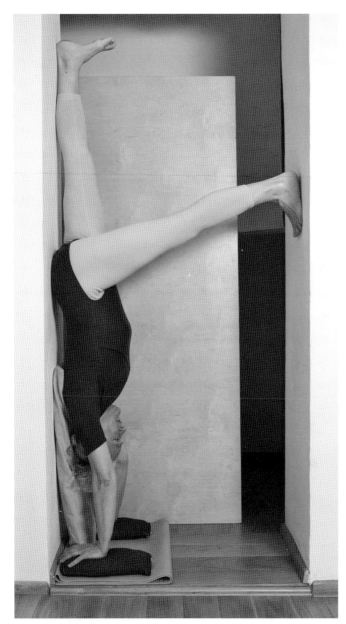

Figure 7.91

29. Sālamba Śīrṣāsana (Figure 7.95)

Meaning of the āsana and its name

Sālamba means supported, śīrṣa is the head. Sālamba Śīrṣāsana is headstand supported by the arms and hands. In classical yoga texts Sālamba Śīrṣāsana is called the king of all āsanas (Haṭha-Yoga-Pradīpikā, chapter III: Sinh 2006). It is beneficial for almost all physical and mental aspects. Reversing the position of the body helps to reverse habits that are an obstacle for health. Nevertheless some cautions

are necessary. As with all other āsanas, the benefits only come if the āsana is practiced correctly. Therefore it should only be learned under the guidance of a qualified teacher. Before learning Sālamba Śīrṣāsana all the standing poses, Uttānāsana, Adho Mukha Śvānāsana, Sālamba Sarvāṅgāsana, and Halāsana should be mastered. Sālamba Śīrṣāsana should always be followed by Sālamba Sarvāṅgāsana, either immediately or with other āsanas in between.

Getting into the posture

1. Prepare a folded mat or blanket as a comfortable and safe head support.

2. Kneel in front of this head support.

3. Place your elbows in one line on this support; to measure the distance of the elbows at shoulder width, put your fingers around your elbows; leave the elbows there, release the hands from the elbows.

4. Maintaining the alignment of the elbows, interlock your fingers so that the pits are together, and the tips of the thumbs are touching.

5. The little fingers and little finger sides of the wrists are firmly on the floor.

6. The hands are like a cup for the head.

7. Place the crown of your head on the floor; the cup formed by the hands is completely touching the back of the head, but not underneath the head.

8. The knees are close to your elbows.

9. Stay calm in this position for a few breaths.

10. Keeping your wrists perpendicular to the floor, your middle lower arms firmly on the floor, maintaining the distance of the elbows and the crown of your head still, lift your shoulders away from the floor.

11. Let your toes point towards your head, the heels off the floor; maintaining the adjustments of point 10, straighten your knees (Figure 7.92).

12. To learn how to stabilize the lifting of the shoulders to protect the cervical spine, lift your right leg, then your left leg as far as possible, holding each side for 1–2 breaths; repeat 2–3

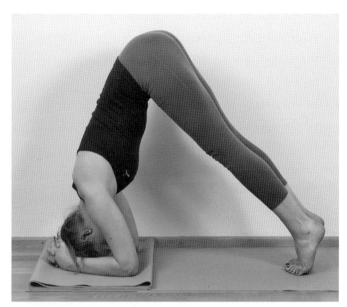

Figure 7.92

which you can feel as a strong lifting towards your tailbone; if necessary, bend your knees.

14. Maintaining this inner lifting against gravity, and with your sitting bones moving towards the ceiling, lift your feet off the floor, bend your knees; move your heels towards your buttocks and your knees upwards to face the ceiling (Figure 7.94).

15. Constantly control the correct action of your hands, lower arms, shoulders, and the position of your head exactly on the crown, and maintain your neutral lumbopelvic position while you straighten your legs up vertically; the feet are between plantar flexion and dorsiflexion (Figure 7.95).

times (Figure 7.93). Once you are able to perform this while maintaining the adjustments of point 10, you are ready to proceed with point 13 to build up the final posture.

13. Maintaining the adjustments of point 10, walk your feet towards your head till the line from the crown of your head to your tailbone is vertical,

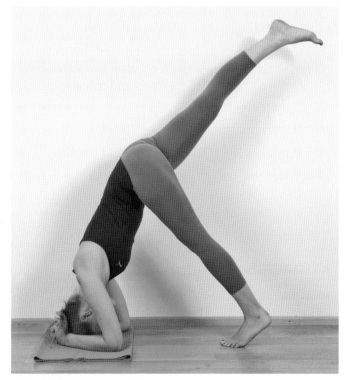

Figure 7.93

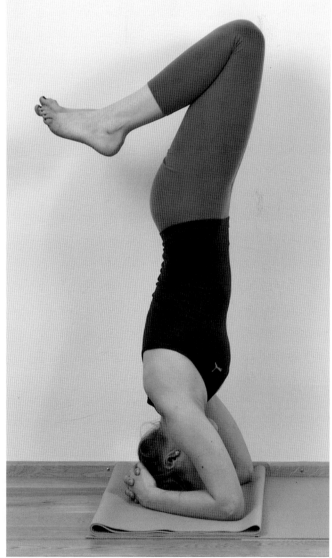

Figure 7.94

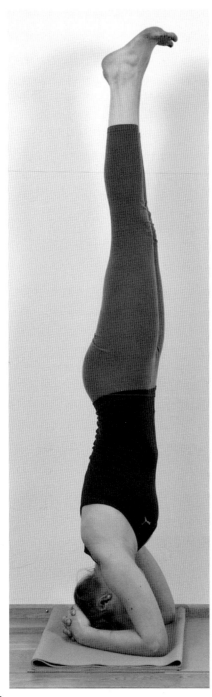

Figure 7.95

4. Combine the lifting of your shoulders with slightly moving your costal arches backwards.

5. Slightly pull your lower abdomen inwards; feel how this lengthens your lumbar spine.

6. Maintain the neutral lumbopelvic position while stretching and straightening your legs more.

7. Keep your legs together.

8. Breathe naturally.

Being in the posture: refined work

1. Slightly press the thumb side of your hands on the back of your head.

2. Slightly move your elbows together to lift your shoulders more.

3. Move your shoulder blades away from the floor and slightly inwards.

4. Feel the inner lifting from the crown of your head to your tailbone, so that your head feels light and calm.

5. Slightly move your groin backwards, your sacrum and tailbone forwards.

6. Lengthen your inner legs through your inner heels.

7. Lengthen the back of your legs through your heels.

8. Lengthen the front legs through the back of the feet, slightly moving the feet away from the shins.

9. Keep the feet in between dorsiflexion and plantar flexion.

10. Constantly adjust the details so that you have not much weight on your head and a subtle, relaxed length in your throat and neck.

11. Keeping your wrists perpendicular, your middle lower arms firmly on the floor, the crown of your head calm, lift your shoulders away from the floor.

Being in the posture: basic work

1. Keep your wrists and lower arms firm.

2. Move your upper arms upwards as if starting to stretch your elbows.

3. Keep your shoulders lifted, to relax your neck and throat.

Finishing the posture

In the beginning hold for 5–10 breaths; with practice increase up to 5 minutes, or even longer.

Keep your wrists perpendicular, your middle lower arms firmly on the floor, the crown of your head light and still, and your shoulders lifted away from the floor. Keep your trunk straight.

With an exhalation bend your knees and slowly bring first your feet down to the floor, then your knees. If you cannot keep your trunk straight while coming down with both legs simultaneously, bring one straight leg down, then the other one. Bend your knees to the floor, bring your buttocks towards the heels, release your hands, rest your chest on your thighs, your arms on the floor and your forehead on the floor or on a folded blanket if necessary. Stay calm for 3–5 breaths or longer.

Suggestions for modifications using props

- Practice close to a wall, the interlocked fingers almost touching the wall, and the heels touching the wall. To practice with the wall support you can swing one leg upwards first with the second leg following (Figure 7.93).

- Practice in a corner, with the interlocked fingers as close as possible to the corner. The elbows are at shoulder width, both elbows at the same distance from the wall without touching it. Check that both hips and heels touch the wall equally.

- Have somebody help you to get up and down and control you while you are in the posture.

30. Supta Pādāṅguṣṭhāsana
(Figure 7.96)

Meaning of the āsana and its name

Supta means lying down, pāda is the foot, and aṅguṣṭha is the big toe. Supta Pādāṅguṣṭhāsana is a supine pos-

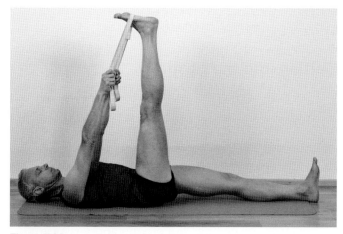
Figure 7.96

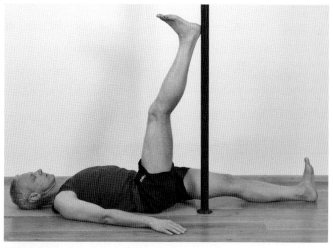
Figure 7.97

ture where one big toe is caught to move the leg in different directions (Iyengar 2001). We emphasize the effect of stretching the legs, therefore we show the version where a belt is used around the sole of the foot and the leg is moved upwards. In this way the leg stretch can be practiced with a completely relaxed spine.

Getting into the posture

1. Lie on the floor; use a folded blanket underneath your head if necessary.

2. Keep your left leg straight, the center of the heel on the floor, and the toes pointing exactly towards the ceiling.

3. Bend your right knee towards your chest.

4. Put the belt around the sole of your right foot, close to the ball of the foot; hold one part of the belt with each hand; you can also try with the belt around the heel, which emphasizes the lengthening of the leg.

5. Keeping your hips and your shoulder blades equally on the floor, and the left leg unchanged, straighten your right leg perpendicularly as you inhale, adjust the length of the belt accordingly.

Being in the posture: basic work

1. Keep your left heel with its center on the floor; push the left thigh to the floor.

2. Move your right outer hip away from the waist until your hips are completely symmetrical.

3. If you cannot keep the right leg perpendicular with the knee stretched, ease away from full extension of the knee, as in Figure 7.97.

4. Keeping the pelvis symmetrical, move the front thighs towards the back of your thighs.

5. Breathe naturally.

Being in the posture: refined work

1. Adjust the position of the hands on the belt so that both shoulders are relaxed.

2. Relax your neck and throat.

3. Keep the center of the left heel and the left calf on the floor.

4. Slightly move the left inner thigh towards the floor.

5. Move the center of the right front thigh towards the back of the thigh; feel the lengthening of the back of the thigh.

6. Adjust the hips so that you feel both symmetrically on the floor.

7. Slightly lengthen the back of your right foot to move the ball of the foot and the toes a little higher; make this movement so subtle that the back of the right leg releases and you can move the right leg closer towards the trunk and still keep the knee stretched.

Finishing the posture

Hold for 5–10 breaths. Bend your right knee; release the belt; stay relaxed lying on your back; straighten your right leg along the floor in line with the right side of your trunk. Repeat for the left leg.

A nice method to change the side is to synchronize the stretching of the right leg on the floor with bending the left knee to the chest.

Suggestions for modifications using props (Figure 7.97)

This method is useful if it is not possible to straighten the lifted leg.

1. Lie on your back, the right leg lifted, the right heel on a column or door frame.

2. Start in a position where the upper leg is not completely straight.

3. Press your heel to the column with one-third of your full strength. Hold for 2–3 breaths.

4. Release and it is very likely you will be able to move your heel slightly higher, to stretch your knee a little more.

5. Starting from the newly reached level repeat points 3 and 4 twice.

6. Lie with both legs straight on the floor for a few breaths; feel the difference between the two legs.

7. Repeat points 1–5 for the left leg.

8. To finish stay calm lying on your back for a few breaths.

9. If there is no door frame or column available, use a wall and raise both legs at the same time.

31. Sālamba Sarvāṅgāsana (Figure 7.100)

Meaning of the āsana and its name

Sa means together with; alamba is a support; sarvāṅga means all parts of the body, the whole body. Sālamba Sarvāṅgāsana is called "the queen or mother of the āsanas. It soothes and nourishes the whole body" (Mehta et al. 1990, p. 108). When practicing the posture, it is important to use sufficient support to maintain the natural curve of the cervical spine, to be relaxed in the neck and throat. Before learning Sālamba Sarvāṅgāsana, the following āsanas should be learned in this sequence (Iyengar & Iyengar 2003):

- Setu Bandha Sarvāṅgāsana (shoulder bridge; see Chapter 6, exercise 3.9)
- Viparīta Karaṇī
- Half Halāsana (see Figures 7.104 and 7.105)
- Halāsana.

Getting into the posture

1. Lie with your back on three or four precisely folded blankets, the shoulders one hand width away from the end of the blankets, the head resting on the floor; you may like to use a thin blanket underneath your head.

2. Maintaining the neutral lumbopelvic position, turn your arms out so that the palms are facing towards the ceiling, and elbows and wrists are touching the sides of the body (Figure 7.98).

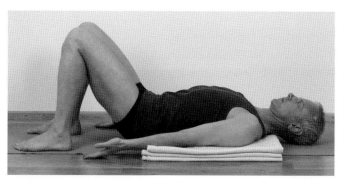

Figure 7.98

7. Move the hands as close as possible towards the shoulders, fingers slanted towards the hips, thumbs to the front; lift the trunk, bring your sternum closer to the chin.

8. Keep your nose, sternum, and navel in one line.

9. Adjust your pelvis so that the sitting bones are moving upwards and the lumbar area is lengthened; contract your buttocks so that the sacrum and tailbone are going inwards and straighten your legs upwards.

10. Stretch upwards from your armpits to your feet; the feet are between plantar flexion and dorsiflexion (Figure 7.100).

3. Keeping your head relaxed, move your shoulder blades closer together, to lift your upper thoracic vertebrae off the blankets about 1 cm.

4. Perform the following steps to go up into the posture so that your head and throat, eyes and ears are relaxed and you can breathe naturally.

5. As you exhale bend your knees – keeping your knees and feet together – towards your chest; lift your pelvis and your back off the floor.

6. Bring your elbows closer together, push them into the blankets, and bring your hands on your back (Figure 7.99).

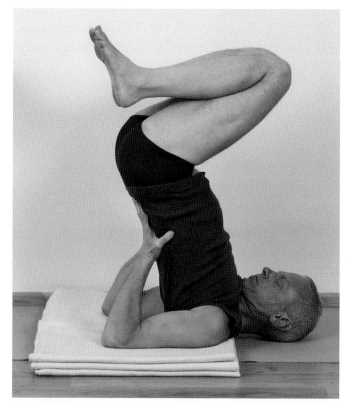

Figure 7.99

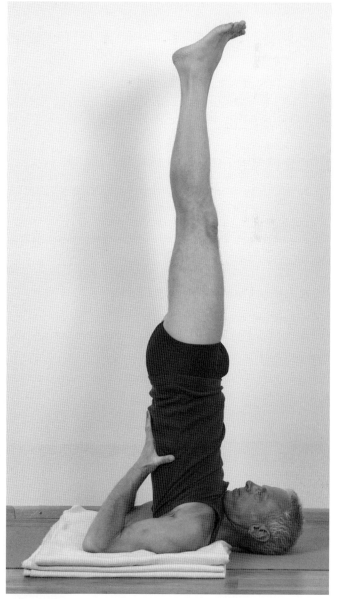

Figure 7.100

Being in the posture: basic work

1. Keep your elbows together at shoulder width.

2. Walk your hands further down towards the shoulder girdle; press your palms into your back to lift yourself more from the armpits to the heels.

3. Keep your throat relaxed.

4. Lift your navel.

5. Contract your buttocks to move your sacrum and tailbone inwards to lengthen your lumbar area.

6. Slightly move your front thighs towards the back.

7. Lengthen your inner legs through your inner heels, your outer legs through your outer heels.

8. Lift from your groins to your toes.

9. Breathe naturally.

Being in the posture: refined work

1. Move your upper arms closer together so that the outer elbows and outer upper arms come closer to the floor.

2. Lift your spine against gravity.

3. Contract your pelvic floor for a few breaths to lengthen your lumbar area more.

4. Lengthen the skin of your inner legs towards the inner heels, the skin of your outer legs towards the outer heels.

5. Keep the back of your head on the floor so that you get a subtle activity in your neck, and from there you get an impulse for the lifting of the posture.

6. Relax your eyes; look towards your chest.

Finishing the posture

Stay 5–10 breaths in the beginning; with practice increase to 2–3 minutes, later up to 5–10 minutes. Exhale, bend your knees towards your head; straighten your arms backwards on the floor. Gradually lower your back and pelvis. Keeping the knees bent, rest your feet on the floor.

Stay for a few breaths with your back on the blankets and your head resting on the floor.

Hold your head with your hands and slide down from the blankets in the direction of the head with a caterpillar movement (see Chapter 6, exercise 2.3); relax lying on your back for a few breaths.

Suggestions for modifications using props

- Put a belt around the upper arms close to the elbows (Figure 7.101).

- Have a bolster behind the blankets to start and finish with the pelvis on the bolster (Figure 7.101).

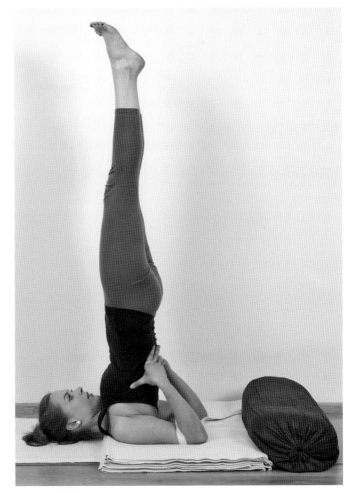

Figure 7.101

- Have a chair behind the blankets; hold the chair with your hands, and rest your feet on the chair; this is an easy and safe method to lift your pelvis and trunk, and is suitable for beginners (Figure 7.102).

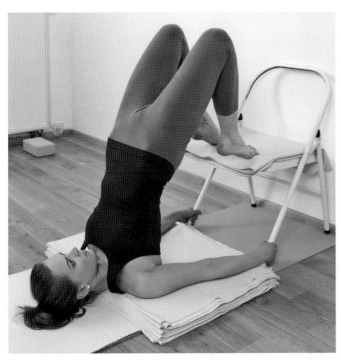

Figure 7.102

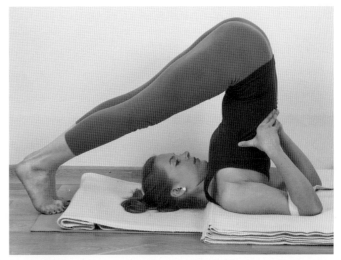

Figure 7.103

32. Halāsana (Figure 7.103)

Meaning of the āsana and its name

Hala means plough; Halāsana is evocative of the shape of a plough. Performed correctly, Halāsana is a very calming posture.

Getting into the posture

1. Start with Sālamba Sarvāṅgāsana, getting into the posture, points 1–8.
2. Relax your neck and throat.
3. Keep your trunk lifted; with an exhalation straighten your legs to bring your toes onto the floor (Figure 7.103).
4. Keep the knees and feet together; walk with your feet, so that the trunk is vertical.

Being in the posture: basic work

1. Keeping your neck and throat relaxed, push yourself up from your upper arms and elbows; press your palms into your back to support lifting the trunk.
2. Tilt your pelvis backwards; lift your sitting bones and groins; move the sacrum inwards.

3. Lift your navel away from the sternum.
4. Push yourself up from your toes to lift your thighs and shin bones further away from the floor to lengthen the front of your trunk, so that your diaphragm can move easily.
5. Relax your face.
6. Breathe naturally.

Being in the posture: refined work

1. Release your hands from your trunk; have the lower arms and hands vertical; bring your elbows closer together, and your hands further apart to turn your arms outwards slightly, to lift yourself more from the outer elbows and outer upper arms.
2. Put your hands onto your back again.
3. Lengthen your back and lengthen from your sternum to your groin.
4. To lengthen the back walk your feet a short way from your head as long as you can lengthen the front of your trunk and your eyes, face, throat, and neck are relaxed, and your breath is subtle.
5. Look towards your sternum.

Finishing the posture

Stay for 5–10 breaths in the beginning; with practice increase to 3–5 minutes. Put your arms and hands on the floor, opposite the head. Slightly bend your knees, lift your feet off the floor, and gradually lower your back, pelvis, and legs to the floor. Relax lying on your back for a few breaths.

Suggestions for modifications using props

- Rest your knees on a chair, with the feet on the back of the chair (Figure 7.104).

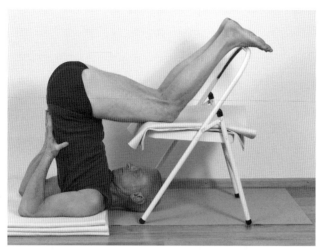

Figure 7.104

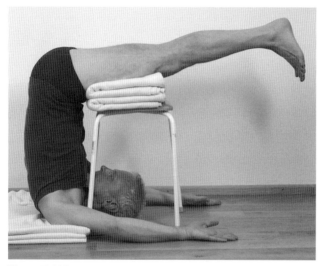

Figure 7.105

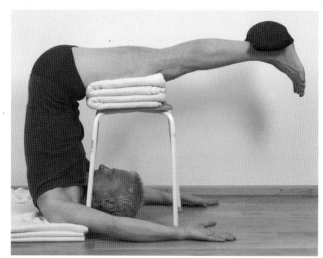

Figure 7.106

- Put the tips of your toes on a chair.
- Rest your thighs on a stool with legs straight. The stool is supporting your legs up to the groin (Figure 7.105). Adjust the height of the stool with one or two folded blankets if necessary to have the optimum height for your trunk. Rest your arms around your head. If your knees can take it, put a weight, e.g., a sandbag, on the heels, to improve the stretch for your trunk (Figure 7.106).

Variation (Figure 7.107)

1. Start in Sālamba Sarvāṅgāsana.
2. Lower your legs over your head nearly horizontally.
3. Find a balance on your shoulders without straining the neck.
4. Take your hands away from your back to move the arms sideways.
5. Balancing carefully without straining the neck, lift the palms of your hands to your knees.
6. Now stretch your arms, get a good balance on the shoulders, and put the weight of the legs into the hands.
7. Now the legs are fully supported by the stretched arms.
8. Concentrate on your breathing.

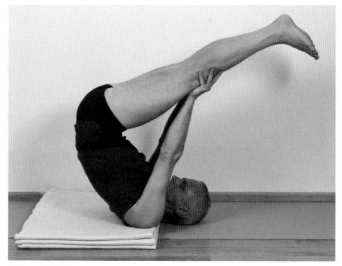

Figure 7.107

9. Stay for 5–10 breaths or longer, if comfortable.

10. To come down lower your legs, bring your arms on the floor opposite your head, and come down as from Halāsana.

33. Viparīta Karaṇī (Figure 7.108)

Meaning of the āsana and its name

Viparīta Karaṇī means inverted lake. This gentle inversion is particularly beneficial for the transport of fluids in the body. It is a helpful substitute, if stronger inversions are not possible.

Getting into the posture

1. Place a bolster one hand width away from the wall.

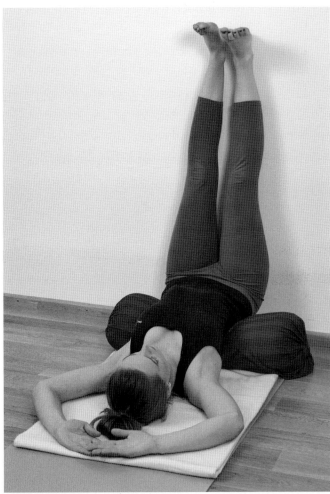

Figure 7.108

2. Lie on your right side with the trunk at right angles to the wall, your right hip on the right third of the bolster, the buttocks and the feet on the wall, the knees bent towards the chest.

3. Turn on your back; if necessary, shift yourself to the center of the bolster so that the pelvis and the lumbar area are in the center of the bolster, and the upper back, shoulders, and head are on the floor; also having the floating ribs on the bolster can be very relaxing.

4. Straighten your legs upwards, knees and feet together, the buttocks and the backs of the legs on the wall; if it is not possible to straighten the legs, practice the posture with the bolster further away from the wall.

5. If the buttocks and backs of the legs are not against the wall, slightly bend your knees, lift your pelvis off the bolster, and walk on your shoulders closer towards the wall until your buttocks and backs of the legs are touching the wall.

6. Rest your arms sideways in line with your shoulder girdle or relaxed around your head.

Being in the posture: basic work

1. Keep your legs together and straight, with the center of the heels touching the wall.

2. Rest your pelvis on the bolster so that the buttocks are slightly dropping towards the floor between the bolster and the wall.

3. Adjust your arms so that the front of your chest is long and wide.

4. Adjust your head so that your neck and throat are relaxed.

5. Close your eyes and breathe naturally.

Being in the posture: refined work

1. Keep your legs completely straight.

2. Drop your groin between the lower abdomen and the thighs.

3. Keep your abdomen soft.

4. While inhaling feel the inner movement from your diaphragm to your pelvic floor.

5. While exhaling feel the inner movement from your pelvic floor to your diaphragm.

6. Feel the lightness of your breath in the chest.

7. Relax your face, eyes, ears, mouth, and tongue.

8. Feel the subtle flow of breath in your nostrils, evenly left and right, evenly with inhalation and exhalation.

9. Look towards the center of your chest.

Finishing the posture

Stay in the posture for 2–3 minutes; with practice you may wish to increase to 5–10 minutes.

Method 1

Hold the back of your head with your hands with interlocked fingers; slide down from the bolster with a caterpillar movement, until you are lying on the floor with your whole back.

Method 2

Lift your pelvis off the bolster, push the bolster to the side, and gently lower your back to the floor vertebra by vertebra.

Once your whole back is lying flat, support your head with a pillow if necessary, and bend your knees towards your chest to relax for a few breaths.

Suggestions for modifications using further props

• To get this posture right is a very individual process that needs experimenting and finetuning.

• If you need more height or a larger support, put one or two folded blankets over the bolster.

• If the bolster is too high, only use one or two folded blankets or support the upper back with a folded blanket.

• To get an easier relaxation put a belt around your ankles.

34. Śavāsana (Figure 7.109)

Meaning of the āsana and its name

Śava is a corpse. Śavāsana means complete stillness in the body and mind. No energy is used; all the systems can recover. B K S Iyengar calls it the best antidote to the stresses of modern civilization. Śavāsana looks simple, but it is one of the yoga postures that needs the longest practice.

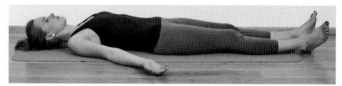

Figure 7.109

Getting into the posture

1. Sit upright with both legs straight, the palms on the floor.

2. Lean backwards, and bring your lower arms and elbows onto the floor.

3. Move your shoulders back, gradually lowering your back onto the floor.

4. Bring both shoulder blades evenly onto the floor.

5. Hold the back of your head with your hands, fingers interlocked, thumbs hooking around the lower ridge of your skull.

6. Gently lengthen your head away from the neck, keeping your throat relaxed.

7. Place your head exactly in line with the spine and on its center on the floor, so that you are looking towards your body.

8. Slide your shoulder blades slightly away from the head.

9. Let your shoulders go towards the floor.

10. Rest your arms beside your body so that the armpits are free and the palms are facing up to the ceiling; if this is not possible, put your hands on your abdomen.

11. Relax your abdomen towards the floor.

12. Release your legs to turn outwards; the outer edges of the feet are coming closer towards the floor.

Being in the posture: basic work

1. Close your eyes gently so that the pupils are not disturbed.
2. Feel the back of your head on the floor.
3. Release your upper neck towards the floor.
4. Relax your face, your forehead, cheeks, lips, and chin.
5. Keep your nose in the center.
6. Look towards the center of your chest.
7. Your shoulders are broad and sinking into the floor.
8. Relax your arms onto the floor, the thumbs moving closer towards the floor.
9. Relax your palms and fingers.
10. Relax your middle ribs and the area of your navel.
11. Relax your abdomen and lumbar area.
12. Let the back of your pelvis rest on the floor.
13. Keep your buttocks relaxed.
14. Relax your thighs and your calves towards the floor.
15. Let the outer edges of the feet sink more towards the floor.
16. Breathe naturally and evenly.

Being in the posture: refined work

1. Relax your eyes; learn to keep your eyes soft during not only exhalation, but also inhalation.
2. Release your forehead from the center to the sides.
3. Keep the skin of your face soft; keep your temples soft.
4. Release your cheeks away from the sides of your nose.
5. Keeping your mouth closed and the lips soft, gently release your upper teeth from your lower teeth and your lower teeth from your upper teeth.
6. Release the outer corners of the mouth towards the sides.
7. Keep your tongue soft.
8. Release your tongue away from the palate; feel the relaxation of your jaw joints and your ears.
9. Let your breath be so subtle and smooth that the nostrils are hardly feeling it.
10. During exhalation and inhalation your whole body and mind are calm.
11. Experience the calming effect of the exhalation, particularly at the end of exhalation.
12. Without moving the head adjust it so subtly that the neck and throat are relaxed.
13. Feel your inhalation from your inner chest to the skin above your clavicles.
14. Keep this area relaxed as you exhale.
15. Keep your abdomen and lumbar area soft.
16. Keep your groin soft.
17. Relax your front thighs towards your back thighs.
18. Relax your shins towards your calves.
19. Feel both heels equally on the floor.
20. Keep your feet relaxed.
21. Be aware that the floor is carrying you.
22. Feel the relaxation in your skin, your eyes, ears, mouth, and nose. Feel the inner calmness. Let the breath be subtle and smooth. Be aware of the inhalation and exhalation and the tiny pauses between inhalation and exhalation and exhalation and inhalation. Get deeper into the inner calmness in these pauses.

Finishing the posture

Stay in Śavāsana for 5–15 minutes. In the beginning you may fall asleep easily. With increasing practice you will stay awake in deep relaxation, recovering more than when falling asleep.

Method 1

Slowly open your eyes, remain still for a few breaths; maintaining the silence of your mind, turn to one side, remain still for a few breaths; then turn to the other side, remain still for a few breaths, and come back to sit.

Method 2

Feel your breath in your nostrils as a subtle link between your inner body and the outer world. Maintaining the silence of your mind, turn to one side, remain silent for a few breaths; then turn to the other side, remain silent for a few breaths, and come back to sit.

Method 3

Bend your legs one after the other; rest the soles of your feet on the floor. Feel the contact of your feet with the floor. Slowly bring your hands onto your chest for a few breaths. Remove your hands from your chest; let the arms rest on the floor beside your body. Maintaining the silence of your mind, turn the whole body to one side; remain silent for a few breaths; then turn to the other side; remain silent for a few breaths. Finally come back to a sitting position with the help of your hands and arms.

Suggestions for modifications using props

• Support the head with a folded blanket.

• Support the knees with a rolled blanket or a bolster (Figure 7.110).

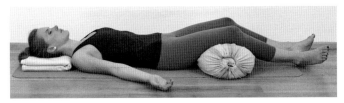

Figure 7.110

• Rest your lower legs on a chair.

• Put a dark-colored scarf folded four times over your eyes.

• Cover yourself if necessary, to be warm enough.

• Any method of positioning patients on the treatment couch comfortably is also suitable to support Śavāsana if necessary.

Combinations and sequencing of āsanas

As discussed in Chapter 4, the steps of learning and practicing must be small enough to follow, to retain motivation, and to avoid injury. On the other hand the effects of practicing should be felt, understood, and convincing. As āsanas are more complex tasks, this means that sufficient preparation is necessary. Elementary steps have to be learned first before proceeding to more complex āsanas or new positions. Most of the basic exercises are suitable preparation for certain āsanas. Depending on which area and aims you need to particularly focus on, you can choose the relevant basic exercises for preparation. Among the āsanas the standing poses are a good preparation for most other āsanas and are recommended for beginners. Next the sitting āsanas and forward bends can be introduced, then the twists. Only then should inversions and back-bendings be learned (Iyengar & Iyengar 2003). In the description of Sālamba Śīrṣāsana and Sālamba Sarvāṅgāsana the important prerequisites for learning these āsanas are discussed. Using props helps us to learn and improve the precision of these āsanas. With increasing practice the props can gradually be reduced.

A balanced program contains all directions of movement. Each direction should be prepared sufficiently and built up gradually. This applies particularly for the directions where there may be restricted movement. The movement directions and cycles should not be mixed; there should not be any "jumping" between different directions. When practicing asymmetrical āsanas there should be a centered, symmetrical position in between and at the end. Each program should finish with relaxation and calming (Weiss & Zugck 2009).

There are many ways of constructing a program for particular emphasis:

- Sequences with a dynamic, warming-up emphasis. This could be a combination of standing poses performed quickly or twists and back-bends. There are sequences of jumpings (Mehta et al 1990) which are not covered in this book.

- Sequences to relax and recover (see Chapter 5, Resting poses for preparing prāṇāyāma).

- Sequences with the emphasis on one group of āsanas, for example some standing āsanas prepared with some basic exercises, finished with a forward-bending āsana and a relaxation.

- Selecting basic exercises and āsanas to focus on a special area of the body.

- Combining a general program to cover the whole body.

Examples of sensible combinations are:

- standing and sitting āsanas
- standing āsanas and inversions
- forward bendings and twists
- backward bendings and twists
- forward bendings and inversions.

It is recommended that you start each cycle with a few minutes of sitting to prepare the mind for the practice and to finish with relaxation.

The selection of basic exercises to prepare āsanas follows directly from the diagnosis and the aims of exercise (see Chapter 3).

These hints give many possibilities of combining basic exercises and āsanas that are well suited to the individual situation. If practice is based on a thorough diagnosis and medical investigation and applied with mindfulness, a pleasant practice with good results is very likely.

The following are some examples of how to apply these considerations:

1. For Pārśvottānāsana the stretch of the back of the legs can be prepared through the modified Supta Pādāṅguṣṭhāsana (Figure 7.97).

2. For all standing poses the awareness and strength of the arches of the feet can be prepared through exercise 10.4 (Chapter 6).

3. For Adho Mukha Śvānāsana and all other āsanas with an emphasis on stretching the legs, the stretch of the back of the legs can be prepared through modified Supta Pādāṅguṣṭhāsana.

4. Awareness of the hands can be prepared through exercise 6.4 (see Chapter 6).

5. Elbow strength for Adho Mukha Śvānāsana and Adho Mukha Vṛkṣāsana is prepared through the four-point kneeling variations (Chapter 6, exercise 6.7).

References

Iyengar, B.K.S., 2001. Light on Yoga. Thorsons, London.

Iyengar, B.K.S., 2002a. The Tree of Yoga. Shambala, Boston, MA.

Iyengar, B.K.S., 2002b. Light on the Yoga Sūtras of Patañjali. Thorsons, London.

Iyengar, B.K.S., 2005. Light on Life. Rodale, Emmaus, PA.

Iyengar, B.K.S., Iyengar, G.S., 2003. Basic Guidelines for Teachers of Yoga. YOG, Mumbai.

Mehta, S., Mehta, M., Mehta, S., 1990. Yoga. The Iyengar Way. Dorling Kindersley, London.

Sinh, P., 2006. Haṭha Yoga Pradīpikā: Explanation of Haṭha Yoga. Pilgrims, Kathmandu.

Weiss, B., Zugck, K., 2009. Āsana Lehrbrief. Fernlehrgang Yoga-Lehrer/in SKA. Sebastian Kneipp Akademie für Gesundheitsbildung, Bad Wörishofen.

Further reading

Francina, S., 1997. The New Yoga for People over 50. Health Communications, Deerfield Beach, FL.

Iyengar, B.K.S., 2001. Yoga – The Path to Holistic Health. Dorling Kindersley, London.

Mehta, M., 2004. Yoga Explained. Kyle Cathie, London.

CHAPTER 8

Yoga in everyday life

Introduction

One of the most important therapeutic aspects of yoga is to integrate what you have learned into everyday life. Yoga practice should not be restricted to going to a class or receiving instruction from a therapist and practicing at home. Rather it should be naturally integrated every day in an ongoing way to enjoy continuing success.

We all have many family, work, and social duties. Often things happen unexpectedly or duties take much longer than planned. Out of the blue, situations arise when we wanted just to relax: the phone rings and our mother-in-law has been admitted to hospital or our child is ill and we have to come and help immediately. Or our tax return needs to be handed in today but the computer breaks down. Then, instead of practicing yoga, it is the computer – otherwise ever so useful – that consumes hours and hours of our time. All these types of event make us feel that there is not enough time to look after ourselves and to practice yoga.

There is time if the spirit of yoga is integrated into everything we do throughout the day. So many things learned from the therapeutic yoga described in this book can be applied at any time and in any situation: mindfulness, awareness, feeling the breath, correcting and finetuning the posture, and gentle movements with the feet, hands, or shoulders. The Yoga-Sūtras (see Chapters 1 and 2) teach us the importance of not accumulating unnecessary things and of controlling our desires, calming the mind, and becoming free from constant distractions. This helps us to organize a disciplined, clearly structured day that starts with getting up early enough, creating extra time for our own development. In Chapter 2 we also learned from the Yoga-Sūtras that our state of mind can be influenced by consciously cultivating a positive attitude. This ancient wisdom tells us that it is possible to fulfill all of life's duties while still feeling relaxed inside.

If we integrate this spirit of yoga into our everyday life, it can help us to be less affected by stressful situations and to maintain a good, healthy posture and natural breathing throughout. Of course it is also important to find sufficient occasions for actual practice. Below we will look at practical aspects relating to our surroundings and the best adjustment of our posture. Also included are short programs to practice in everyday life. If time is short or the surroundings are not suitable for some of the exercises, you can practice only parts of a suggested program.

To make our daily yoga practice successful lifestyle and diet are important. The furniture, which chair we use in the office, the height of our desk and computer screen, how we sit in our spare time, in the car, on a bike, what sports we play, how much effort we put into them – all these factors contribute to the results of yoga therapy. Furthermore our bed, mattress, pillow, and the shoes we wear play an important role. Nowadays there are so many possibilities which need to be tailored for individual use, so we will not give specific endorsements here. However we do recommend that you respect the importance of these factors and consult an expert when you come to buying or changing any of this equipment.

Selections from practice that are suitable for integration into many areas and situations

Exercise: Breathing and listening

To calm the sensory organs and the mind in noisy surroundings, this simple perception exercise can be practiced even if you only have a short time:

Sit on a chair or on the floor in a position of your choice so that your spine is upright. Close your eyes and keep them closed till you finish the practice. Be aware of your whole body; feel the contact with the floor and your clothes. Accept everything that your senses are perceiving; be completely open to these perceptions. Probably sound will be the most dominant perception. Be aware of all sounds, no matter whether people are speaking, birds are singing, the telephone rings, a car is passing by, there is noisy construction work going on, or anything else. Listen carefully without judging, without asking where the sounds are coming from, but be aware that you are listening. Remain as an observer without becoming involved. In this way your perception connects the object with your sense organs, while your inner observer is not affected by it.

Focus on a particularly dominant sound, then move your awareness to a different one, and then to a few more different ones. Now listen to as many different sounds as possible at the same time. Expand your perception to the most distant sound; listen to even more subtle sounds. Expand your perception further and further: this helps to keep your thoughts calm. You perceive the sounds directly without your mind judging. Now pull your perception inwards to your breath, just below the nostrils. Sounds from outside are excluded now. Be with your breath for some time. As long as time allows you can switch between awareness of the outer sounds and your breathing.

Quiet breathing in a good sitting posture

Quiet breathing in a good sitting posture can be practiced as follows, even if time is very short. In this case correct your sitting posture and practice a few breaths consciously.

Sit in a firm and comfortable position on the floor with the legs in a simple cross-legged position or sit on the front half of a chair. Find the balance for your pelvis between tilting it forwards and backwards so that your spine is lifting without effort. If the chair is too high for you to sit and correct yourself well, put a suitable item, for example a book, underneath your feet. If the chair is not high enough, use a folded blanket, properly adjusted, underneath your buttocks. Rest your hands on your thighs, palms facing upwards, so that your elbows and shoulders move slightly backwards and downwards. This will probably settle the hands and arms well after most working positions.

Keep your chest lifted; slightly bend your head, chin towards the throat, keeping the throat soft. If this causes stress in the neck or throat, keep your head upright. Keeping the mouth closed, slightly lift the upper teeth and the palate away from the lower jaw. Keep your pelvis slightly tilted forwards when you pull your lower abdomen towards the lumbar spine and the diaphragm. Maintaining this stable pelvic position, lift your side ribs, sternum, and upper ribs. All these adjustments in posture prepare you for correct breathing. Feel the slow soft flow of breath in your nostrils first. Slightly lifting yourself from your lower abdomen, feel the inhalation from your lumbar area and costal arches to your middle and upper chest. Be aware of the lifting of your upper chest at the end of inhalation and maintain this lift while you exhale. This gives you a good upright posture for exhaling and calms the exhalation. Practice for 5–10 minutes. If you have less time you will benefit from doing even a few breaths like this.

Conscious standing

Conscious standing with some fine adjustments can be integrated whenever you have to wait or queue up. To perfect the following fine adjustments, you need comfortable shoes. The foot work may need to be modified slightly.

1. Stretch your toes; rest your toes straight on the soles of your shoes.

2. Distribute your weight evenly between the left and right foot, and the front and hind feet, putting slightly more weight into the heels.

3. Balance between lifting the inner and outer ankle, the inner and outer arches of your feet, keeping the base of the toes on the sole of the shoes, and lengthen your toes.

4. From this position feel the upward movement against gravity in your legs.

5. Straighten your knees, ease off a tiny bit, make your quadriceps muscles firm, and pull your kneecaps up.

6. Move the front of your thighs towards the back of your thighs, and the groin slightly backwards.

7. Adjust your pelvis to the neutral position; lift from your lower abdomen.

8. Maintain the neutral pelvic position while you lift your chest.

9. Relax your shoulders.

10. Gently turn your arms inwards; feel the space between the shoulder blades.

11. Gently turn your arms outwards; feel the space in your front chest and the subtle stretch over your upper ribs and clavicles.

12. Let your arms hang naturally.

13. Maintaining the position of the chin, slightly move the back of your head backwards parallel to the floor and away from the neck.

14. Relax your face as if smiling slightly.

15. Breathe naturally.

You can combine the upward movement from the arches of your feet with the upward movement from your knees, pelvis, through your spine, chest, and head. Add any of the fine adjustments described in points 1–15 as appropriate.

Conclusion

The exercises with their fine adjustments explained above can be practiced in many settings. Even if you cannot practice yoga in between classes, improving your sitting or standing posture as often as possible is of tremendous value for your health. Posture significantly affects bodily function. In a compressed trunk the fluid transport and nerve supply to all tissues and organs are compromised. A poorly lifted spine also affects the functions of the central and autonomous nervous system. Good posture improves the function of all connected tissues and organs.

Examples for integrating the spirit and practice of yoga into everyday life

In bed

To relax, lie on your back and use a support for your head and a bolster underneath your knees, if necessary (see Chapter 7, āsana Śavāsana with props).

Then be aware of your breath. Feel the slow soft breathing in your nostrils first. Then feel the inhalation from your lumbar area and costal arches to your middle and upper chest. Be aware of your upper chest lifting at the end of inhalation and maintain this lift when you exhale. This renders the exhalation slower and subtler. In particular observe the end of your inhalation and the end of your exhalation and the pause between the exhalation and the new inhalation, the inner calmness of this moment.

Before you get up in the morning it can be very helpful to start with a few basic exercises to stimulate the body and mind gently. The following program selected from Chapter 6, or part of it, would be suitable:

- Feel your breath for a few cycles.

- Move your eyes (Chapter 6, exercise 5.10).

- Do side-lying rotation (Chapter 6, exercise 3.2).

- Carry out rhythmic relaxation (Chapter 6, exercise 1.3).

- Straighten your legs either on the bed or perpendicularly and perform the foot movements as explained in Chapter 6 (exercise 10.3).

- Before getting up, lie on your side with bent legs, close to the edge of the bed. Let your feet drop to the floor and at the same time push yourself up to sit with the help of your upper hand.

- Before standing up remain seated for a few breaths: feel your feet on the floor, and the inner lift from your pelvis.

In the bathroom

- Standing in front of the sink, perform the weight-bearing exercises for the feet, as explained in Chapter 6 (exercises 10.6, 10.9, and 10.10).

- While brushing your teeth, stand on one foot or perform Vṛkṣāsana (see Chapter 7).

- While looking into the mirror practice some of the exercises for the head:

  - relaxed jaw (Chapter 6, exercise 5.7)

  - moving your tongue (Chapter 6, exercise 5.8)

  - moving your eyes (Chapter 6, exercise 5.10)

- While drying yourself after your bath or shower you can also integrate a few movements:

  - Stand on one foot to dry the other one; also stand on one foot while putting on your socks.

  - All-embracing shoulder work (Chapter 6, exercise 4.11): instead of the belt, use your towel between your hands; keep it loose enough so that you have some range of movement and you can dry your upper back at the same time.

Housework and gardening

Even if your muscles are well trained and you are aware of your movements, much of the work in the house and garden needs special attention as to how you engage your body. Moving economically and performing the movements so slowly that they can be reversed at any time helps to avoid injury. This is supported by being centered in the working position, and avoiding leaning over. For vacuum cleaning, ironing, opening bottles or glasses, using a broom or spade or lawn mower, this means holding these objects as close as possible to the center of the body. When making the bed or cleaning the bathtub, avoid leaning over as much as possible. You can use a long-handled brush to clean the bathtub. If you support yourself with the other hand on the edge of the tub, you will greatly reduce the stress on your back. When you have different tasks to do in one day, change around often, so that you do not spend too long on one type of work: for example, alternate between cleaning, watering the flowers, and desk work. If your knees can cope, squatting is a healthy posture for shorter work on the floor, and is very relaxing for the pelvis, the abdomen, and the back.

Going out

Whenever you do not have to carry anything swing your arms while walking, as described in Chapter 6 (exercise 4.1). If you are using carrier bags, distribute the weight evenly between both hands. Every now and then perform a few steps, consciously feeling the change of contact with the floor in the front and rear foot respectively. Adjusting the neutral lumbopelvic position improves the lifting of your spine and chest and gives you a gentle, functional pelvic floor training.

If you have to wait in line, practice conscious standing, as explained in the exercise above.

Driving a car

It is inadvisable to exercise during driving, so it is all the more important to adjust the seat and the steering wheel so that your posture is comfortable and well lifted. This gives some of the effects of practicing yoga and improves breathing. A good back support can be made from a rolled towel or a long pillow between the spine and the back of the seat, as shown in āsana Baddha Koṇāsana (see Chapter 7). When you are waiting at a red light you can carry out some head movements:

- mobile head on the spine (Chapter 6, exercise 5.3)
- gentle side-bending (Chapter 6, exercise 5.5).

Putting the palms of your hand above your head on the car roof at shoulder width apart, walk the hands backwards along the roof as far as you can maintain a neutral lumbopelvic position. Make sure to put them back on the steering wheel in time.

Traveling in a bus, train, or plane

Change your sitting posture often; walk around as much as possible.

While in your seat, a variety of exercises can be performed without disturbing your neighbours. If possible take off your shoes.

Some examples are:

- weight-bearing foot exercises, performed seated (Chapter 6, exercise 10.6)
- Achilles tendon alignment (Chapter 6, exercise 10.8)
- correcting your sitting posture, as explained above, recommending a good sitting posture for quiet breathing

- finetuning rotation (Chapter 6, exercise 2.8)
- scapular movements (Chapter 6, exercise 4.2)
- mobile head on the spine (Chapter 6, exercise 5.3)
- gentle side-bending (Chapter 6, exercise 5.5)
- use any available time to practice quiet breathing, as described earlier in this chapter, even if it is only for a few breaths.

In the office

First of all your chair, desk, and the height and direction of your computer screen need to be adjusted to you individually, so that your surroundings create good posture. All exercises recommended for sitting in a bus, train, or plane are also suitable for an office chair.

If the back of your office chair is suitable, do the exercise leaning over the back of the chair (Chapter 6, exercise 3.7). For the shoulders, spider monkey 1 (Chapter 6, exercise 4.3) will be useful, as will turning the head (Chapter 6, exercise 4.5) and all-embracing shoulder work (Chapter 6, exercise 4.11).

For the wrists and hands, do the following exercises:

- carpal tunnel stretch (Chapter 6, exercise 6.3)
- strong and flexible wrists, the variation with the arms on the table (Chapter 6, exercise 6.4)
- elevating the arms (Chapter 6, exercise 4.8).

For relaxing the eyes:

- moving your eyes (Chapter 6, exercise 5.10)
- palming (Chapter 6, exercise 5.11).

For relaxing the neck:

- turn and bend (Chapter 6, exercise 5.4)
- gentle side-bending (Chapter 6, exercise 5.5).

A good office stretch is shown in āsana Uttānāsana, modifications using props (see Chapter 7, Figures 7.34, 7.35); if you can remove your shoes or you are wearing comfortable ones, include some foot exercises. Also develop the habit of standing when you are on the phone or straighten your legs horizontally under your desk. Another useful habit is to swing your arms or slightly pull your lower abdomen inwards and upwards when you go to the toilet.

In an occupation with hard physical labor or many asymmetrical positions

If you are working in such a job or are a young mother carrying your baby around it may not be possible to balance between both sides. Learning to use your body economically will help to some degree. If possible, keep changing the side of your body you are using. It is particularly important to use your spare time to center your position and relax, but also to keep the muscles in good shape.

In your spare time

Our spare time is when we have the best chance of looking after ourselves and our health. Most of us do not have much spare time, so it is all the more precious. Sometimes it may be necessary to take a nap, but this should not take up all your time. We need good time management skills to make the best use of our free time. And it is important to select what we do in our spare time carefully, so that we avoid falling into the same stressful routine we have at other times.

If you like to read, try to lie over a big bolster, as explained in Chapter 6, exercise 2.4. Position your back and head support high enough so that you can read comfortably. When watching TV change your sitting posture occasionally; also sit cross-legged on the floor. If you are taking a course in your spare time and have to learn by heart, you will be surprised how easily this comes while walking.

Think about further opportunities when you can include yoga practice. It is lovely to practice together with friends. Why not start an afternoon get-together by doing a little yoga? 20 to 30 minutes of common yoga practice are quite sufficient. Just try it: invite your friends. Even if they are shy at first, they will appreciate it because they will feel the benefit.

Conclusion

We have considered possibilities for integrating the spirit and the practice of yoga into everyday life. These are only a few examples: there are countless variations. Which particular exercise you choose is less important: it is more important to start to practice. It is up to you to make the first move; no one else can do it for you. Start with short periods of practicing, with a few exercises. Even if there are times in your life when you think it is impossible to include any practice, do not give up. Start with a small program. If you cannot find any other time, get up 10 minutes earlier. It is not so difficult to do this, and you will feel the benefit from 10 minutes' practice each morning.

It is definitely possible to integrate your personal development, the yoga path, with the challenges of life, so that you can enjoy a successful family and work life and still be relaxed.

There is no way to achieve knowledge and ability quickly. It is a lifelong process that requires a willingness to become involved in study and practice, to work with diligence and dedication. Reading a book like this can initiate change, but only through practicing the concrete details will change really happen. This may require a modification of lifestyle, altering unhealthy habits, revising our diet, balancing activity and rest, including mindfulness in any form of practice, and constantly striving for a positive mental attitude.

There is good evidence for the effects of therapeutic yoga. Empirical and clinical observations have been available for a long time, and since the mid 20th-century a great deal of research on the effects of the practice of yoga has been undertaken. Much more research should be carried out in the future.

Interdisciplinary work among physicians, manual therapists, and yoga teachers can be further developed.

We have a tremendous capacity to correct the posture, improve the functions of the body, and refine the understanding, awareness and sensitivity of both ourselves and the people around us. Likewise we should practice with an attitude of admiration and deep respect for the miracle of creation that is expressed by our body and our life. However, we should also respect the limits of what we are able to do. In the last years of his life, Werner Heisenberg, Physics Nobel laureate, gave lectures on science and philosophy. While speaking in Munich sometime in the late 1960s, he said that in spite of everything science has proved, we must respect the fact that we can only go so far. Beyond this limit only God is able to go.

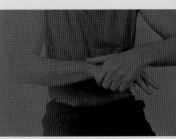

Index